INTRODUCTION TO STERILIZATION AND DISINFECTION

INTRODUCTION TO STERILIZATION AND DISINFECTION

JOAN F. GARDNER MSc(Melb) DPhil(Oxon)

Formerly Senior Lecturer, Department of Microbiology,
University of Melbourne

MARGARET M. PEEL BSc(Qld) DipBact(Lond) PhD (Lond) AAIMLS

Senior Bacteriologist, Microbiological Diagnostic Unit,
Department of Microbiology, University of Melbourne

Foreword by J.C. Kelsey MA MD(Cantab) DipBact(Lond) FRCPath

Formerly Deputy Director, Public Health Laboratory Service,
London

Churchill Livingstone ▦

MELBOURNE EDINBURGH LONDON AND NEW YORK 1986

CHURCHILL LIVINGSTONE
Medical Division of Longman Group Limited

Distributed in Australia by Longman Cheshire Pty Limited,
Longman House, Kings Gardens, 95 Coventry Street, South
Melbourne 3205, and by associated companies, branches and
representatives throughout the world.

© Longman Group Limited 1986

First published 1986

ISBN 0-443-02796-X

British Library Cataloguing in Publication Data
Gardner, Joan F.
    Introduction to sterilization and disinfection.
    1. Disinfection and disinfectants   2. Sterilization
    I. Title   II. Peel, Margaret M.
    614.4'8   RA761

Library of Congress Cataloging in Publication Data
Gardner, Joan F.
    Introduction to sterilization and disinfection.
    Includes index.
    1. Disinfection and disinfectants.   2. Sterilization.
I. Peel, Margaret M.   II. Title.   [DNLM: 1. Sterilization. WA
240 G227i]
    RA761.G37   1986   614.4'8   85–16652

Produced by Longman Singapore Publishers (Pte) Ltd.
Printed in Singapore

Foreword

It gives me great pleasure to write a foreword to the book by Joan Gardner and Margaret Peel.

This book will be a welcome addition to the literature on this important subject. Dr Gardner has been involved in sterilization and disinfection for nearly as long as I have been. I first got involved in the subject quite by accident and I did not think that we would become involved both in making medical history and making friends all over the world. I was wrong and I am now very glad to give a little help in promoting what is not only a science, but also a very real art.

Ramsgate 1986   J.C. Kelsey

Preface

The presentation of sterilization and disinfection in this book has been tailored to the requirements of hospital staff who hold positions of responsibility in the supply and use of sterile equipment and pharmaceuticals and also in the broader field of infection control. A balance has been sought between principles and practice, the number of references cited in the text being reduced in order to avoid undue interruption for the reader. The book is also intended to provide background information for engineers whose duties include the maintenance and servicing of sterilizers and ancillary equipment, for manufacturers of such equipment and for companies that produce sterile medical devices or chemical disinfectants.

The proper use of chemical disinfectants and a sound knowledge of the conditions that determine whether the solutions fulfil their intended purpose of killing microorganisms are important to all who rely on the products for control of microbial contamination in situations ranging from hospitals, dental surgeries and other health services to community-based services such as podiatry and hairdressing.

This new, enlarged book has been developed from a former publication (Rubbo S.D., Gardner J.F. 1965 A review of sterilization and disinfection. Lloyd-Luke, London). Like its predecessor, it is designed for use as a textbook in specialized courses for microbiologists and for post-basic education or training of hospital staff. It should also be suitable as a reference text for students reading for medical, dental or science degrees in universities and other tertiary education institutions.

Melbourne 1986

J.F. Gardner
M.M. Peel

Acknowledgements

Many colleagues in various countries have given valuable assistance in the preparation of this book. Those in the United Kingdom include Dr J.C. Kelsey and Mrs I.M. Maurer of the Public Health Service, and Mr A. Bishop, Mr R.P. Cowtan, Mr R. Montgomery and Miss S.B.R. Scott, who provided information about official policies of the U.K. regulatory authorities. Others have made the results of their own research freely available in personal consultations; they include Dr E.J.L. Lowbury, Dr G.A.J. Ayliffe, Dr V.G. Alder, Professor R. Knox, Mr J.K. Pickerill, Mr K.M. Henfrey and the late Dr J.H. Bowie. Mrs E. Holmes, Miss M. Jenkins and other sterile supply department managers also gave of their special expertise.

Dr C.W. Bruch, the late Mr R.R. Ernst, Dr C.R. Phillips and Mr P.M. Borick (U.S.A.) and Dr E.A. Christensen (Denmark) provided information about regulations and recommended practices in their respective countries. This also applies to Dr R. Sen (India), Dr Prakorb Boonthai and Miss Pien Poonsuwan (Thailand), the late Dr M. Kelan, the late Dr A. Wardojo and Dr Marda (Indonesia).

In the authors' home country, Australia, Dr P.A. Wills and Dr D. Sangster made an important contribution to Chapter 8 (radiation sterilization) and Mrs J. Sherrard to the chapter on steam sterilization (Ch. 6). Within the University of Melbourne, Mrs S. Boxshall, Miss J. Cook, Miss E. Duff, Mrs J. Feary, Mrs M. Gierveld, Mrs J. Hesline, Ms A. Pottage and Miss N. Puglielli performed the essential functions of typing and illustrating the manuscript. Professor A.J. Pittard made the services of the Department of Microbiology freely available for the project.

Last but by no means least, thanks are due to the Rowden White Foundation for financial support which facilitated personal interviews with specialists outside Australia.

J.F.G.
M.M.P.

Contents

1

Sterilization, disinfection and the microbial target

The principles and practice of methods used for killing, removing or excluding microorganisms to assist in the prevention of infectious disease comprise the subject of this book. Their applications in hospitals, health clinics and microbiological laboratories will be described in detail and, when appropriate, reference will be made to the commercial production of sterile pharmaceuticals and processed foods.

In this chapter, the difference between sterilization and disinfection is explained and other relevant terms defined. This is followed by a summary of the essential prerequisites for sterilization and disinfection. A brief description of microorganisms is provided for readers who might not be familiar with their nature, activities and distribution.

STERILIZATION

The term 'sterile' refers to the inability of living organisms to reproduce. Sterility of microorganisms is synonymous with death because their activities are usually undetectable in the absence of multiplication. Articles that are free of living organisms are also termed sterile; as the presence of a single microorganism renders an article unsterile, terms such as 'almost sterile' or 'partially sterile' should not be used.

Sterilization is a process that kills or removes all types of microorganisms, including resistant bacterial spores. However, for reasons that will be explained in Chapter 2, it is impossible to guarantee that every microorganism exposed to a particular treatment has been killed or that every article has been sterilized. It is therefore realistic to define sterilization as a process that provides an acceptably low probability (e.g. one chance in a million) that any microorganism will survive the treatment.

It is important to know when sterilization, which may involve severe treatment of equipment and materials, is required. It is essential for articles that enter the blood or tissues, such as surgical instruments, syringes, needles and solutions for injection or intravenous infusion. Diagnostic instruments that come in contact with delicate mucous membranes, such as those lining the urinary tract or peritoneal cavity, should also be used in a sterile condition. Sterile culture media, containers and laboratory apparatus are essential for microbiological research and investigation, including the diagnosis of infectious disease. It is also necessary to ensure that discarded cultures are sterilized before cleaning or disposal of the containers.

Microorganisms that are sterile or dead cannot cause infectious disease but Gram-negative bacteria or their liberated cell wall constituents can cause serious febrile (pyrogenic) reactions if they are introduced into the blood or tissues in large numbers. Sterile solutions intended for parenteral use must therefore be pyrogen-free.

DISINFECTION

A disinfection process is intended to kill or remove pathogenic (disease-producing) microorganisms, with the exception of bacterial spores. Spores can be killed only by a sterilization process. Terminal disinfection of used equipment which may be contaminated with harmful microorganisms is commonly referred to as 'decontamination'. Antisepsis is not synonymous with disinfection; this term should be reserved for the prevention of infection by topical application of antimicrobial agents to injured tissue.

Disinfection is adequate for the preparation of many articles intended for use in patient care. These include bedpans, urinals, clinical thermometers and, if necessary, eating and drinking utensils. Floors, walls, tables, trolleys and work benches require disinfection as well as cleaning if contamination with blood, tissues, exudates or microbial cultures has occurred. Disinfection by chemical agents is the only method applicable to the skin of hands, operation sites and injection sites for killing transient contaminants or reducing the resident microbial flora to a low level.

Disinfection by pasteurization, boiling or chemical agents does not make surgical instruments safe to use. Its use as a substitute for sterilization cannot be justified; when this is unavoidable because a costly instrument, in short supply, is heat-sensitive and insufficient time is available for the slower process of gas sterilization a broad spectrum disinfectant, such as glutaraldehyde, should be chosen. The person responsible should be fully aware of the risk involved.

Definitions

Activation	Initiation of a chemical or biological process (e.g. germination of bacterial spores).
Airborne infection	Infection caused by inhaling airborne dust, fibres, droplets or droplet nuclei carrying microbial contaminants.
Antimicrobial	Adjective describing an agent or action that kills or inhibits the growth of microorganisms.
Antisepsis	Prevention of infection by topical application of biocidal or biostatic agents to injured tissues.
Antiseptic	A chemical agent used for antisepsis.
Asepsis	Prevention of microbial contamination of living tissues or sterile materials by excluding, removing or killing microorganisms.
Autoclave	A vessel fitted with a self-closing door; not descriptive of modern steam sterilizers but continued usage (as noun or verb) is often convenient.
Bactericide	A chemical or physical agent that rapidly kills vegetative (non-sporing) bacteria.
Bacteriostat (Bacteristat)	An agent that prevents multiplication of bacteria.
Biocide	A physical or chemical agent that kills some or all types of microorganisms (often used in the inexact sense).
Buffered solution	An aqueous solution containing chemicals which maintain a specified pH value.
Commensals	Non-pathogenic microorganisms that are living and reproducing as human or animal parasites.
Contact infection	Infection transmitted by direct personal contact or indirectly by contaminated droplets or fomites (inanimate objects).
Contamination	Introduction of microorganisms to sterile articles, materials or tissues.

Contamination level (Bioburden)
The number, or density, of microorganisms on a particular object or surface, or in a specified volume of liquid or air.

Culture medium
A nutrient solution or agar gel for isolating and identifying microorganisms.

Decontamination
Disinfection of used articles to make them safe to handle.

Detergent-sanitizer
A cleaning solution containing an antibacterial agent.

Disinfection
A process that is intended to kill or remove pathogenic microorganisms, with the exception of bacterial spores.

Disinfectant
An agent that is used for disinfection.

DNA
Deoxyribonucleic acid; nuclear material which determines inherited characteristics and controls metabolism of living organisms.

Droplets
Rapidly sedimenting particles of liquid (10–1000 μm) expelled from the respiratory tract.

Droplet nuclei
Particles (0.5–12 μm) which arise from dehydration of small airborne droplets and are capable of wide airborne dispersal.

D value
The time of exposure to heat or chemicals, or the dose of ionizing radiation, that kills 90 per cent of the viable cells in a microbial population.

Fomites
Inanimate objects, other than food, that may harbour and transmit microorganisms.

Fungicide
An agent that kills fungi and their spores.

Fungistat
An agent that inhibits fungal growth.

Germicide
A colloquial term, usually referring to chemical disinfectants; biocide or bactericide are recommended alternatives.

Heat penetration time
The additional time required for all of the articles in a steam or dry heat sterilizer to reach the selected sterilizing temperature after it has been reached in the chamber.

Heat shock
A sublethal heat treatment that may be applied to bacterial spores to kill residual vegetative forms or induce spore germination.

Holding time
The time for which all of the articles in a steam or dry heat sterilizer must be held at the selected sterilizing temperature.

Inactivation
Death of microorganisms, destruction of enzyme activity or 'neutralization' of the antimicrobial activity of a disinfectant.

Inactivation factor
Reduction of a microbial population by a specified biocidal treatment, usually expressed to nearest factor of 10.

Infection
Growth of organisms in the tissues of a host, with or without detectable signs of injury.

Infectious disease
The harmful result of infection by microorganisms.

Isolator
An enclosure for protecting infection-susceptible patients or germfree animals from microbial contamination.

Laminar air flow (unidirectional)
System in which the entire body of air in a confined area moves with uniform velocity along parallel flow lines.

Pasteurization
A process that kills non-sporing microorganisms by hot water or steam at 65–100°C.

Pathogenic microorganism
A species that is capable of causing disease in a susceptible host.

Plenum
A chamber upstream from the air filters in a ventilation system.

Preservation
Prevention of microbial spoilage of foods, pharmaceuticals or industrial materials.

Preservative
A chemical agent used for preservation.

Pyrogens
Heat-stable substances in the cell walls of Gram-negative bacteria that cause a febrile reaction if introduced into the blood or tissues.

Relative humidity (RH)
The amount of water vapour in air, steam or other gaseous atmospheres, expressed as a percentage of the maximum amount that is possible at the existing temperature.

RNA
Ribonucleic acid; controls protein synthesis.

Safety cabinet
A completely or partly enclosed work bench, usually ventilated, for containment of harmful microorganisms or protection of aseptic manipulations.

Sanitization
A process that reduces microbial contamination to a low level by the use of cleaning solutions, hot water or chemical disinfectants.

Spores (bacterial)
Thick-walled resting cells formed by certain Gram-positive bacteria (*Bacillus* and *Clostridium*), capable of survival in unfavourable natural environments and often highly resistant to heat and chemicals.

Spores (fungal)
Unicellular or multicellular reproductive cells, capable of survival in dry conditions and resistant to chemicals but not highly resistant to heat.

Sporicide
An agent that kills bacterial spores.

Sterilant
An agent that kills all types of microorganisms.

Sterile
Term applied to organisms that are incapable of multiplication or articles that are free from living organisms.

Sterilization
A process that is intended to kill or remove all types of microorganisms, with an acceptably low probability of an organism surviving on any article.

Sterilization time
The time for which sterilizing conditions are maintained in a steam, hot air or gas sterilizer.

Thermal death time
The time required to kill a specified fraction (e.g. 90 per cent or 99.999 per cent) of a microbial population at a specified temperature.

Tuberculocide
An agent that kills *Mycobacterium tuberculosis* and related acid-fast bacteria.

Vegetative bacterium
A bacterium that is in the growth and reproductive phase.

Viable microorganism
A microorganism that is capable of multiplication in favourable conditions.

Virucide
An agent that renders viruses non-infective.

ESSENTIAL PREREQUISITES FOR STERILIZATION AND DISINFECTION

The efficiency of sterilization and disinfection depends on:

1. Biocidal action
2. Effective contact between biocidal agent and the microorganisms
3. Appropriate biocidal agent and apparatus
4. Severity of treatment.

Biocidal action

Biocidal action implies death of microorganisms, as indicated by their failure to multiply in any situation. It must be distinguished from reversible inhibition of multiplication (biostasis), from which the organisms may recover on return to favourable conditions. Biocidal action is essential for sterilization and disinfection. A biocidal agent is one that is capable of killing microorganisms. The term is sometimes restricted to agents that kill all types of microorganisms but is also used in a less exact sense to imply that some organisms are killed. Biocidal action against microorganisms of a specified type is termed bactericidal, sporicidal, virucidal or fungicidal.

Effective contact

Effective contact between a biocidal agent and its microbial target requires penetration of the physical or chemical agent to all sites at which the organisms may be located.

Saturated steam

Steam under pressure reaches the outer surfaces of solid objects and penetrates into accessible cavities and packed cotton textiles if the air has been completely removed. It cannot penetrate into nonaqueous liquids and impervious solids. Effective contact involves condensation to water. The latent heat that is released brings the articles rapidly to the sterilizing temperature and the film of moisture ensures that conditions are optimum for biocidal action. Wrapping materials must be permeable to steam and also to the removal of air.

In sterilizers that rely on gravity for the downward displacement of air by steam, the articles must be packed and loaded to facilitate drainage of the heavier air from trays, bowls, tubes and textiles. Flexible tubes should not be tightly coiled.

Gaseous chemicals

Gas sterilization by ethylene oxide requires penetration of the chemical agent and also of water vapour, which is essential for biocidal action. Ethylene oxide is highly diffusible, passing through many materials including thin polyethylene films.

Dry heat

Dry heat sterilization does not involve penetration of vapours but the articles must be heated to the sterilizing temperature by conduction or convection. Metals are good conductors but glass and oily materials are poor conductors of heat.

Ionizing radiation

The penetrating power of sterilizing radiations depends on the type of radiation and the energy level. Electromagnetic gamma radiation penetrates deeply into large cartons containing materials of unit density. Accelerated electrons have greater energy than gamma radiation but have less penetrating power because they are particulate.

Chemical disinfectants

Effective contact between the solutions and the articles to be disinfected depends on the nature of the articles and the condition of the microorganisms. Contact is unlikely to be achieved if the microorganisms are located in pores or crevices or are protected by hardened deposits of organic or crystalline material. The complex, lipid-rich cell walls of Gram-negative bacteria, especially *Pseudomonas* species, present a barrier to the entry of some bactericidal agents into the cells. The wetting power of disinfectants is enhanced by alcohol or detergents.

Appropriate agents and apparatus

Biocidal agents that are used for sterilization are

Table 1.1 Biocidal agents for sterilization

Agent	Applications	Apparatus
Saturated steam	Wrapped articles	Prevacuum sterilizer, 134°C
	Unwrapped instruments and utensils	Downward displacement sterilizer, 132–134°C
	Aqueous liquids	Downward displacement sterilizer, 121°C
Dry heat	Metal articles, glassware, oils	Hot air oven, 160°C
Gaseous chemicals	Heat-sensitive instruments and medical devices	Ethylene oxide sterilizer or Low-temperature steam and formaldehyde sterilizer
Ionizing radiation	Medical devices	^{60}Co installation or Electron accelerator

Table 1.2 Biocidal agents for disinfection

Agent	Applications	Apparatus
Hot water	Heat-sensitive instruments	Temperature-controlled water bath, 75°C
	Anaesthetic apparatus	Washing machine, 75°C
	Blankets and linen	
	Mopheads	
	Eating and drinking utensils	
Low-temperature steam	Heat-sensitive instruments	Low-temperature steam and formaldehyde sterilizer (without the formaldehyde)
Ultraviolet radiation	Room air	Germicidal lamps
Formaldehyde vapour	Contaminated rooms	Electrical vaporizer
Chemical disinfectants	Articles not required in sterile condition	Suitable containers
	Decontamination of used articles	
	Skin and mucous membranes	

listed, with main applications and types of sterilizers, in Table 1.1. Physical and chemical agents of disinfection are presented in a similar way in Table 1.2.

Steam sterilizers

Pressure steam sterilizers are specially designed for porous loads (comprising all wrapped articles), unwrapped instruments and utensils, or aqueous liquids. Prevacuum sterilizers, with mechanical air removal, are required for efficient sterilization of porous loads. The downward displacement type may also be used but is more liable to error and the cycle is longer. Downward displacement steam sterilizers should be used for unwrapped instruments and utensils and also for bottled liquids. The provision of a spray-cooling system for liquids reduces the time required for sterilization and minimizes the deterioration of heat-sensitive ingredients.

Gas sterilizers

Sterilizers for heat-sensitive equipment are de-signed for the removal of air by mechanical evacuation, vaporization of the chemical agent (ethylene oxide or formaldehyde) and maintenance of the relative humidity required for biocidal action.

Dry heat sterilizers

Dry heat sterilization is usually carried out in hot air ovens with forced air convection. Direct flaming is used to sterilize some laboratory bench tools such as inoculating loops. Incineration of waste material is also a form of dry heat sterilization; the design of incinerators is critical as live microorganisms escape with the effluent if burning is incomplete.

Radiation installations

Radiation sterilization is virtually restricted to industrial installations because of the complexity of the equipment and the essential safety precautions. A cobalt-60 (^{60}Co) gamma radiation source or an electron accelerator may be used.

Chemical disinfectants

Chemical disinfection does not require complex apparatus. Containers should be of suitable shape and size and filled with sufficient solution to ensure that the articles are completely immersed and that cavities are free from trapped air. The selection of an appropriate disinfectant is based on its range and degree of bactericidal activity (determined by an approved method), its compatibility with the articles to be disinfected and other materials with which it may come in contact during use.

Bacterial filtration

The physical removal of bacteria from liquids and air is accomplished by filters of appropriate pore diameter and retention efficiency. Suitable filter holders and other accessories are required. Membrane filters which have an average pore diameter of 0.22 μm or 0.45 μm and act as mechanical sieves are most suitable for filtration of liquids. Fibrous filters have a greater bacterial load capacity but the flow rate is slow and the quality of the solution may be affected by adsorption of solutes, alteration of pH or addition of fibres. Fibrous filters in the form of packed columns or thin paper sheets, are commonly used for air filtration but membrane filters are suitable for some applications. The fibrous sheets have a large surface area and are used in conventional or laminar flow ventilation systems; each sheet is pleated and all the edges are sealed into a frame to form a compact unit. HEPA (high-efficiency particulate air) filters are 99.97–99.997 per cent efficient for retention of particles with a diameter of 0.3 μm.

Severity of treatment

Heat sterilization processes are defined by time at a specified temperature. Recommended times for steam sterilization are 15 minutes at 121°C and 3 minutes at 132–134°C (Working Party on Pressure-Steam Sterilizers, 1959). These represent the minimum holding times for which the whole of the material treated must be held at the selected sterilizing temperature to kill the microbial contaminants. They are based on the resistance of *Bacillus*

stearothermophilus spores to moist heat. In dry heat sterilization, a holding time of 60 minutes at 160°C allows for the possibility of a 10°C variation in temperature within the oven.

The parameters of a gas sterilization process are more complex. The conditions required for sterilization in a hospital ethylene oxide process operated within a temperature range of 45–60°C are:

ethylene oxide:	400–1000 mg/litre
relative humidity:	70 per cent
time:	4 hours

A radiation sterilization process is described by a single value, the minimum absorbed dose. A minimum dose of 25 kGy (2.5 Mrad) is commonly used in the commercial production of medical devices but is increased if the contamination level of the articles exceeds the level for which the dose has been calculated.

The efficiency of chemical disinfection depends on the concentration and the time for which the solution is in contact with the articles or surfaces to be disinfected.

THE MICROBIAL TARGET

The rational selection and correct performance of procedures that are intended to kill, remove or exclude harmful microorganisms requires knowledge of their nature and distribution, their capability of survival in different conditions and their resistance to physical and chemical biocidal agents.

The term 'microorganism' embraces a wide range of primitive life forms; most of them are unicellular. but they have little else in common except the need of a microscope to observe them. Microorganisms are widely distributed in outdoor and indoor environments, on the human skin and in the mouth, upper respiratory tract, large intestine and parts of the urogenital tract. They are rarely harmful in these situations but are likely to cause disease if they gain access to organs or tissues that are normally sterile. Despite their small size and primitive nature, microorganisms present a formidable challenge to the methods that are used to prevent or control the spread of infection. The major groups and some of the distinguishing

Table 1.3 Types of microorganisms

Group	Affiliates	Growth habits	Sources
Bacteria	Neither plants nor animals	Free-living or parasitic	Soil, water, organic materials, man, animals, plants
Viruses	Subcellular particles	Obligate intracellular parasites	Human, animal, plant or bacterial hosts
Fungi (moulds and yeasts)	Some resemblance to plants, but not photosynthetic	Free-living or parasitic	Decaying organic matter, soil, fruit juices, plants, animals, man
Protozoa	Animals	Free-living or parasitic	Soil, water
Algae	Green plants	Free-living	Sea, fresh water, soil

characteristics, together with their relationship to higher forms of life, are listed in Table 1.3.

Bacteria

Structure and composition

The bacteria will be described in more detail than other microorganisms. They are neither plants nor animals; the single cells differ from these higher forms of life in that the nuclear DNA is not confined within a membrane and does not break up into chromosomes during cell division. Bacterial DNA is a single circular, tightly coiled molecule, bearing the genes that determine the characteristics and metabolic processes of the particular species. Bacteria also lack cytoplasmic particles called mitochondria, which are sites of enzymes concerned with respiration and other metabolic activities in animal cells. The delicate cell membrane, composed of proteins and lipids, acts as a semipermeable barrier, regulating the entry of essential nutrients and preventing loss of vital constituents from the cells. The nuclear material, cytoplasm and membrane are enclosed in a rigid cell wall that is unique to bacteria. The wall contains a lattice-like compound called peptidoglycan. It maintains the shape and integrity of the bacterium and a step in its synthesis is the specific target of the bactericidal action of the penicillin and cephalosporin (ß-lactam) antibiotics.

Some bacteria have additional structures that are located outside the cell. Flagella are long, thin hair-like processes. They arise in the cell membrane and their external movement confers motility on the bacterium. Other bacteria may have a capsule of viscous carbohydrate or protein material which can prevent the uptake of the organisms by phagocytic cells. Capsulated bacteria are non-motile. The structure of a bacterial cell is shown in Figure 1.1.

Morphology and staining

The term morphology embraces the shape, size and arrangement of bacteria as seen in tissues or in laboratory cultures. Variation in the shape of the cells is limited by their unicellular nature to two main types: spherical cocci (*sing.* coccus) and rod-shaped bacilli (*sing.* bacillus). The cocci are round or oval and approximately one micrometre (μm) in diameter. They may be arranged in clusters, chains or pairs but also occur singly. Bacilli exhibit greater variation as the cells vary in width (0.2–2.0 μm) as well as in length (2–10 μm). Spirochaetes are long cells (up to 20 μm) in which a thin strand of protoplasm is wound around an axial filament

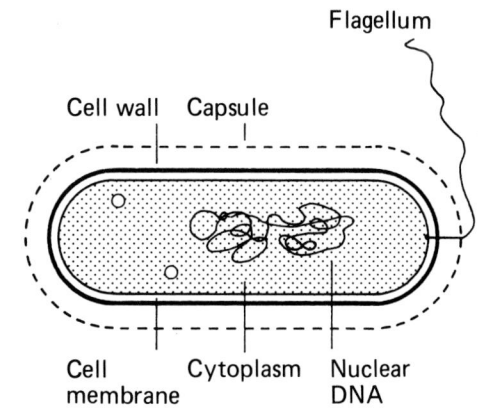

Fig. 1.1 Structure of a bacterial cell. Note: flagella and capsules are mutually exclusive.

and enclosed in an outer sheath. Most of the basic bacterial forms recognized today were observed and drawn in the seventeenth century by the Dutch draper Antonie van Leeuwenhoek when he examined material from around the teeth with simple, high quality lenses which he made.

Clinical specimens and laboratory cultures containing bacteria are prepared for microscopic examination by spreading a sample thinly on a glass slide. The dried smear must be stained with a suitable dye to render the cells visible. Basic dyes, such as crystal violet, methylene blue and carbol fuchsin (red) serve this purpose by combining with nucleic acids in the cells. However, Gram's stain is routinely used for most purposes because it also differentiates between the Gram-positive and Gram-negative bacteria. The stain may be performed as follows:

1. Stain with crystal violet (30 seconds), rinse
2. Mordant with iodine solution (30 seconds), rinse
3. Decolourize with acetone (a few seconds), rinse
4. Counterstain with neutral red or dilute carbol fuchsin (30 seconds), rinse and blot dry.

Both groups of bacteria take up the purple stain. The Gram-positive species retain it when treated with acetone and appear purple when the slide is examined. Gram-negative species are decolourized by acetone and are counter-stained red to render them visible. Tissue, pus, sputum and other material of human or animal origin also stain red.

The Gram stain reaction is attributable to differences in the structure and chemical composition of bacterial cell walls. The peptidoglycan in Gram-positive bacteria constitutes 50–100 per cent of the cell wall material and is a closely linked lattice which contracts on treatment with acetone, retaining the dye-iodine molecules that have been formed within the cell. Gram-negative bacteria have only 5–10 per cent of peptidoglycan in their cell walls and the open lattice does not contract sufficiently to retain the purple dye (Salton, 1963; Beveridge & Davies, 1983). A comparison of important properties that differ in Gram-positive and Gram-negative bacteria is given in Table 1.4.

The genus *Mycobacterium*, which includes the species that causes tuberculosis, has a high lipid content, including wax. It is stained by treatment with hot concentrated carbol fuchsin (red) or fluorescent auramine-rhodamine (golden) for 10 minutes. Species of *Mycobacterium* are termed acid-fast bacilli (a.f.b.) because they retain the primary stain on treatment with acid alcohol. Gram-positive and Gram-negative bacteria, tissue cells and tissue debris are decolourized and are counterstained with methylene blue or a green dye.

Growth and multiplication

In common with other living organisms, bacteria require sources of carbon, hydrogen, nitrogen, oxygen, sulphur and phosphorus for growth and reproduction. Water is also essential. Many bacteria have additional requirements for trace metals and vitamins. Certain soil bacteria which can utilize carbon dioxide and atmospheric nitrogen are essential for the continuation of life on earth because they convert these elements to forms that can be used by plants and animals. Most bacteria, including human and animal parasites, require organic carbon such as carbohydrate. Organic nit-

Table 1.4 Comparison of Gram-positive and Gram-negative bacteria

Characteristic	Gram-positive bacteria	Gram-negative bacteria
Cell wall composition	50–100% peptidoglycan; polyalcohol and polysaccharide complexes	5–10% peptidoglycan; lipid-protein-polysaccharide complexes (pyrogens, or endotoxins)
Toxins	Potent, specifically acting exotoxins may be produced (diphtheria, tetanus, botulism)	Non-specifically acting endotoxins (cell wall lipo-polysaccharide)
Resistance to drying	Good	Poor
Susceptibility to chemical disinfectants and antibiotics	Susceptible to a wide range	Susceptibility restricted to a narrower range

rogen, such as amino acids, is also commonly required. Most bacteria will grow on a suitable artificial culture medium in the laboratory. Basal media are prepared from meat extracts but added blood or serum may be required to isolate some pathogenic bacteria. Liquid media are solidified to a gel by the addition of agar for isolation of microorganisms in pure culture.

When a culture medium has been inoculated with material containing bacteria, it is incubated at the optimum temperature for the likely species (usually 37°C in medical bacteriology) and in the presence or absence of oxygen, as appropriate. Aerobic bacteria require oxygen for growth and strict anaerobes grow only in the absence of oxygen. Many bacteria grow in the presence or absence of oxygen; these are described as facultative. Incubation times for the development of bacterial colonies on an agar medium or of turbidity in a liquid medium range from less than 24 hours to several days. The human strain of *Mycobacterium tuberculosis* requires 3–6 weeks to produce visible growth.

The growth of bacteria is measured by the rate of multiplication because the cells alter little in size during the growth cycle. They multiply asexually by binary fission, a process in which a cell divides into two similar daughter cells. The DNA is replicated to provide a copy of the nuclear material for each daughter cell. The mother cell divides after a septum consisting of cell membrane and cell wall material has been formed across the centre of the cell. When a small number of cells of a fast-growing species of bacterium is inoculated in a suitable medium and incubated in suitable conditions, cell division may occur at 20 minute intervals doubling the population each time. The number of bacteria reaches a maximum at 10^8–10^{10} per millilitre of a broth culture; exhaustion of oxygen or an essential nutrient, or the accumulation of metabolic waste products slows and eventually terminates multiplication. Multiplication could be sustained indefinitely in living tissues if the bacteria are supplied with nutrients by the blood, which also removes their waste products. Termination may be brought about by the host defence mechanisms or antibiotic treatment.

Although bacteria are isolated as pure cultures in the laboratory for investigation and identifica-

tion, natural populations are mixed. The type of nutrients and amount of moisture determine which types of microorganisms predominate in a given ecological situation. Non-pathogenic Gram-positive cocci and bacilli constitute the normal resident bacterial flora of the skin, but streptococci predominate in the mouth and Gram-negative bacilli in the bowel.

Bacterial spores

Bacterial forms that are not killed by boiling water have been a subject of research since their discovery a hundred years ago. The resistant spores have apparently evolved as a response to adverse conditions; each vegetative cell usually produces only one spore and only a small proportion of the cells in a population may sporulate. *Bacillus* (aerobic) and *Clostridium* (anaerobic) species are the only bacteria that have the capacity to produce spores; their natural habitat is the soil and they are disseminated by dust to indoor as well as outdoor environments. Diseases caused by spore-forming bacteria include tetanus, anthrax, gas gangrene and other wound infections. Botulism food poisoning is caused by *Clostridium botulinum*; if spores survive the food canning process they can germinate and grow in the anaerobic conditions within sealed cans containing non-acid foods, producing their lethal toxin.

The production of a spore commences with the formation of a membranous septum towards one end of the rod-shaped mother cell. The smaller compartment develops into a spore which contains a copy of the nuclear material. The DNA, cytoplasm, cell membrane and cell wall of the vegetative cell constitute the vital spore core which is reduced in volume by loss of water to the mother cell during maturation of the spore. The involvement of a low moisture level in the heat resistance of spores is discussed in Chapter 4, which also contains a diagram of a mature spore. The spore core is enveloped by a wide cortex and one or more outer spore coats. When the integuments have been completed the remains of the mother cell degenerate.

The return of a resistant spore to a vegetative cell is stimulated by conditions that are not always understood. The process is initiated by activation, which involves a change in the physical state of the spore components. Activation is brought about by chemicals in the natural environment but may be accomplished by sublethal heat or the addition of calcium and dipicolinic acid in the laboratory. Germination follows activation; uptake of water activates the spore enzymes, the integuments are broken down and heat resistance and other spore characteristics are rapidly lost. The outgrowth of a vegetative cell completes the process of germination.

Nomenclature

Each bacterium is given two official names. The first is the genus and starts with a capital letter; the second identifies the species. The proper name is italicized in books and published papers and is usually underlined in typed manuscripts. Colloquial names, such as staphylococci, streptococci, gonococci, coliform bacilli and tubercle bacilli, may be used but are not italicized and do not have capital letters. Subdivision of species, such as *Staphylococcus aureus* and *Salmonella typhi*, is unnecessary for the diagnosis of disease but may be of assistance in tracing the source of an epidemic. Some genera and species that are representative of well-known Gram-positive and Gram-negative bacteria are listed in Table 1.5.

Contamination, infection and disease

Microorganisms that are present in situations where they are not multiplying are termed contaminants. Gram-positive bacteria and bacterial spores are common on dry surfaces and airborne particles because they are not readily killed by drying. Gram-negative bacilli, such as coliforms and pseudomonads, die rapidly in dry conditions but survive in damp or wet situations; they may multiply in water if it contains impurities that are adequate for growth.

Bacteria that are growing in a close association with another form of life are parasites. Some parasites exist in a stable relationship with their human host and constitute the normal flora of body surfaces and adjoining mucous membranes. These relatively harmless bacteria are termed commensals. Pathogenic bacteria can also be found in some healthy individuals, who are referred to as carriers (for example, of staphylococci, streptococci or typhoid bacteria). Colonization by parasites constitutes infection. Disease is the harmful result of infection. A pathogenic microorganism is

Table 1.5 Nomenclature of bacteria (examples of genera and species mentioned in this book)

Group	Genus	Species
Gram-positive cocci	*Staphylococcus*	*S. aureus*
	Streptococcus	*S. pyogenes*
Gram-positive bacilli	*Corynebacterium*	*C. diphtheriae*
	Bacillus	*B. anthracis*
		B. subtilis
		B. stearothermophilus
	Clostridium	*C. perfringens*
		C. tetani
Gram-negative cocci	*Neisseria*	*N. meningitidis*
		N. gonorrhoeae
Gram-negative bacilli	*Escherichia*	*E. coli*
	Klebsiella	*K. pneumoniae*
	Proteus	*P. vulgaris*
	Salmonella	*S. typhi*
		S. typhimurium
	Shigella	*S. sonnei*
	Pseudomonas	*P. aeruginosa*
		P. cepacia
Acid-fast bacilli	*Mycobacterium*	*M. tuberculosis*
Spirochaetes	*Treponema*	*T. pallidum*
	Leptospira	*L. icterohaemorrhagiae*

one that is capable of causing disease in a susceptible host. Opportunistic pathogens cause disease in individuals with immune deficiencies that are inherited or caused by certain diseases or by treatment with immunosuppressive or cytotoxic drugs. These organisms are frequently Gram-negative bacteria, such as *Klebsiella*, *Proteus* and *Pseudomonas*.

Viruses

Structure and composition

Viruses are subcellular particles, termed virions. They were initially detected as infective agents that passed through bacterial filters. They cannot be seen by the ordinary light microscope but their shape and structure is revealed by the electron microscope. Virus particles range in size from 20–200 nanometers (nm) and may be brick-shaped, bullet-shaped, spherical, helical or icosahedral.

The infective component of the virion is the nucleic acid core; this may be DNA or RNA but they do not both occur in the same virus. The core is enclosed in a protein coat, the capsid, which determines the external shape of the particle. Viruses which have an outer lipid envelope are termed lipophilic; they are inactivated by organic solvents, such as ether, and many chemical disinfectants. The non-enveloped (hydrophilic) viruses are killed only by strong chlorine disinfectants and aldehydes. All viruses are killed by boiling water but the time required has not always been precisely determined.

Reproduction

Viruses are obligate intracellular parasites because they do not contain all the enzymes required for their own replication. They multiply within specific host cells in animals, plants or bacteria. When a virus particle attaches to the surface of the host cell it is taken up into the cytoplasm, where its components are dismantled by the host cell enzymes. The liberated viral nucleic acid programmes the host cell to synthesize new viral protein and nucleic acid which are then assembled to form new virus particles. These are liberated by the disintegrating host cell. The lipid envelope, when present, is acquired from the membrane of the host cell. For one virus particle that enters the host cell, a large number may be discharged. Viruses survive for varying periods outside their host cells but cannot reproduce until they invade a new cell.

Nomenclature

A binomial system is not yet in use. Viruses are characterized by the type of nucleic acid (DNA or RNA), the presence or absence of a lipid envelope, or by the route of infection (respiratory or alimentary tract), or by an intermediate host, such as a species of insect. Some groups of viruses, with examples, are listed in Table 1.6.

Mycoplasmas, Chlamydiae and Rickettsiae

These organisms are intermediate in size between

Table 1.6 Nomenclature of viruses

Group	Nucleic acid	Lipid envelope	Diseases (examples)
Adenoviridae	DNA	Absent	Pharyngitis
Arenaviridae	RNA	Present	Lassa fever
Coronaviridae	RNA	Present	Colds
Hepadnaviridae	DNA	Absent	Hepatitis B
Herpesviridae	DNA	Present	Cold sores, chicken-pox/shingles, genital herpes
Orthomyxoviridae	RNA	Present	Influenza
Paramyxoviridae	RNA	Present	Measles, mumps
Picornaviridae	RNA	Absent	Hepatitis A, poliomyelitis, colds
Reoviridae	RNA	Absent	Gastroenteritis (including rotavirus infections)
Retroviridae	RNA	Present	Acquired immune deficiency syndrome (AIDS)

the bacteria and viruses (0.3–0.5 μm). They are now recognized as bacteria because they contain both DNA and RNA, have the cell wall peptidoglycan that is characteristic of bacteria, and multiply by binary fission. Chlamydiae are Gramnegative but the mycoplasmas and rickettsiae are difficult to stain by any method. Mycoplasmas have defective cell walls but can be grown on laboratory media. They cause atypical pneumonias, formerly thought to be viral in origin. Chlamydiae are obligate intracellular parasites because they cannot produce the energy that is necessary for growth and must derive it from the host cell. They are released as elementary bodies, which survive until they are taken up by another cell. The group includes organisms causing trachoma, inclusion conjunctivitis of the newborn, non-specific urethritis, and psittacosis (a disease of birds which can be transmitted to man). They are susceptible to broad spectrum antibiotics. The rickettsiae are obligate intracellular parasites because their cell membrane is defective, allowing vital constituents to leak out. One species causes epidemic typhus, a human infection with an arthropod vector, the body louse.

Fungi

These ubiquitous organisms are usually saprophytes, growing on non-living organic matter. They are known principally as causes of spoilage in foods, textiles, painted surfaces and many other materials. However, some cause human and animal disease, usually in individuals whose resistance to infection is impaired.

Morphology

The filamentous fungi, commonly called moulds, are multicellular organisms with complex life cycles that involve the production of spores by sexual or asexual processes. The spores of terrestrial fungi are shed into the air in large numbers. Their primary function is reproduction of and dissemination of the species. They withstand dry conditions but are much less resistant to heat than are bacterial spores.

The yeasts are unicellular fungi. Some produce spores but they reproduce mainly by budding from the vegetative cells. Some yeasts form filaments in addition to single cells. Unlike the filamentous fungi, yeast cells can be examined as stained smears. The round or oval cells are Gram-positive and are usually about 5 μm in diameter (cf. spherical bacteria, 1 μm).

Conditions for growth

Fungi flourish in tropical and temperate climates. They are usually grown in the laboratory at 25–30°C but pathogenic species may grow better at 37°C. The filamentous fungi are strict aerobes but yeasts can grow aerobically or anaerobically. Glucose peptone agar and malt extract agar are commonly used culture media. Atibiotics may be added to the medium to facilitate the isolation of fungi from pathological specimens by preventing overgrowth by bacteria and common saprophytic fungi.

Fungal infections

Fungal diseases may be superficial or systemic, depending on the organism and the route of infection. Species of filamentous fungi belonging to the genera *Microsporum*, *Trichophyton* and *Epidermophyton* cause tinea, or ringworm, which is restricted to the skin, hair and nails but may occur at various body sites. The filament-forming yeast, *Candida albicans*, infects the skin and mucous membranes, causing oral thrush and infections of the nail beds. It also causes serious blood-borne systemic infections. Systemic fungal infections may involve the lungs, brain and kidneys. Aspergillosis is a mild or severe infection of the lungs, caused by species that are widely distributed in the environment. Tissue invasion by *Candida* or *Aspergillus* species frequently occurs in patients with terminal cancer. The conditions that predispose individuals to fungal infection cannot always be identified but they include extremes of age, diabetes, imbalance of the normal bacterial flora of the body by treatment with antibiotics, and treatment with steroids, cytotoxic agents or immunosuppressive drugs.

Protozoa

These single-celled forms of animal life occur in

aquatic environments and in the soil. They do not possess a rigid cell wall but may have an external skeleton of secreted minerals. Most are motile by means of hair-like processes (flagella or cilia) or by amoeboid movement. Some protozoa produce non-motile cysts which are resistant to drying and chemical agents. Protozoa causing human disease include *Leishmania*, *Trypanosoma* (sleeping sickness), *Trichomonas* (vaginitis), *Toxoplasma*, *Giardia* (intestinal infection), *Pneumocystis* (pneumonia), *Plasmodium* (malaria) and amoebae (amoebic dysentery or meningitis).

Algae

These primitive green plants will not figure prominently in this book because they are not a major cause of disease in man or animals. However, their growth in fresh or sea water exposed to sunlight presents problems of control in some situations because algae are not susceptible to many antibacterial agents. Algae occur in fresh and salt water and include large seaweeds as well as the unicellular forms. They are also found in soil. The microscopic forms multiply by binary fission, a process in which each cell splits to produce two similar daughter cells. The mature cells vary in shape and may produce spores. Diatoms are algae which contain silica in the cell wall.

REFERENCES

Beveridge T J, Davies J A 1983 Cellular responses of *Bacillus subtilis* and *Escherichia coli* to the Gram stain. Journal of Bacteriology 156: 846–858

Salton M R J 1963 The relationship between the nature of the cell wall and the Gram stain. Journal of General Microbiology 30: 223–235

Working Party on Pressure-Steam Sterilisers 1959 Sterilisation by steam under increased pressure. A report to the Medical Research Council. Lancet i: 425–435

FURTHER READING

Block S S (ed) 1983 Disinfection, sterilization, and preservation, 3rd edn. Lea & Febiger, Philadelphia

Braude A I, Davis C E, Fierer J 1982 Microbiology. Saunders, Philadelphia

Lowbury E J L, Ayliffe G A J, Geddes M, Williams J D (eds) 1981 Control of hospital infection, 2nd edn. Chapman and Hall, London

Maurer I M 1978 Hospital hygiene, 2nd edn. Arnold, London

Parker M, Stucke V 1982 Microbiology for nurses, 6th edn. Bailliere Tindall, London

Russell A D, Hugo W B, Ayliffe G A J (eds) 1982 Principles and practice of disinfection, preservation and sterilisation. Blackwell, Oxford

White D O, Fenner F J 1985 Medical virology, 2nd edn. Academic Press, New York

2

Efficiency of sterilization

Sterilization is a process that is intended to kill all types of microorganisms. A particular article is either sterile or unsterile (an all or none state) but, when all of the items that are treated by a particular process are considered, there is always a chance that some contaminants may survive and a proportion of the articles will remain unsterile. An efficient process is one that has been designed to achieve an acceptably low proportion (e.g. one per million) of surviving microorganisms and unsterile items.

Efficiency is built into the design of the process by determining the severity of treatment (e.g. time at a specified temperature) that is required to kill the types and numbers of microbial contaminants on the articles to be treated. The process must be validated by appropriate physical, chemical and biological tests and monitored regularly during routine operation to ensure that the intended conditions for sterilization are achieved throughout the load in the sterilizer and are maintained for an adequate time. This chapter deals with:

Designing the process
Testing the process
Testing the product.

DESIGNING THE PROCESS

The following information is required for calculation of the conditions that will sterilize the articles for which the process is designed:

1. Rate of biocidal action
2. Initial contamination level
3. Sterility assurance.

Rate of biocidal action

Determination of death rates

The rate at which a biocidal agent reduces the number of viable cells in a microbial population is determined by counting the survivors in samples obtained after graded exposures to heat, radiation or chemical vapour in specified conditions. The viable counts are usually performed by preparing serial dilutions of each sample and spreading a volume of each dilution (in duplicate) on nutrient agar plates. Each colony that develops on incubation is assumed to represent a single viable microorganism or a small cluster. The volume and dilution are taken into account when the number of viable cells or spores in the original sample is calculated.

If the initial count and the sample counts are plotted on a logarithmic scale against the exposure time and a line is drawn through the separate points, a death rate curve is obtained. A straight line represents a constant (logarithmic or exponential) death rate. Nonlogarithmic death rates are represented by curves which show initial or final lags in the killing rate.

The range of time or dose over which reliable counts can be obtained for preparation of a death rate curve limits the experimental determination of killing rates to a level of about 200 survivors per ml. Extrapolation of the death rate to lower survivor levels may be valid when the available curves do not deviate from linearity but extrapolation of

nonlinear curves may result in an underestimate of the conditions required for sterilization.

Logarithmic death rate

A hypothetical series of viable counts which shows that a constant proportion (not a constant number) of microorganisms is killed in each unit of time or dose is contained in Table 2.1; the corresponding logarithmic curve is illustrated in Figure 2.1.

In this stylized example, a tenfold reduction in the number of survivors, corresponding to 90 per cent kill, has occurred in each minute of exposure to the specified conditions. As the initial count was 10^4, the population would be reduced to a single

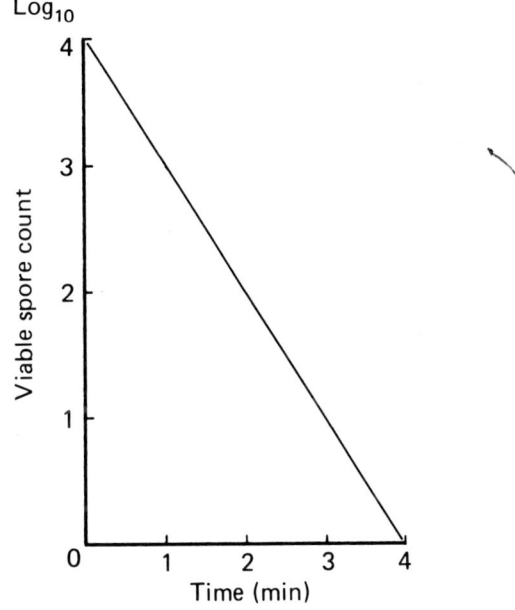

Fig. 2.1 Logarithmic (linear) death rate curve.

Table 2.1 Set of survivor counts illustrating logarithmic death rate

Time of exposure (min)	No. surviving (at commencement of time unit)	% Killed (in each time unit)	% Killed (cumulative)
0	10 000	0	0
1	1000	90	90
2	100	90	99
3	10	90	99.9
4	1	90	99.99
5	0.1 (1/10 ml)	90	99.999
6	0.01(1/100 ml)	90	99.9999

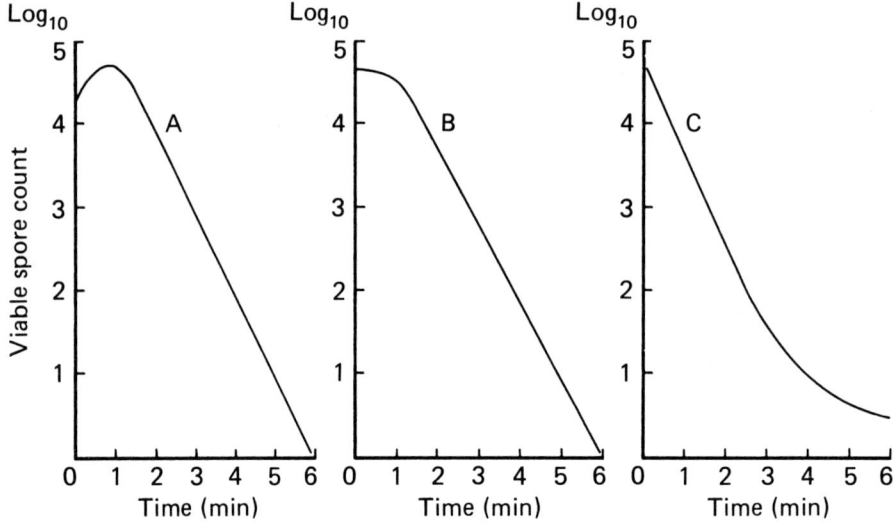

Fig. 2.2 Types of nonlogarithmic (nonlinear) death rate curves.

survivor in 4 minutes. Further reduction would be expressed as the probability of a microorganism surviving (e.g. 10^{-1}, 10^{-2}, and so on) as the duration or severity of treatment increases.

Nonlogarithmic death rates

A survivor curve that is nonlinear over part or all of its length indicates that the death rate is not constant. The deviations usually take the form of an initial or final lag; a curve that shows a lag at each end is described as sigmoid. Some common types of nonlogarithmic death rate curves are illustrated in Figure 2.2.

The anomaly in curve A is an initial increase in viable count. This is followed by a regular logarithmic killing rate. This type of curve is usually associated with heat-resistant bacterial spores, such as *Bacillus stearothermophilus*, which are activated for germination as they approach the sterilizing temperature. This results in early counts that are higher than the initial count obtained on the untreated spore preparation. The rate of activation exceeds the rate of killing until the peak of the hump has been reached; beyond this point, killing increases until the true logarithmic rate is established (Shull et al, 1963). If this type of curve were obtained for a non-sporeforming microorganism, it would suggest that clumped cells were being dis-

persed in the early stage of the killing process.

The flat shoulder in curve B, if obtained for a spore population, would indicate that the number of spores activated balances the number that are killed. A similar curve for non-sporing bacteria may be explained by clumping of the organisms; each clump registers as a colony-forming unit until the last survivor in the clump has been killed and a logarithmic death rate may become apparent.

Curve C shows the type of lag that is often observed when the death rate is slow (e.g. at a relatively low temperature or radiation dose, or when the bacteria are treated with a solution of chemical disinfectant). Terminal lags may be explained in various ways (Cerf, 1977). They might represent the combined logarithmic death rates of two or more species of microorganisms; the steeper part of the curve would correspond to a relatively sensitive population that was present in larger numbers initially, while the lag corresponds to a more resistant species. The latter would determine the outcome of the process although it may be a minor component of the original population. Evidence for this explanation was provided by Bond et al (1970) who studied mixed soil isolates containing heat-sensitive and heat-resistant spores. The separate killing curves were logarithmic but the nonlinear curve was reproduced when they were recombined.

Tailing curves are rarely accounted for by variation in the resistance of individual cells in a homogeneous population because the same curve is obtained if the survivors are cultured and retested. However, a true lag in the killing rate may occur if the biocidal agent causes a gradual change in the microorganisms that hinders its access to the cellular target. The hardening of the protein coat of a virus by prolonged treatment with formaldehyde protects the nucleic acid core, preventing the desired loss of infectivity (Gard, 1957). However, a similar tailing may also be attributed to protection by particulate matter in the virus suspension (Salk & Gori, 1959).

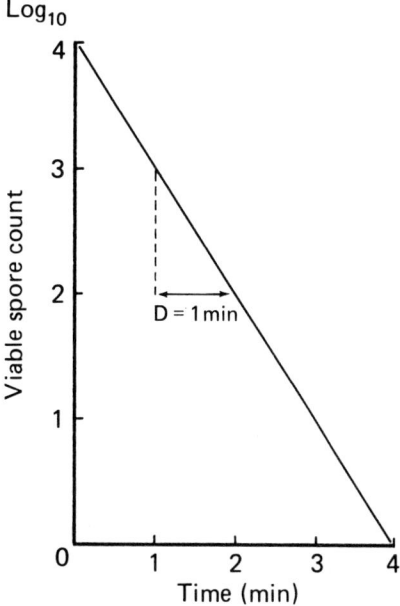

Fig. 2.3 Constant D value (Decimal Reduction Time) for a logarithmic death rate curve.

D value

A quantitative expression of the death rate is required to describe the activity of a biocidal agent against different microorganisms, or to compare the resistance of different microorganisms to a particular agent. The rate constant K, which is used to describe logarithmic chemical reaction rates, has also been applied to the death rate of microorganisms by use of the formula:

$$K = \frac{1}{t} \log_{10} \frac{N_o}{N_t} \text{ , where t is time,}$$

N_o is the initial viable count and N_t the viable count at time t.

However, the D value, which is based on killing time instead of killing rate, is now commonly used as a measure of biocidal activity. The D value, or Decimal Reduction Time, is the time required to effect a tenfold reduction in the number of viable microorganisms, which is equivalent to 90 per cent kill. When the D value refers to sterilizing radiation, it is expressed as a dose.

When the D value is constant, as in a logarithmic killing rate, it may be multiplied by a figure corresponding to the number of tenfold reductions which are required to provide sterility assurance. The derivation of a D value from a logarithmic death rate curve is shown in Figure 2.3.

It is difficult to estimate a useful D value for designing a sterilization process from a nonlogarithmic death rate curve unless the observed deviation can be explained and accounted for as, for example, when an initial shoulder or hump is followed by a logarithmic killing rate. When the curve does not include a linear section of significant length, an average D value may be calculated from the equation (Stumbo, 1973):

$$D = \frac{t}{\log N_o - \log N_t} \text{ , where t is the relevant}$$

time, N_o is the initial viable count and N_t is the viable count at time t.

However, the value derived in this way from a tailing curve is likely to be too low. Other formulae have produced D values which are approximately twice as great as those derived from experimental death rate curves (Schalkowsky & Wiederkehr, 1968).

Initial contamination level

The initial contamination level (also termed the bioburden) refers to the number of microorganisms on articles or in liquids prior to sterilization. Knowledge of the average contamination level is an essential component of process design because it influences the severity of treatment that will be needed to meet the requirement for sterility assurance.

An approximate estimate of the number of microbial contaminants in a liquid can be estimated by the plate count method that was outlined in a previous section. If the number is too low for accurate determination by this method, a sample of the liquid may be passed through a membrane filter. Colonies develop on the surface of the membrane when it is incubated in contact with an appropriate solid or liquid medium. Microorganisms on solid objects must be collected by immersion in, or rinsing with a diluent, which may contain a suitable nonionic dispersing agent. Counts are performed on the resulting suspension as above. Contamination levels are always likely to be underestimated because no single culture medium or set of conditions will grow all types of microorganisms.

It is not necessary to isolate and identify the types of contaminants in detail but it may be important to determine the highest level of resistance in the natural population. Bacterial spores are most resistant to heat but viruses, fungal spores and certain types of vegetative bacteria may have greater resistance to sterilizing radiation. The most resistant types or species in a population of natural contaminants can be isolated by submitting samples of the product to treatment of decreasing severity until survivors are recovered. When a sterilization process is designed, it is generally assumed that all of the contaminants have the maximum resistance level although bacterial spores may constitute only about 1 per cent of the microorganisms in soil or dust.

Sterility assurance

Sterility assurance is expressed as a calculated probability that a microorganism will survive a sterilization process and thereby render a proportion of treated articles unsterile. The level of sterility assurance required varies with the intended use of the articles. A likelihood that one article per million processed may be unsterile (10^{-6} probability of a surviving organism) is generally acceptable for medical equipment. A more rigorous standard of 10^{-12} for the probability that a spore of *Clostridium botulinum* will survive is applied to the heat treatment of non-acid canned foods. A standard of 10^{-4} was the subject of international agreement for the sterilization of space exploration vehicles designed to seek evidence of extraterrestrial life on the planet Mars; this was considered adequate because fewer than 10 vehicles are likely to land on the planet, intentionally or accidentally, in the foreseeable future.

Determination of sterilizing conditions

When the appropriate D value and the initial contamination level are known, and the desired level of sterility assurance has been specified, conditions for sterilization can be calculated by the method illustrated in Figure 2.4.

If the acceptable probability of a surviving microorganism is 10^{-6} and each article carries a single contaminant before sterilization, an exposure equivalent to 6 times the D value would meet the requirement of no more than one unsterile article per million processed. In this example, where the hypothetical D value is 1 minute, 6 minutes would be required. The articles in batch A, with a con-

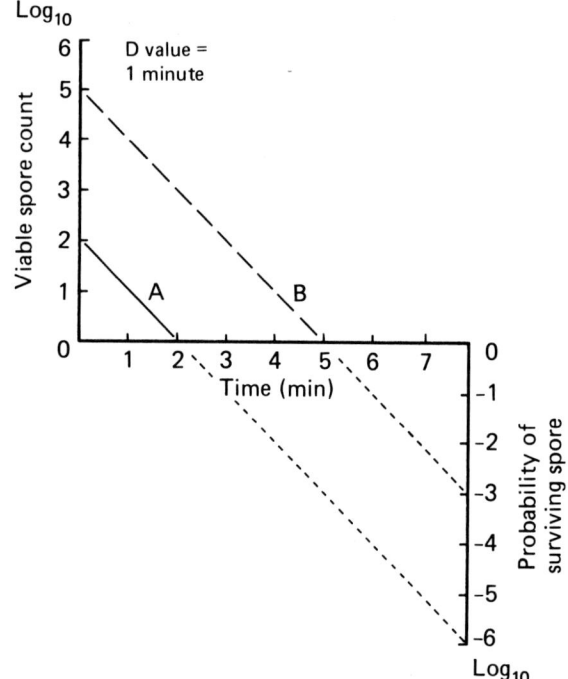

Fig. 2.4 Relationship between D value, initial contamination level and level of sterility assurance.

tamination level of 100 organisms per unit, will require an additional 2 minutes and those in batch B, with 10^5 organisms per unit, an additional 5 minutes. Thus, those in batch B, which may have been manufactured in unhygienic conditions, will require a total of 11 minutes, compared with 8 minutes for batch A, to provide the required level of sterility assurance.

The following examples will serve to illustrate the application of the design calculations to sterilization practice.

1. Linen packs with a contamination level of 10^4 are to be sterilized by steam at 121°C. If the D value for *B. stearothermophilus* is 1.8 minutes at this temperature, the minimum holding time will be the sum of 7.2 minutes (4D) plus 10.8 minutes (6D), making a total of 18 minutes.
2. The D value of gamma radiation for spores of *Bacillus pumilus* is approximately 0.3 megarad (Mrad) and the proposed minimum dose is 2.5 Mrad. This dose is equivalent to 8D and will be adequate for the sterilization of articles that carry no more than 100 microorganisms.
3. The heat treatment of non-acid canned foods of a type which is likely to be contaminated with spores of *C. botulinum* is based on a D value of 0.21 minutes at 121°C. If each can contains a single spore, 2.52 minutes (12×0.21) will be the minimum treatment required. In practice, this is extended to 4 minutes to ensure safety and keeping quality.

These examples underline the importance of minimizing initial contamination levels in order to ensure that requirements for sterility assurance are met. A sterilization process that has been designed for articles with a certain contamination level may be inadequate if the contamination level increases. This may occur as the result of a change in raw materials or factory hygiene. With medical devices and pharmaceutical products, a periodic assessment of contamination levels should be conducted in order to detect any increase above the level for which the process was originally designed. Surveillance of the materials and methods used in production plays an important part in drawing attention to the need for investigation. Medical devices and pharmaceuticals that are manufactured and sterilized commercially are subject to regulations based on an official Code of Good Manufacturing Practice (GMP). These codes provide guidelines for hygienic production, covering the quality of raw materials, cleaning and disinfection of the processing equipment and hygiene in the factory environment, including the provision of defined clean room conditions for aseptic filling of pharmaceuticals into the final containers. The health of employees is also included. Quality control procedures for sterile pharmaceuticals are also subject to the requirements of a national Pharmacopoeia.

The contamination of raw materials depends on the type, source and the treatment used in their preparation. Plastic devices that are moulded by heat emerge from the machine in sterile condition but acquire a small number of microbial contaminants during assembly and packaging. On the other hand, starches and resins used as raw materials for pharmaceuticals, may be so heavily contaminated that they require pretreatment to reduce the number of microorganisms before they are added to the formulation.

The regulations for commercial production do not apply to sterilization within hospitals and laboratories. The determination of the initial contamination level of a wide variety of articles which are sterilized in relatively small numbers is impracticable. In these situations, low contamination levels must be ensured by thorough cleaning (with disinfection if necessary) and careful handling before sterilization.

TESTING THE PROCESS

The purpose of carrying out a sterilization process is to deliver the intended biocidal treatment to the whole of the material to be sterilized. Achievement of this objective depends on the design and performance of the sterilizing apparatus, the nature of the articles to be sterilized, and the methods used for packaging the articles and loading them into the sterilizing chamber. Physical, biological and chemical methods are used to demonstrate the efficiency of the process. They are performed at sites in the sterilizing chamber and within packs or bottles that present the greatest challenge to penetration of the biocidal agent.

Some tests are performed by the operator of the sterilizer and others by the engineer who is responsible for its maintenance and repair. The assistance and advice of a microbiologist may be required in the performance and interpretation of biological tests and for evaluating the end result of a testing programme.

Physical tests

Sterilizer performance

Tests for the performance of steam and gas sterilizers involve observation of temperature, pressure and vacuum gauges and also of stage timers throughout an automatically controlled sterilization cycle. Temperature and pressure readings should be taken at least 3 times during the sterilizing stage of autoclaves and ovens (Department of Health and Social Security, 1980). Recorded charts should be examined carefully and kept until all other tests have been completed. Gauges and recorders should be calibrated at regular intervals against standard instruments.

Leak rate tests

Prevacuum steam sterilizers are tested at least once a week for the rate of air leakage into the evacuated chamber during the air removal and drying stages. The test is usually performed in the drying stage when all parts of the sterilizer are hot. The chamber should be evacuated to 80–90 kPa below atmospheric pressure. After the pressure gauge reading has stabilized, it should not increase by more than 133 Pa, or 1 mm Hg, per minute (Department of Health and Social Security, 1980). Ethylene oxide sterilizers and low-temperature steam and formaldehyde sterilizers should be tested in a similar way. Ethylene oxide sterilizers, which are usually operated above atmospheric pressure in hospitals, should also be tested for outward leakage of the chemical vapour.

Thermocouple tests

Temperatures at selected sites in the chamber or within the load of a dry heat, steam or gas sterilizer are measured by thermocouples. These are insulated leads containing two wires of different composition (e.g. copper and constantan) which are fused together at one end to form a temperature-sensitive junction. The other end is connected to an instrument outside the sterilizer, where the temperature from each lead is recorded continuously on a chart. The leads should enter the chamber of a steam or gas sterilizer through a pressure-tight thermocouple port which is usually located in the door. Fine leads may be inserted in the door closure but tight pressure on the seal is required to prevent leakage of steam or gas. In hot air ovens, which operate at atmospheric pressure, thermocouples may be inserted through the door closure but a thermocouple port is preferred.

Several thermocouples are used in a test; one should be placed in the chamber drain of a steam sterilizer; other sites may also be monitored if the chamber is large. Leads are inserted into one or more test packs or bottles which are located at positions in the chamber where residual air is most likely to accumulate. When leads are placed in packs, care must be taken to avoid creating a path for entry of steam. Several leads are required to monitor temperature distribution in a hot air oven and others are inserted into packs or containers. Thermocouples provide the only means of determining the heat penetration time for packs and bottles in steam and dry heat sterilizers. In ethylene oxide sterilization, temperature measurements are required to determine the time taken for the load to reach the temperature that is controlled by the jacket; the other parameters of ethylene oxide concentration and relative humidity are more important in determining efficiency of sterilization but cannot easily be measured.

Air removal test

Although it involves the use of a chemical indicator the Bowie-Dick Autoclave Tape test (Bowie et al, 1963; Department of Health and Social Security, 1980) is more properly classed as a physical test. It was designed for routine performance in prevacuum steam sterilizers to demonstrate removal of air and penetration of steam. A cross is made with autoclave tape on a sheet of steam-permeable paper and the sheet is placed at the midpoint of a horizontal stack of cotton towels that are used to make the standard test pack. The pack is subjected to a sterilization cycle in which the sterilizing stage is limited to 3.5 minutes. When the indicator sheet is recovered, it is inspected for uniformity of colour change; a paler area, usually in the centre, shows that the pack contained sufficient air to interfere with sterilization. A uniform colour change demonstrates that steam penetration was satisfactory; it does not provide information about the temperature reached in the pack or the time for which it was maintained. A thermocouple test is required for this purpose.

Measurement of radiation dose

A radiation sterilization process is described by a single parameter, the amount of energy absorbed by the material treated. Sterilizing doses are measured in megarad (Mrad) or kilogray (kGy). Dose distribution in the large load of material within the irradiation chamber is measured by placing small strips or cylindrical pieces of red, yellow or colourless Perspex at various sites. The Perspex darkens in proportion to the dose, which is determined by reading the colour change in a spectrophotometer or a white light photometer. Each batch of Perspex dosimeters must be standardized against a reference dosimeter. Dosimetry is repeated as required to monitor changes in dose rate which occur as the output of the ^{60}Co source decreases, or to determine the time required to deliver the prescribed dose to materials of different density.

Chemical indicators

Chemical indicators take the form of solutions or solids that are sealed in tubes or sachets, and dye patterns which are printed on paper strips or directly on the outside of wrapping materials. The chemicals undergo a specified colour change on exposure to a particular sterilizing agent. The indicators may be intended for placement within packs or for external use only.

Internal indicators

These are designed for placement within packs at sites in the sterilizer which are likely to be least accessible to penetration of steam or chemical vapours, or slowest to reach the temperature in a hot air oven. They should be used in conjunction with thermocouples and biological indicators. The chemicals are intended to undergo the full colour change only if sterilizing conditions have been maintained for the specified time. However, there are no official standards for chemical indicators and the change sometimes occurs before conditions for sterilization have been fulfilled. Different types of indicators are required for steam, dry heat, ethylene oxide and steam with formaldehyde processes. The following types of internal indicators are available:

1. Sealed tubes containing a red liquid which changes to yellow, brown and finally to green. Browne's tubes are available for steam sterilization at 120°C (16 minutes) and 135°C (3 minutes). Other types respond to hot air sterilization at 160°C (60 minutes) and 180°C (16 minutes)
2. Pellets in sealed tubes which fuse and change colour (e.g. to red). Diack Controls may be used for steam sterilization at 121°C and Vac Controls at temperatures above 130°C
3. Sachets made from plastic and metal foil containing a substance which displays a colour change that progresses along the length of the sachet. The change is observed through a transparent slit. The colour must reach a marked point on the scale; this type of indicator is used for steam sterilization and has the advantage that the extent of under-exposure or over-exposure can be measured
4. Strips or rectangular pieces of absorbent paper with a band of dye or a pattern of spots which change colour in turn, the last indicating over-exposure. Different types of indicators are required for steam, dry heat, ethylene oxide and steam with formaldehyde processes
5. Sachets made from thin plastic film containing an acidified solution of magnesium chloride and a pH indicator (Royce & Bowler, 1959). Reaction with ethylene oxide produces alkalinity and the colour change occurs when a certain amount has been absorbed.

Chemical indicators should not be used as the sole criterion of sterilization efficiency but routine use of internal indicators can provide immediate evidence of gross deficiency in steam penetration or in ethylene oxide concentration.

External indicators

External indicators are intended only to distinguish packs which have been through a sterilization cycle from those which have not been processed. They do not confirm sterilizing conditions in the chamber or the load.

Paper bags, or pouches made from joined webs of paper and plastic, are prepared commercially for use in steam or gas sterilization. They bear printed patterns which change colour on exposure to the sterilizing agent. Adhesive tapes which are commonly used to fasten paper or cloth wrappings also incorporate a chemical indicator, usually as diagonal stripes which darken or change in colour during the sterilization process. Different types of indicators are required for steam, dry heat and ethylene oxide. Adhesive discs which change colour during exposure to gamma radiation are fixed to the outer cartons and may also be provided on the primary or secondary packaging. They indicate that the packs have been irradiated but do not provide evidence of the dose.

Biological indicators

A biological indicator is a standardized preparation of bacterial spores, presented in a suitable manner for placement at strategic sites in test packs. Biological indicators may be used to monitor sterilizing conditions within test packs but the realistic nature of the tests must be weighed against the inherent variability of living microorganisms. They should not be used as the sole criterion of sterilization efficiency. A brief outline of the methods used in the preparation and standardization of biological indicators will assist understanding of their use as indicators and the significance of results. The species of spore-forming bacteria that are commonly used in the different sterilization processes are listed in Table 2.2.

Preparation

The bacterium is grown on a solid or liquid medium under conditions that produce a high yield of spores. The spores are harvested, treated to eliminate the remaining vegetative cells and washed until they are free from medium constituents and cell debris. The resistance of the suspension to the relevant sterilizing agent is determined. Minor variations between batches of spores can be adjusted by varying the number of spores inoculated onto the units of biological indicator. Water-soluble polymers, such as polyethylene glycol and methyl cellulose, may be added to the suspension to bring the level of resistance to that of naturally occurring microbial contaminants (Doyle, 1971).

The suspension is inoculated on small units of absorbent paper or other suitable material and dried under controlled conditions. The number of spores per unit varies between 10^4 and 10^6. Two packaging methods are commonly used:

1. Each spore paper is placed in a transparent glassine envelope in which it will remain during the test. The envelopes are placed in outer

Table 2.2 Species of spore-forming bacteria used as biological indicators

Process	Species	Incubation temperature °C	Importance in test programme
Steam above atmospheric pressure	B. stearothermophilus	56	Low
Dry heat	B. subtilis var. niger	37	Low
Ethylene oxide	B. subtilis var. niger	37	High
Subatmospheric steam and formaldehyde	B. stearothermophilus	56	High
Gamma radiation	Bacillus pumilus	37	Low

paper packets which may be divided into two compartments, one sealed and one open; the single unit in the sealed compartment is retained for use as untreated control and the two in the open compartment are used in the test.

2. Individual spore papers are placed in plastic sachets or capsules which also contain the culture medium in a thin glass vial. The vial is broken by pressure on the outside of the pack after the test cycle has been completed. The medium is released to engulf the spore paper and the pack is incubated intact.

The first method involves a risk of accidental contamination when the paper is transferred to culture medium in a separate container; however, contaminants will not significantly interfere because only *B. stearothermophilus* will grow above 50°C and *Bacillus subtilis* var. *niger* is easily recognized by the orange colour of the growth on agar and on the surface of liquid medium.

Standardization

The United States Pharmacopeia (1980) specifies D values for spores which are used to prepare biological indicators; these are listed in Table 2.3.

The performance of the spore papers may be tested by exposing them in groups (e.g. 10, 20 or 100 units) to the intended sterilizing conditions. Specially designed sterilizing chambers are described in American Standards prepared by the Association for the Advancement of Medical Instrumentation (1981, 1982). They are called Biolo-

gical Indicator-Evaluator Resistometer (BIER) vessels. Heating and cooling times are very short and a means of inserting the samples after sterilizing conditions have been established may be provided.

The aim of the test is to determine the maximum exposure that results in at least 99.5 per cent of the indicators showing growth and the minimum exposure that is required for at least 90 per cent to be sterilized. The curve in Figure 2.5 represents a hypothetical result for *B. stearothermophilus* indicators in steam at 121°C. There is a high probability of positive culture until 5 minutes and a high probability of negative results after 15 minutes. In the 10 minute interval between 'total

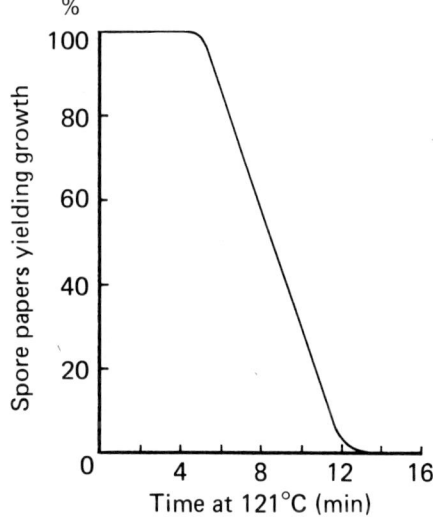

Fig. 2.5 A dose-response curve for *B. stearothermophilus* spore papers to steam at 121°C.

Table 2.3 D values for spores used as biological indicators (from United States Pharmacopeia XX, 1980)

Species	Sterilization process	D value
B. stearothermophilus	Steam: 121°C	1.5 min
B. subtilis var. *niger* ('B globigii')	Ethylene oxide, 54°C, 50% RH:	
	600 mg/1	3 min
	1200 mg/1	1.7 min
	Dry heat:	
	121°C	60 min
	170°C	1 min
B. pumilus	Radiation:	
	Dry conditions	0.15 Mrad (1.5 kGy)
	Wet conditions	0.2 Mrad (2.0 kGy)

survival' and 'total kill', the proportion of positive and negative cultures varies with the time of exposure (partial survival zone).

A sensitive indicator would have a narrow zone of partial survival but no biological indicator is capable of giving a sharp end point. Resistance of the spore papers may be expressed as an 'LD$_{50}$' value, which is the time that corresponds to 50 per cent of positive and 50 per cent of negative cultures (Kelsey, 1961), or as the time required for at least 90 per cent of the papers to yield negative cultures. The aim is to ensure that the chance of obtaining a positive culture after exposure to adequate sterilizing conditions is extremely low. However, spores are not biological thermometers and it is inevitable that positive cultures will occasionally occur although the sterilizer has performed satisfactorily. It has been recommended that biological indicators for use in ethylene oxide sterilizers should be standardized at a temperature above 50°C and a relative humidity close to 50 per cent (Oxborrow et al, 1983).

The stability of biological indicators within the expiry date specified by the manufacturer may be influenced by environmental temperature and relative humidity. The indicators should be stored in a cool, dark place at or below 20°C and the manufacturer's instructions should be strictly observed. Reich & Morien (1982) demonstrated that storage at a relative humidity below 20 per cent decreases the resistance of *B. stearothermophilus* indicators to heat but increased the resistance of *Bacillus subtilis* spore papers to ethylene oxide, so that they no longer conformed to the requirement of the United States Pharmacopeia. They recommended that storage of both types of indicators below 20 per cent or above 60 per cent RH should be avoided.

Incubation

After the sterilization cycle has been completed, the biological indicators are recovered and cultured, together with an unexposed control. A good quality nutrient broth, such as trypticase soy broth, is used. Bromcresol purple is sometimes added so that early growth may be detected by acid production but it is necessary to demonstrate that the concentration used does not inhibit germination of the spores (Cook & Brown, 1960). The temperature of incubation is 37°C for *B. subtilis* var. *niger* and 56°C for *B. stearothermophilus*. If a water bath is used for incubation at the higher temperature, the culture bottles should be well-sealed and placed in fixed racks and the water level should not be so high that it can wet the screw caps. The water should be changed frequently and the water bath sterilized (Joynson, 1975). The unexposed spore strip should yield growth in 24 hours and those that have been used in a test are likely to show growth within 3 days if they contain surviving spores. However, incubation should be continued for 7 days before a negative result is recorded. Shorter incubation times are recommended by some manufacturers; they may be adequate if they have been used in the standardization process.

Results

The significance of the result of a biological indicator test depends on the number of units used. A result obtained with a single unit is meaningless because there is a chance of obtaining a positive or negative culture at any point in the partial survival zone. If a single unit has a 1 in 10 chance of producing a positive culture despite exposure to sterilizing conditions, two units will reduce the probability to 1 in 100 and three will reduce it to 1 in 1000.

Role of biological indicators

Biological indicator tests should be accompanied by measurement of the sterilization parameters. Their use in steam sterilization and hot air sterilization is usually not required because reliable measurements of temperature and time are sufficient. However, their use is essential in ethylene oxide and formaldehyde sterilization processes because the complex parameters cannot be measured in the packs. Five to 10 units should be used in each test until confidence in the sterilizer and the packing methods has been established. Two units should then be used in each cycle unless positive cultures are obtained. In that event, the mechanical performance of the sterilizer must be investigated and the humidity and gas concentration in the chamber checked.

Testing programmes

Qualifying tests

A combination of the appropriate test methods is used when a new sterilizer has been installed or on recommissioning after repairs or modifications. The sterilizing department supervisor, the maintenance engineer and the microbiologist are involved in the performance and interpretation of the tests. Some are repeated at quarterly, half-yearly or yearly intervals as part of a planned preventive maintenance (PPM) programme.

Routine tests

Routine tests are carried out to confirm efficiency in the day to day operation of the sterilizer. They must be convenient to perform so that they do not interfere with the production of sterile supplies, but sensitive enough to give early indication of a fault. Temperature, pressure and vacuum readings are sufficient in steam sterilization but biological and chemical indicators are required in gas sterilization.

The tests required for dry heat, steam and gas sterilizers will be described in more detail in the relevant chapters; a summarized testing programme is set out in Table 2.4.

TESTING THE PRODUCT

The performance of sterility tests on a limited sample of the final product is a less sensitive method for testing the efficiency of sterilization than are tests on the sterilization process, which have been described in the preceding section. However, sterility tests must be performed on pharmaceutical products that are sterilized in bulk by filtration and then filled aseptically into the final containers. The frequency of testing, or the number of samples tested, may be reduced when the initial contamination level of the product is known and it is sterilized in the final containers by a process that has been monitored by approved methods. The same principles apply to sterile medical devices. The limitations of product sterility tests are:

Table 2.4 Testing efficiency of sterilization

Type of sterilizer	Qualifying tests	Routine tests
Dry heat sterilizer	Sterilizer function Thermocouple test	Observation of temperature readings
Instrument sterilizer	Sterilizer function Thermocouple test	Observation of temperature and pressure readings
Porous load sterilizer (prevacuum type)	Sterilizer function	Observation of temperature, pressure and vacuum readings
	Leak rate test	Leak rate test (weekly)
	Bowie-Dick tape test	Bowie-Dick tape test (daily)
	Thermocouple test	
	Chemical indicator ⎫ optional Biological indicator ⎭	
Bottled liquid sterilizer	Sterilizer function Thermocouple test	Observation of temperature and pressure readings
Ethylene oxide sterilizer	Sterilizer function Thermocouple test Biological indicator	Observation of temperature, pressure and vacuum readings Biological indicator (each cycle) Chemical indicator (each cycle)
Steam and formaldehyde sterilizer	Sterilizer function Thermocouple test Biological indicator	Observation of temperature and vacuum readings Biological indicator (each cycle) Chemical indicator (each cycle)
Gamma radiation installation	Measurement of absorbed dose and dose distribution Biological indicator	Dosimetry (as required) Biological indicator (optional)

1. Sample size
2. Culture methods
3. Antimicrobial action
4. Accidental contamination.

Limitations of sterility tests

Sample size

A batch or lot is a homogeneous collection of sealed containers or packages, prepared in such a manner that the risk of contamination is the same for all of the items. It may be a single sterilizer load or the products of a continuous process, such as radiation sterilization or an aseptic filling operation, over a specified period. The sterility of a whole batch could be guaranteed only if all of the material were tested. In practice, the likelihood of all the items in the batch being sterile is determined by testing a sample containing a relatively small number of items. The sensitivity of a sterility test depends on the:

1. Per cent of contaminated items in the batch
2. Number of items tested.

The relationship between the per cent of unsterile items in the batch and the probability of accepting a contaminated batch as sterile when 10 or 20 items are tested is shown in Table 2.5. The quantity of a powder or liquid from each container that is tested also influences the sensitivity of the test. The amount or volume of material tested, and the sensitivity of the test, is increased by use of the membrane filtration method for soluble powders and liquid products.

Ernst et al (1969) reported the results of 12 separate sterility tests on a batch of sterilized material in which 5 per cent of items had been subsequently inoculated. Each test was done on a sample of 20 items. Approximately 4 per cent of the 240 samples yielded positive cultures, but 7 of the 12 separate tests failed to detect the contamination. It is generally recognized that product sterility tests are reliable only for detecting a high per cent of unsterile items, such as might be expected from a faulty sterilization process. The United States Pharmacopeia (1980) permits reduction of the number of items in a sample if the material has been sterilized in the final sealed containers and the sterilization process has been monitored by approved methods.

Culture methods

No single medium or condition of incubation will recover all types of microbial contaminants. Thioglycollate broth, incubated at 32–37°C, is widely used because it will support the growth of anaerobic bacteria. It will also grow many aerobes and facultative anaerobes, but the low oxygen tension is unfavourable to *Bacillus* species if the bacteria are few in number and have been damaged by the treatment received (Doyle et al, 1968). Soybean casein digest medium is commonly chosen for growing fungi and bacteria that have a low optimum temperature range (20–25°C).

Antimicrobial action

Sterility tests are performed on antibiotics that have been sterilized by filtration and subsequently dispensed into the final containers, where they may be freeze-dried before sealing. Other pharmaceuticals that have been prepared in this way, or are intended for repeated use, also contain an antimicrobial agent, such as an organic mercurial, a phenol, a quaternary ammonium compound or chlorhexidine, to kill or inhibit the growth of contaminants that enter the product after the container has been opened. Antimicrobial action in the culture medium may be prevented by dilution of the samples, by chemical inactivation or by use of the membrane filtration method.

Solutions of penicillin are filtered and the membrane filter is washed with a diluent that contains

Table 2.5 Relationship between per cent of contaminated items, number of items in the sample, and sensitivity of sterility tests

Unsterile items (per cent)	Probability of drawing 20 sterile items	Probability of drawing 10 sterile items
0.1	0.90	0.99
1.0	0.82	0.90
2.0	0.67	0.82
5.0	0.36	0.60
6.7	0.25	0.50
10.0	0.12	0.35

an appropriate amount of the enzyme penicillinase. As inactivators are not available for other antibiotics, their removal must be accomplished by washing alone. Quaternary ammonium compounds and chlorhexidine may be inactivated by including lecithin and a nonionic detergent in the culture medium. Mercurial preservatives are inactivated by thioglycollate medium but not by soybean casein digest medium. Phenolics, such as chlorocresol, may be added directly to the culture medium if the dilution factor is sufficient to inactivate them.

Accidental contamination

The accidental introduction of contaminants to samples, culture media or equipment during the performance of a sterility test results in false positive cultures which necessitate repetition of the test and may cause costly recalls of industrial products. Contamination cannot be prevented completely but the risk can be reduced to a very low level by suitable selection and training of staff, the provision of sterile outer wear (gowns, headgear, overshoes and gloves) and an ultraclean working environment. Clean room conditions of the Class 100 standard (not more than 3.5/litre, or 100/ft^3, of airborne particles 0.5 μm or more in diameter) are recommended. This necessitates the use of a laminar flow room or a Class II laminar flow cabinet, located in a room with a clean air supply.

All equipment brought into the testing area must be sterile and the outer surfaces of the containers or packs to be tested should be chemically disinfected. Ethyl alcohol is commonly used because it leaves no residue. Containers that have been sealed under vacuum should be opened by piercing the rubber closure with a sterile hypodermic needle attached to a bacterial filter. Packages containing solid articles should be inspected for integrity before they are opened aseptically and the article is transferred to the culture medium with sterile forceps. Transfer forceps should not be sterilized by alcohol flaming because the temperature on the metal surface may be only 124°C although the air temperature 3 mm away is 205°C (Doyle & Ernst, 1969). Large or complex articles, such as dressings or intravenous sets, present an added risk of contamination if they must be dismantled or aseptically cut into pieces for testing.

The rate of accidental contamination in a testing laboratory may be estimated in the long term from the accumulated results of negative controls. Accidental contamination rates below 0.1 per cent can be achieved by skilled workers in favourable conditions.

Methods of testing

Direct method

Aqueous liquids and water soluble powders may be added directly to the culture media, but a preliminary test is required to determine whether they contain antimicrobial agents. The sample and culture medium are mixed in the usual proportions and inoculated with a small number of organisms that are sensitive to the antimicrobial agent. Failure to grow within 48 hours indicates a need to increase the volume of medium or decrease the amount of sample, within permitted limits, until growth is demonstrated. The direct method may also be used for devices that are small enough to be immersed in not more than a litre of medium. Larger devices may be dismantled or cut into pieces aseptically if this is feasible. Contamination of tubular devices is most likely to be detected if they are filled with sterile culture medium which is incubated in situ.

Membrane filtration method

This technique requires more elaborate apparatus and a high level of skill but it is the method of choice in most situations. It overcomes the problem of antimicrobial action in the culture medium because the membrane and the microorganisms retained on its surface can be washed thoroughly with a diluent or treated with an appropriate inactivator. Membrane filtration is also used for testing oily substances and large volumes of liquid, such as intravenous solutions or a diluent which has been used to recover microbial contaminants from large objects.

Membrane filters with a diameter of 47 mm and an average pore diameter of 0.45 μm are used. Membranes with hydrophobic edges are required to avoid retention of antimicrobial substances between the sealing surfaces of the filter holder. Filtration apparatus with a closed reservoir and receiver is essential. The units should be sterilized by autoclaving with the membrane in place and the system must be tested for integrity before use (see Ch. 9). The membranes are wetted with a sterile diluent before the sample is filtered, except with oils for which a dry sterile membrane is required.

The liquid samples may be pooled and filtered through one membrane, which is divided aseptically for addition to each of the culture media. Alternatively, the pooled liquid may be divided into equal parts by an automatic pumping device and distributed to separate filter units.

Aqueous solutions and oils are filtered directly and the membrane is washed with a diluent containing polysorbate 80. Water soluble powders are dissolved in a suitable diluent, which is also used for washing the filter. Ointments are dissolved in isopropyl myristate which has been sterilized by filtration through a membrane of 0.22 μm average pore diameter and tested against a strain of *Pseudomonas aeruginosa* to demonstrate that it is free from toxicity. Penicillin may be inactivated by the addition of a high concentration of penicillinase to the solution or a lower concentration to the diluent used for washing the filter.

Controls

Positive and negative controls should be included in each working session. Tests on 10 samples to which 10–20 bacteria have been added constitute a positive control, and a similar number of samples which have been sterilized by a severe process is used as the negative control.

All culture media must be tested for sterility by incubation under the conditions that will be used in the test. Growth-promoting ability must also be demonstrated by inoculation with fewer than 100 cells of recommended species of bacteria and yeasts. The membrane filtration method must be tested to demonstrate effective removal or inactivation of antimicrobial agents. Ten to 20 viable microorganisms are added to the final rinse and the membrane is cultured in an appropriate medium for each species used. Growth should be detected within 48 hours. Media that have been

used in a sterility test should be incubated for 14 days; 20–30 per cent of positive cultures may be missed if incubation is terminated after 7 days. An additional test for the ability of the media to support growth may be performed at the end of the normal incubation period by adding microorganisms and incubating for a further 48 hours. This is referred to as a 'stasis test'.

Results

The sample tested, and the batch it represents, passes the sterility test if no growth occurs in any culture vessel. If occasional growth is observed, repetition of the test may be permitted. The report on a sterility test cannot state that the whole batch is sterile; it demonstrates only that the incidence of contaminated units is below the level that the sampling system used is capable of detecting. The decision to accept a batch of sterilized material should be undertaken by a responsible microbiologist who understands the limitations of sample size. Sterility testing is laborious and requires a high level of skill. It should never be undertaken by persons, however well qualified, who lack the necessary training, equipment and environmental conditions. Neither should it be performed on an inadequate number of samples.

REFERENCES

Association for the Advancement of Medical Instrumentation 1981 Standard for BIER Steam Vessels. AAMI BSV-3/81
Associated for the Advancement of Medical Instrumentation 1982 Standard for BIER/EO Gas Vessels. AAMI BEOV–3/82
Bond W W, Favero,M S, Petersen N J, Marshall J H 1970 Dry-heat inactivation kinetics of naturally occurring spore populations. Applied Mircobiology 20: 573–578
Bowie J H, Kelsey J C, Thompson G R 1963 The Bowie and Dick autoclave tape test. Lancet i: 586–587
Cerf O 1977 Tailing of survival curves of bacterial spores. Journal of Applied Bacteriology 42: 1–19
Cook A M, Brown M R W 1960 Preliminary studies of the heat resistance of bacterial spores on paper carriers. Journal of Pharmacy and Pharmacology Supplement 12: 116T–118T
Department of Health and Social Security 1980 Sterilizers Health Technical Memorandum 10. HMSO, London
Doyle J E 1971 Sterility indicator with artificial resistance to ethylene oxide. Bulletin of the Parenteral Drug Association 25: 98–104
Doyle J E, Ernst R R 1969 Alcohol flaming – a possible source of contamination in sterility testing. American Journal of Clinical Pathology 51: 407–408
Doyle J E, Mehrhof W H, Ernst R R 1968 Limitations of

thioglycolate broth as a sterility test medium for materials exposed to gaseous ethylene oxide. Applied Microbiology 16: 1742–1744

Ernst R R, West K L, Doyle J E 1969 Problem areas in sterility testing. Bulletin of the Parenteral Drug Association 23: 29–39

Gard S 1957 Chemical inactivation of viruses. In: Wolstenholme G E W, Millar E C P (eds) Ciba Foundation Symposium on the nature of viruses. Churchill, London, p 123

Kelsey J C 1961 The testing of sterilizers 2 Thermophilic spore papers. Journal of Clinical Pathology 14: 313–319

Joynson D H M 1975 Sterilization by steam. Journal of the Association of Sterile Supply Administrators 4 (1): 4

Oxborrow G S, Placencia A M, Danielson J W 1983 Effects of temperature and relative humidity on biological indicators used for ethylene oxide sterilization. Applied and Environmental Microbiology 45: 546–549

Reich R R, Morien L L 1982 Influence of environmental storage relative humidity on biological indicator resistance, viability, and moisture content. Applied and Environmental Microbiology 43: 609–614

Royce A, Bowler C 1959 An indicator control device for ethylene oxide sterilisation. Journal of Pharmacy and Pharmacology Supplement 11: 294T–298T

Salk J E, Gori J B 1959 A review of theoretical, experimental, and practical considerations in the use of formaldehyde for the inactivation of poliovirus. Annals of the New York Academy of Sciences 83: 609–637

Schalkowsky S, Wiederkehr R 1968 Estimation of microbial survival in heat sterilization. In: Sneath P H A (ed) Sterilization techniques for instruments and materials as applied to space research. Cospar Technique Manual Series, Manual No. 4 p 87–100

Shull J J, Cargo G T, Ernst R R 1963 Kinetics of heat activation and of thermal death of bacterial spores. Applied Microbiology 11: 485–487

Stumbo C R 1973 Thermobacteriology in food processing, 2nd edn. Academic Press, New York, ch 7, p 74

United States Pharmacopeia 1980 20th rev. Mack Publishing Company, Easton, p 1039

3

Preparation and packaging for sterilization

Effective contact between the biocidal agent and the microbial contaminants is the essential prerequisite for sterilization. Access of the biocidal agent to all areas where the contaminants may be located depends on the types of articles and the methods of cleaning, wrapping and packing that are used to prepare them for sterilization. Packaging materials and package design are also important in the maintenance of sterility during storage and transportation of the sterilized articles and at the time when the packages are opened for use. The preparation of articles for sterilization will be discussed under the following headings:

  Decontamination
  Cleaning and maintenance
  Packaging materials
  Package design
  Package testing
  Maintenance of sterility.

DECONTAMINATION

Decontamination, or terminal disinfection, is the 'make-safe' treatment of used equipment and materials that may be contaminated with pathogenic microorganisms. Procedures used for decontamination vary according to the types of contaminants present; careful cleaning is often adequate but disinfection or sterilization by an appropriate method may be necessary.

Assessment of risks

The risks posed by most pathogenic microorganisms can be avoided by taking appropriate precautions in the transportation and cleaning of the contaminated equipment. However, hepatitis B virus causes particular concern in hospitals and microbiological or biochemical laboratories because it is transmitted by blood or blood products and a minute quantity may contain an infective dose. Special care must be taken with instruments and equipment that have been soiled with blood. The type of hazard that was formerly associated with smallpox virus might now be extended to the rare cases of viral haemorrhagic fevers or Creutzfeld-Jakob disease.

Used medical and laboratory equipment is frequently contaminated with pathogenic bacteria. However, these rarely present a major hazard to those handling them if appropriate precautions are taken (Mitchell, 1974). *Mycobacterium tuberculosis* and antibiotic resistant strains of *Staphylococcus aureus* might merit special attention, to be decided in the actual situation. Haemolytic streptococci should also be treated with caution. Opportunistic pathogens such as the pseudomonads are unlikely to affect healthy persons, although they may constitute a serious risk to hospital patients with naturally or artificially depressed immune systems. Routine precautions should be observed, regardless of the microorganisms involved, when medical or laboratory equipment is cleaned manually.

Instruments and utensils

If decontamination is considered necessary, it may be carried out in the ward or operating theatre suite or, preferably, in a central service department where the equipment will be cleaned and resterilized. Treating the articles at the site of use involves a risk that the bacterial contaminants will be spread by nurses' hands or other means. If possible, the articles should be sent to the sterilizing department in a covered tray or other suitable container that prevents leakage or drying of biological material (Mitchell, 1974). Immersion in a chemical disinfectant solution for transport is rarely necessary. In the sterilizing department, the articles may be boiled, treated in a washing machine (Cowtan, 1974) or an instrument washer-sterilizer (Perkins, 1969), where they are cleaned by a suit-

able detergent (Barrie, 1974) and disinfected by heat. Staff who handle soiled equipment should wear plastic aprons, rubber gloves and eye protection. If a chemical disinfectant is used, a clear soluble phenolic would be suitable as this does not precipitate or coagulate proteins.

Syringes and needles

Reusable syringes which have been used for aspirating blood, pus or other exudates should be autoclaved before they are disassembled for cleaning (Darmady et al, 1965). Syringes used for routine injections are not considered to be hazardous.

Anaesthetic machines

Most components of the breathing circuit can be disinfected in a washing machine fitted with jets to circulate the cleaning solution and hot rinsing water through the tubes (Bennett et al, 1968; Talbot, 1974). Apparatus constructed entirely from autoclavable components should be used for tuberculosis patients.

Bedpans and urinals

These ward utensils are usually emptied, cleaned and disinfected in the ward service area. Efficient cleaning is the main factor in making them safe for reuse; this can be done most efficiently in a flusher-sanitizer where the cleaned utensil is disinfected by hot water or steam at 98–100°C (Daley et al, 1971). If the pan flusher does not operate at a pasteurizing temperature, the cleaned articles may be disinfected by immersion in freshly prepared sodium hypochlorite or an alternative disinfectant.

Textiles

Used hospital bedclothing and surgical linen should be disinfected by heat in the washing machine cycle. Items that are classed as infected should be placed, with minimum handling, in special marked bags that are sewn with alginate thread (Rogers & Slater, 1961). The thread dissolves in hot water and the materials are released within the washing machine. If the machine does not incorporate a pasteurizing stage, a quaternary ammonium disinfectant may be included in the penultimate rinse. Hospital blankets should be laundered regularly (e.g. fortnightly, or when there is a change of bed occupant) by a process that includes disinfection at 65°C for 10 minutes or 71°C for 3 minutes (Kelsey & Wagg, 1969). A high-temperature laundering process which includes disinfection at 98–100°C for one minute, is used in Australia for blankets that withstand this treatment (Pressley & Morris, 1962; Standards Association of Australia, 1962).

Laboratory apparatus and cultures

Used pipettes are placed immediately in a tall jar that contains sufficient disinfectant to immerse them completely. A phenolic formulation or a sodium hypochlorite solution (1000 p.p.m.) may be used for bacteria (Maurer, 1972). Sodium hypochlorite (5000 p.p.m.) or formalin (20 per cent v/v) should be used for tissue cultures containing viruses. Ideally, all discard containers that have been used at the laboratory bench should be autoclaved before they are emptied. If this has not been done, the empty containers should be sterilized or disinfected before they are refilled with disinfectant.

Clinical specimens and laboratory cultures must be sterilized before those in single-use containers are discarded or the reusable containers are cleaned. They should be collected in leakproof bins or bags for transport to a steam sterilizer. A long sterilization time, at least 60 minutes, is required because the impervious transport containers trap air. The fused residue from single-use petri dishes may safely be placed in an incinerator or garbage bin; direct incineration of live cultures is less satisfactory because microorganisms may escape from the chimney if burning is incomplete (Barbeito & Gremillion, 1968).

CLEANING AND MAINTENANCE

Cleaning is a prerequisite but not a substitute for sterilization. It serves several purposes:

1. Reduction of microbial contaminants
2. Removal of tissue debris, blood and other organic soiling material, thus promoting contact between the biocidal agent and the remaining contaminants
3. Avoidance of cumulative deterioration of instruments and utensils.

The role of meticulous cleaning in ensuring a low contamination level of equipment used in hospitals and laboratories is comparable with the observance of Good Manufacturing Practice in the industrial situation. It is especially important to avoid the presence of Gram-negative bacteria that, dead or alive, contain pyrogenic substances in their cell walls. Pyrogens cannot be easily removed or destroyed if they have been adsorbed on the surfaces of equipment or containers.

The principal types of equipment which are cleaned in hospital sterilizing departments are surgical instruments, a small number of reusable syringes, and bowls. Complex instruments, such as endoscopes, are usually cleaned in the operating theatre suite. Tubing made from rubber or synthetic materials should be used once only and then discarded because it is difficult to clean and internal cleanliness cannot be verified. Presterilized surgical gloves, syringes and needles are now available commercially; this relieves the sterilizing department of tedious and time-consuming procedures. Laboratory glassware in the form of bottles, flasks, test tubes and pipettes, and polypropylene or polycarbonate containers are cleaned for reuse, usually in a special service area.

The following cleaning methods are used (Darmady et al, 1965):

Manual cleaning
Mechanical cleaning
Ultrasonic cleaning.

Manual cleaning

This time-consuming method is suitable only for small scale work or for items requiring individual treatment because of their size, shape or complex design. These may include delicate articles, such as fine cutting instruments, and complex equipment, such as endoscopes and dental handpieces, which must be dismantled and cleaned by specially trained staff. Jugs, bowls and trays are also cleaned manually.

The articles are rinsed in cold water to remove blood; if it has dried or coagulated, a warm solution of a blood solvent may be required. A soft brush may be used to assist cleaning. It must be sterilized or disinfected at the end of each session to prevent colonization by Gram-negative bacteria. The choice of a suitable detergent should be advised by the instrument manufacturer; soaps which precipitate in hard water and abrasives which damage smooth surfaces should not be used. Highly caustic detergents are unsuitable for manual cleaning.

Some laboratory equipment is cleaned manually. Screw caps, cotton wool plugs and coagulated material must be removed from bottles and other containers before they are placed in a washing machine. Pipettes may be rinsed by a water jet at the sink; they are difficult to clean if they have been soaked in a disinfectant which precipitates protein. Phenolic formulations, which have a high detergent content, and sodium hypochlorite solutions are suitable. Glassware that is difficult to clean with detergent or is required for critical tests, such as microbiological assays, may be cleaned by soaking in chromic acid. Detergents that have a high level of bacteriostatic activity should not be used for cleaning culture containers because adsorbed residues may inhibit the growth of microorganisms.

Mechanical cleaning

Specially designed machines that include a heat disinfection stage in the washing cycle are available for cleaning surgical instruments, anaesthetic apparatus, hospital ward utensils, laboratory glassware and bedlinen.

Instrument washers may clean separate batches in a closed chamber or perform a continuous process in which the articles pass through a tunnel on a moving belt. They are washed and rinsed by spray jets, usually positioned above and below. Soiled instruments and utensils sometimes require presoaking to ensure a satisfactory result. A washing machine cycle includes the following stages (Keall, 1980):

1. Cold water rinse
2. Hot water wash (e.g. 71°C for 2 minutes)
3. Hot water rinse (e.g. 88°C for 10 seconds)
4. Drying (e.g. 50–75°C) by means of a heater and fan.

Alternatively, instruments may be cleaned in an instrument washer-sterilizer, if this type of machine is available. The instruments are washed in a hot detergent solution which is violently agitated by air or steam. The wash liquid is expelled from the chamber when steam is admitted to raise it to the sterilizing temperature.

Anaesthetic circuit components may be washed in a machine that is fitted with water jets to distribute the cleaning solution and rinsing water to the internal and external surfaces of corrugated tubes, connectors, valves and rebreathing bags. The machine may be located in the operating theatre complex or the central sterilizing department. Bedpan washer-sanitizers are designed to empty the contents, flush the pan with cold water and disinfect it by jets of water or steam at 98–100°C (Daley et al, 1971). Efficiency is critically dependent on placement of the jets. Washing machines that are used to clean and disinfect eating utensils which have been used by patients with tuberculosis, or are to be used by patients who are being isolated from sources of infection, require adjustment of temperature and time to achieve disinfection.

All washing machines require daily cleaning and regular maintenance. Machines should be constructed so that no part retains water between cycles as Gram-negative rods, including possible pathogens, can multiply in stagnant water (Gamble & Bullin, 1969).

Ultrasonic cleaning

Articles for ultrasonic cleaning (Goddard, 1967) are immersed in a suitable detergent and subjected to ultrasonic vibration for a few minutes. This method is similar in efficiency to manual and mechanical cleaning methods but does not remove stains, except those which are caused by the presence of boiler additives in steam sterilizers. Ultrasonic vibration at the frequency used for cleaning does not kill microorganisms and infective aerosols may be produced unless the tank is tightly closed during operation.

Applications

Ultrasonic cleaning is generally used as a supplement to manual or mechanical cleaning (e.g. for weekly treatment of hinged instruments) or to clean delicate tubes and other hollow instruments such as special syringes and needles. Articles made from stainless steel or polypropylene are most suitable for ultrasonic cleaning but glass, polytetrafluoroethylene (Teflon) and chromium plate may be treated. Flaking may occur if the metal plating has been damaged. The method is unsuitable for cystoscopes because the lens cement may be loosened, and for rubber, polyvinyl chloride (PVC) and wood because these materials absorb the vibrations. Different metals, or metals and plastics, should not be included in the same load.

Mechanism of cleaning

Ultrasound is energy in the form of a wave motion, which is above the maximum level of audible sound (16 kHz). Ultrasonic cleaners operate at low frequency (20–25 kHz) or, less commonly, at high frequency (38–40kHz). Electric power is supplied to a generator which converts it to high-frequency oscillations. These, in turn, are converted to mechanical vibrations, which are transmitted to the liquid by transducers fixed to the underside of the cleaning tank. When the ultrasonic vibration passes through water it gives rise to waves of low and high pressure. The low pressure causes the liquid to vaporize with the formation of microscopic bubbles which penetrate into small crevices. In the succeeding wave of high pressure, the bubbles collapse, or implode, creating a vacuum that plucks dirt from the surface of the articles immersed in the cleaning solution. The process is termed cavitation.

Design and operation

A low-frequency ultrasonic cleaner with a high power output (0.44 watt/cm^2) is most commonly used. The bank of transducers below the cleaning tank must be removable for replacement. The cleaning tank is provided with a tightly fitting lid to prevent the escape of audible sound and infectious aerosols. The wire loading basket must be 2.5 cm from the side of the tank, where cavitation intensity is low. A post-rinsing tank is required.

The detergent must be carefully selected and should be effective at a low concentration because ultrasonic vibration may enhance any corrosive effect; Pyroneg is usually satisfactory. A dilute citric acid solution may be used to remove stains on instruments caused by an alkaline detergent (Weymes, 1973).

Articles must be prerinsed or, if dirty, precleaned in an alkaline detergent. Power to the tank should be turned on for 20 minutes after filling in order to expel dissolved air, which decreases cavitation by introducing non-condensable gases into the water vapour bubbles. The basket is loaded with instruments to a depth of about 76 mm and is carefully placed in the tank to avoid reintroducing air into the liquid. Hinged or jointed instruments should be opened. An operating temperature of 55°C is satisfactory; higher temperatures prevent cavitation by forming large vapour pockets instead of small bubbles. Five minutes treatment is usually sufficient; extended times are likely to redeposit the soil unless scum is removed by an overflow system. The water used for post-rinsing may be heated to 90°C, which assists subsequent drying of the instruments. Tubes and cannulae should be jet flushed.

The tank should be emptied daily. Cleaning efficiency may be tested by use of azocarmine, a dye which combines with protein residues; however, this substance may be dangerous to use because it is a potential carcinogen. The method of testing efficiency by artificially soiling instruments with radioactively labelled organic material is unsuitable for routine use. Unglazed ceramic rings that have been marked with a lead pencil give an indication of cleaning performance.

Drying

Instruments and other equipment that has been cleaned manually, mechanically or by ultrasonic treatment should be dried quickly to prevent corrosion and stains. Hot air drying is commonly used but a more rapid process using an organic solvent (trichlorotrifluoroethane) has been described and evaluated (McGuiness, 1977). Instruments are treated first with a solvent preparation containing water and a surface active agent; this dissolves oil, grease and water-soluble contaminants. The articles are then boiled in the liquid at 46°C to remove water and rinsed in pure solvent. This is finally boiled off, producing clean, dry instruments.

Inspection of cleaned articles

Routine inspection of articles for efficiency of cleaning and for need of repair or lubrication are important steps in the preparation of articles for sterilization. If instruments remain soiled after manual or mechanical cleaning, ultrasonic treatment might be successful. All metalware should be free from corrosion because a damaged surface prevents proper cleaning and protects microorganisms from contact with the sterilizing agent (Meredith, 1977). Instruments should be examined for alignment of jaws, tight closure of ratchets, sharpness of blades and points, and correct stiffness of hinges and joints.

The need for lubrication should be assessed carefully because many instruments, especially those with box joints, do not require oiling if they are perfectly clean. Grinding to loosen stiff joints should be unnecessary if the instruments are maintained in good condition and are dipped, after cleaning, in an oil-and-water emulsion lubricant. This permits access of steam to the surfaces and facilitates cleaning after use by decreasing the adherence of soil. The same type of emulsion may be applied to dental and surgical drills before steam sterilization but supplementary lubrication with sterile oil may be required.

The person in charge of the sterilizing process should check the condition of the articles and ensure that they will be sterilized by the most suitable method. Equipment that withstands steam or dry heat sterilization should not be treated by a low temperature gaseous process. Laundered surgical linen should be inspected for freedom from stains, loose fibres and holes. Stains may be caused by oil, rust or bleaching agents but the cause is sometimes difficult to identify. Loose fibres (lint) result from laundering linens with cloth or paper towels that have been carelessly discarded into laundry bags. The significance of holes caused by towel clips during an operation is difficult to assess. All items in which holes have been detected should be rejected but a high rejection rate may overload the laundry facilities. Holes may be repaired with adhesive patches, which are satisfactory if the edges do not lift off. Any hole that is detectable when the material is held against strong daylight or a glass-topped table which is lit from below can provide a passage for microorganisms. Linen that has been packed for sterilization should not be placed in a hot sterilizing chamber until the cycle is due to be started. Articles and wrapping materials to be sterilized by ethylene oxide should also be protected from dehydration while awaiting sterilization.

PACKAGING MATERIALS

The aim of packaging is to protect sterilized articles against recontamination until they are used. The requirements of a packaging material include:

1. Permeability to air, steam and gaseous sterilants (does not apply to dry heat or ionizing radiation)
2. Resistance to penetration by microorganisms
3. Resistance to punctures and tears
4. Good draping quality
5. Freedom from loose fibres and particles (Marotta, 1983).

Closely woven cotton fabric, bleached kraft paper, drapable creped paper and paper combined with transparent plastic film to form a 'window pack' are commonly used in hospital sterilization processes because they are permeable to air, steam and chemical vapours. They do not provide an absolute bacterial barrier but are satisfactory for short term storage of sterilized packs if they are kept in a clean and dry condition. Medical grade paper is free from loose particles but liberates fibres if sealed packs are opened by tearing, cutting or opening a fibre tear seal. Aluminium foil, aluminium tubes, and canisters made from aluminium, steel or copper are used for dry heat sterilization in hot air ovens. Glass and autoclavable plastic containers of a quality that does not liberate particles are used for water and parenteral solutions. A wide variety of synthetic materials is used for industrial packaging of medical devices. The types of packaging materials that are suitable for different sterilization processes are listed in Table 3.1.

Cotton fabric

Closely woven cotton material, such as unbleached calico (muslin in U.S.A.) or balloon cloth, is used for heavy packs that are sterilized in prevacuum or downward displacement steam sterilizers. It is less efficient as a bacterial barrier than is kraft paper, but is more resistant to tearing and will maintain sterility for several weeks in clean, dry, storage conditions. Two layers of cloth or one of cloth and one of drapable paper, separately removable, should always be used. The cloth wrappings should be freshly laundered.

Kraft paper

Kraft paper is the most commonly used packaging material for steam, dry heat and gas sterilization in

Table 3.1 Selection of packaging materials for sterilization

Process	Suitable packaging material
Steam sterilization	Paper Cardboard boxes Cotton cloth Sterilizable cellophane Window packs (paper and heat-stable plastic) Perforated metal boxes with air filters Glass containers for liquids (plastic containers for liquids sterilized commercially)
Dry heat sterilization (hot air oven)	Metal canisters and tubes of aluminium foil Glass tubes, bottles
Ethylene oxide sterilization	Paper and plastic (combined in window pack) Low-density polyethylene (commercial only)
Low-temperature steam and formaldehyde process	Paper Cardboard boxes
Radiation sterilization	Treated paper Polyethylene (including Tyvek) Polyvinyl chloride (PVC)[1] Polypropylene[1] Various laminates, including metal foil

[1] Stability marginal (2.5 Mrad)

hospitals. It is permeable to steam, air and chemical vapours and is an effective bacterial barrier if the packs are stored in clean, dry conditions for relatively short periods. In industrial sterilization the use of untreated paper is limited to materials which are used in a clean, but not necessarily sterile, condition. However, specially treated papers, which may be laminated to plastic film or metal foil, are important components of commercial packaging. The wet strength and water repellancy are improved by impregnating the paper with resins that do not impair its permeability to air and sterilizing vapours.

Bleached kraft paper is the principal type used for hospital packaging procedures. Plain white paper with a glazed outer surface is used for bags but creped paper, which has good draping quality and is not noisy to handle, is preferred for wrapping linen, instrument trays, and ward procedure packs. Bags may be made entirely from paper, or a web of paper may be joined to a web of transparent plastic film to produce a 'window pack'.

Standards are set for the quality of wrapping paper for use in sterilization. Physical properties which are subject to specification include weight, dry and wet bursting strength, dry and wet breaking load, water repellancy, surface absorbency and draping quality. Chemical properties include the pH of the water extract and the content of chlorides and sulphates. The penetration of particles which are 0.5 μm or less in diameter may be determined by tests using a chemical dust, such as dioctyl phthalate or sodium chloride. Microbiological tests are more difficult to standardize.

Cardboard

Cardboard resembles paper in being permeable to air, steam and gases. Lidded cardboard boxes may be used as outer containers for textiles (Nuffield Provincial Hospitals Trust, 1963) in prevacuum steam sterilizers and for cystoscopes which are sterilized by the low-temperature steam and formaldehyde process (Alder et al, 1971). Such boxes should be autoclaved before use to kill bacterial spores and remove bituminous products which might otherwise be deposited on the surface of the endoscopes. Cardboard cartons of appropriate thickness are used as ancillary packaging for commercially produced sterile equipment.

Metals

Aluminium foil may be used as a wrapping material for large articles, such as surgical drills, which are sterilized by dry heat. However, the foil tends to collapse around the article and pinholes may be produced where it creases. Aluminium tubes with crimped foil caps are used for glass syringes (Darmady et al, 1957) and for canisters with perforated lids and felt wad liners for small instruments (O'Grady & Thompson, 1962). Larger canisters, which may be made from aluminium, copper or stainless steel, are used in laboratories as containers for unwrapped pipettes. A plug of filter material may be placed in the mouth of the containers to prevent contamination by airborne bacteria during cooling. Perforated metal containers, described by Thompson & O'Grady (1959) are the subject of a British Standard (BS 3281:1960). The perforated lid and floor of the box are lined with high efficiency filter material. These containers are used in the Bowie-Dick test for air removal from textile packs in prevacuum steam sterilizers. The routine use of metal containers for textiles is not recommended because they are likely to be overpacked.

Glass

Glass tubes, closed with cotton wool plugs or crimped foil caps may be used for dry heat sterilization of glass syringes and needles in a hot air oven, but they are poor conductors of heat. Needles should be supported so that the tip does not contact the wall of the container. Glass bottles, vials and ampoules are used for steam sterilization of aqueous liquids and lidded jars for dry heat sterilization of oils. Glass containers are unsuitable for gas sterilization because they are impermeable to vapours. They are inappropriate for radiation sterilization unless darkening of the glass is desired.

Synthetic materials and laminates

Synthetic polymers (plastics) are widely used, as flexible films and moulded containers, for indust-

rial sterilization of medical devices by ionizing radiation and ethylene oxide. Flexible or semi-rigid plastic are also used for water and aqueous solutions that are sterilized commercially by heat. Plastics provide an absolute barrier to dust and microorganisms, permitting indefinite storage of sterile products if the seals are intact and the packaging material is free from pinholes, punctures and tears. They are robust, transparent and can be heat sealed. However, some materials are unstable to heat or to ionizing radiation.

Polyethylene (polythene)

Although polyethylene is heat-labile, it is widely used for small devices and dressing packs which are sterilized industrially by ethylene oxide or ionizing radiation. Ethylene oxide vapour will pass through a 0.076 mm thickness of low-density polyethylene by dissolving in the film and eluting from the inner surface (Ernst, 1973). However, the impermeability of polyethylene to air and water vapour makes it unsuitable for hospital use except as part of a composite pack, in which a web of the plastic film is joined to a web of permeable paper.

High-density polyethylene is spun as a fine continuous fibre and bonded by heating to produce grades of paper-like material which is permeable to air and vapours (Marotta, 1981a). It is commonly referred to by the brand name Tyvek. Although porous, it is water repellant and provides a satisfactory bacterial barrier for dry articles. It presents some problems in sealing and printing, but these may be overcome by the application of heat-seal lacquer coatings and by the use of inks which are not oil-based. Lacquered Tyvek may be sealed to a transparent polyethylene/polyester laminate to make peelable pouches. As Tyvek is expensive, it is used mainly as breathable lidding material for blister packs, or as a peelable insert in a web of transparent material. A strip may be used to form a breathable seal by joining the edges along one side of a pack. Tyvek has a tendency to electrostatic attraction of dust and fibres; an antistatic grade is unsuitable for sterilization because it it likely to contain pinholes.

Polyester

Oriented polyester film withstands steam sterilization. It is commonly used as a laminate with polyethylene, in which the polyethylene presents a heat-sealing surface and the outer layer of polyester provides a good printing surface.

Polyvinyl chloride (PVC)

PVC has low stability to heat and ionizing radiation. It absorbs a large amount of ethylene oxide which combines with phthalate plasticizer, from which it elutes very slowly under ambient conditions. However, suitable grades are widely used to make moulded bases for blister packs.

Polypropylene and polycarbonate

These heat-stable plastics are extensively used, separately or laminated together, as flexible, semi-rigid or rigid containers for heat sterilization of water and aqueous solutions. A laminate of nylon and polypropylene has also been used (Weymes, 1971). Polypropylene may also be laminated with aluminium foil for packaging wet or oily materials such as skin swabs and wound dressings. Polypropylene film is impermeable to ethylene oxide, moisture and air.

Nylon

Nylon film is heat stable and permeable to steam but is unsuitable for use as a wrapping material in prevacuum and downward displacement steam sterilizers because retention of air delays steam penetration and may cause the packs to burst. It is not stable to irradiation.

PACKAGE DESIGN

The number of layers of packaging material, the type of pack (two-dimensional or three-dimensional), the method of sealing and provision for extracting the articles aseptically are the principal features of package design. Although sterilization processes are designed to reduce the probability of an unsterile article to 1 in 10^6, there may be a 1 in 10^3 chance of contamination occurring when the package is opened.

Number of layers

Individual product package

Individual products which are produced commercially may be enclosed in a single layer of wrapping material, or they may be double-wrapped to reduce the likelihood of contamination when the package is opened to remove the contents (Speers & Shooter, 1966; Hughes et al, 1967). The outer wrap is sealed and provides the bacterial barrier. The inner wrap, which is unsealed, acts as a protective cover during the removal of the article. Moulded plastic shields which cover hypodermic needles, the opening of syringe barrels and connections of intravenous administration sets perform the role of inner wraps as well as giving physical protection. Double wrapping is strongly recommended for urinary catheters, intravenous cannulae and other equipment that will be used in an aseptic environment, such as an operating room or a protective isolation unit (Duncan, 1972). It is unfortunate that the cost of double wrapping may defeat its purpose (Lewis, 1972; Rutter, 1972). If single-wrapped products are purchased to save money, they should be stored in the shelf carton or a clear plastic dust cover until they are used. Single wrapping is adequate for Ryles tubes, oesophageal and suction tubes, urine bags, mouth toilet and rectal examination sets, which do not penetrate to the blood stream or sterile tissue.

Surgical instrument and dressing packs that are sterilized in hospitals are wrapped in two separate layers of paper or cloth; the inner layer provides a sterile field when the pack is opened on a table or tray in the operating room.

Ancillary packaging

In commercial production, the individual packaged products may be packed in shelf storage cartons, each containing a relatively small number of articles. Several cartons are then enclosed in transport cartons, which must withstand predictable risks arising from pressure, rough handling or accidental dropping (Nyström, 1973). All layers of packaging material may be applied prior to industrial sterilization by ethylene oxide or gamma radiation. The transport container, which is soiled and contaminated in the outside environment, should be removed before the contents are taken into a storage area for sterile equipment.

TYPES OF PACKS

The wide variety of package designs may be grouped in three categories:

1. Wrapped packs
2. Formed bags and pouches
3. Moulded blister packs.

Wrapped packs

The large sheets of paper and cloth which are used to wrap textile and instrument packs in hospitals may be folded in two different ways. In the parcel fold used for large packs, the contents are placed parallel to the edges of the wrapping sheets, which are folded to overlap the centre line. The edges are turned back to facilitate aseptic opening. The ends are then turned in and folded, one over the other, and taped in position. Large packs are tied with cord. An envelope fold system is suitable for smaller packs, such as wound dressing trays and ward instrument sets. The tray is placed diagonally and slightly off centre on the wrapping sheet. Three folds are made by bringing the corners to the centre and each corner is turned back to provide a flap for opening. The larger fold is then brought over the top and fastened or tucked in, with a corner protruding.

Bags and pouches

Paper bags may be gussetted to facilitate filling and to separate the broken edges when the article is removed. The glued joints must be as strong as the paper. The bottom of the bag should be folded twice, with each fold glued and a peelable seal may·be provided at the top. A protruding lip or thumb cut assists filling. Window packs that are made by sealing plain or treated paper to a transparent plastic film are used in hospitals as well as in industry. They may be cut from a continuous roll and sealed at both ends, or they may be supplied individually with a peelable seal at one end.

Flat pouches for industrial sterilization may be constructed entirely from plastic films, or from a combination of paper and plastic or paper and metal foil, depending on the sterilization process and the intended use of the article. When a single type of film is used, the package may be formed from a cut length of lay-flat tubing, or from a flat piece of film which is folded and sealed along three edges. When webs of different material are used, the four edges are sealed (Powell, 1973).

Laminates of polyester, nylon or cellulose are suitable for dry articles. Plain or treated paper or spun-bonded polyethylene (Tyvek) is used for one side of the pack if permeability to air, moisture and ethylene oxide is required. Wet devices, such as impregnated sponges or skin swabs, wound dressings, sutures in alcohol, gels and solutions, must be packaged in materials that are proof against leaching or leaking and are solvent and grease resistant, chemically inert and capable of being sealed through a film of the liquid or grease (Marotta, 1982a). Aluminium foil, laminated with plastics such as polypropylene, polycarbonate, nylon, polyethylene or polyester, may be used for swabs, dressings and sutures. An inner layer of pinhole-free polyester is essential for swabs soaked in a povidone-iodine disinfectant because iodine attacks aluminium. A package made from a film and foil laminate, sealed to a polyethylene/metallized polyester laminate, has high resistance to puncturing and is suitable for gels. Polypropylene/polycarbonate laminates have been used for sterilizing water. Transparent, flexible packaging is widely used for intravenous solutions; it has the advantage that air, which may introduce microbial contaminants, is not drawn in as the container empties.

When two-dimensional packs are used for solid articles, sufficient material must be used to ensure that the article does not break through the seal if, for example, a carton is dropped during transport. The extra material adds to the cost of packaging and increases the storage space required.

Blister packs

Blister packs are used industrially to accommodate solid articles in the minimum amount of material.

Tubular semi-rigid packs are used for urinary catheters. The most common form of three-dimensional pack is a moulded tray, conforming to the shape of the contents, with flanges that are sealed to a flat lid. The trays may be made from PVC, polystyrene, polyester, acrylic or cellulosic material. These materials may be laminated to polyethylene to provide a heat-sealing surface. The lid is made from coated Tyvek or treated paper when permeability to air and vapours is required. Advantages of three-dimensional packs are avoidance of stress on the seal, economy of material and decrease in storage space. However, an inner wrap cannot be accommodated (Lewis, 1972; Powell, 1973). The industrial use of blister packs has increased as automated packaging methods have been developed.

CLOSING AND SEALING

Packs that are wrapped in hospitals are fastened with autoclave tape and may also be tied. Paper bags which are not provided with heat-sealing surfaces should be closed by turning in the corners, folding the open edges three times and fastening with autoclave tape; a piece at the centre of the fold is sufficient. Staples must never be used because they perforate the packaging material. Heat sealing is performed by pressing the lacquered surfaces between heated plates; the temperature, pressure and contact time must be accurately set and controlled. Creases may result in faulty seals. Gussetted bags may be difficult to seal because the thickness across the sealing area is uneven. When paper is heat-sealed to polyethylene film, the plastic melts and flows into the paper. Paper to paper and paper to plastic seals may release fibres when opened. These can cause adverse reactions if they gain access to human tissues.

A wider variety of sealing methods is used for industrial packaging. The seals may be plain or they may be crimped parallel with the edge of the pack or at right angles to it. Channels may develop in the seal if the crimping plates are not perfectly aligned. Peelable seals facilitate opening and are less likely to disturb microorganisms on the surface of the pack but the flaps that are provided for opening should be folded or fastened together to prevent access of dust to the sealing area (Powell, 1973). However, a peelable pack made from a single layer of wrapping material is less satisfactory than a double wrapping. The strength of a peelable seal is a compromise between maintenance of package integrity and ease of opening. The effect of the sterilization process on the seal must be taken into account. Heat seals are weakened during steam sterilization but usually return to the normal condition on cooling. Sterilization by ethylene oxide or radiation does not have a significant effect on the seals.

Most peelable seals are of the non-fibre tear type, made from combinations of lacquered or latex coated paper, plastic films, coated metal foil and laminates. Tyvek must be coated for heat sealing to other types of material and cannot be sealed above 150°C because it has a low melting point. It produces a non-fibre tear seal and is commonly used as lidding for blister packs. Polyethylene film and polyethylene/polyester laminates seal readily to many materials, polyethylene acting as the sealant. Polypropylene, polycarbonate and nylon are suitable sealants for aqueous dressings which are sterilized by steam at 120–124°C. Special resin coatings are required for sealing aluminium foil packs containing wet skin cleansing swabs, antiseptic dressings or vaseline gauze. Solvent-resistant, peelable adhesives are used for packs containing sutures in alcohol.

Different methods are used to make breathable seals for packs that are impermeable to ethylene oxide (Marotta, 1981b); however, package integrity may be compromised. A strip of fibrous material may be incorporated in the sealing area, or the unsealed edges may be joined externally by a strip of Tyvek, which may be peeled off to open the pack. Syringes are sometimes packaged in moulded plastic containers, closed by overlapping caps which are spot welded at one point to the base. These cannot be recommended because the maintenance of sterility depends on a tortuous path to the interior of the pack and the effectiveness of the system cannot be proven.

Sealed packs should always be inspected for integrity before they are opened. Faults in fibre tear seals might not be detected before opening unless one web is transparent (Marotta, 1982b).

PACKAGE TESTING

The essential function of a package as a barrier to dust and microorganisms may be lost for a variety of causes which include:

1. Use of poor quality or unsuitable packaging material
2. Failure to establish and maintain the integrity of the pack
3. Lack of provision for opening aseptically.

The functions of physical protection, identification of the contents and labelling with instructions for use must also be taken into account when assessing the efficiency of packaging.

Medical grade paper is manufactured to specifications for physical and chemical properties, resistance to air flow and penetration by chemical dusts. The tests that are described below are concerned with the performance of packaging films as bacterial barriers, the detection of pinholes and the integrity of sealed packs.

Tests for bacterial penetration (Schneider, 1980)

The paper and other porous wrapping materials that are used for steam or gas sterilization processes must be permeable to air, steam and the chemical vapour. Effectiveness as a bacterial barrier cannot be deduced from airflow measurements. Tests for penetration by chemical dusts, such as sodium chloride or dioctyl phthalate (DOP) particles with an average diameter of 0.3 μm, are most reliable. Microbiological methods have been described but the conditions are difficult to standardize and they suffer from problems of reproducibility. Some tests involve inoculating a bacterial culture on one side of the material to be tested and placing the other side in contact with a solid or liquid culture medium for a specified time. The medium is then incubated to detect growth. The sample may be placed between Rodac plates which are filled to the rim with nutrient agar; the uninoculated plate is removed for incubation. In a similar method, the sample is mounted on the rim of a wide-mouth bottle containing nutrient broth and the bottle is inverted to place the sample in contact with an agar plate. In a more elaborate method, a bacterial aerosol is drawn through the

sample at a specified velocity and the bacteria that pass through are collected on a membrane filter for culture and counting. Per cent penetration is calculated from the density of the aerosol and the volume that passed through the paper.

Tests in actual storage conditions are time consuming, extending to weeks or months. Sterilized packs are placed in dusty, draughty conditions and penetration is detected by culturing cotton wool swabs that were placed inside the wrapping material. A simulated storage test in which the material is placed over the mouth of a bottle containing nutrient broth and stored in adverse conditions is also prolonged.

Tests for pinholes

A pinhole in porous material, such as paper or spun-bonded polyethylene, is any aperture that is larger than the normal range of pore diameter. Any opening is significant in nonwoven plastics and metal foil. Pinholes are caused by fold lines or creases in paper and metal foil; they are unlikely to occur when two layers of material are laminated together because the chance of holes at the same place in both layers is remote.

Pinholes in aluminium foil can be detected by holding the sample over a strong light beam in a darkened room. An electric discharge may be applied to films with a low moisture content and openings are detected by sparks. Other methods involve passage of a dye solution through the sample to a piece of white paper underneath, or of ammonia to a filter paper impregnated with ferrous ferrocyanide; the filter paper turns white.

Tests for package integrity

Physical, chemical and microbiological tests for package integrity are designed to reveal a variety of faults. Fifty per cent of faults have been attributed to poor sealing due to faulty equipment or the use of incompatible materials. Seals may be liable to breakage if insufficient material has been used to make the pack or if cartons are dropped during transportation. Punctures, tears or pinholes in the packaging material may be caused by unprotected sharp or rough edges within the pack or by stress during filling. Most of the tests for integrity of sealed packs involve destruction of the pack and can only be carried out on a small number of samples.

A break in the bacterial barrier, such as a faulty seal, a hole or a tear, can usually be detected by inspection. The person who intends to use the article should always inspect the pack before opening it. Physical tests for integrity may be carried out in the following ways (Powell, 1973):

1. A waterproof pack is squeezed under water
2. The pack is placed in a vacuum desiccator; it should distend on evacuation and return to normal when atmospheric pressure is restored
3. A solution of dye is injected into a plastic pack, the hole is sealed and the outside surface is inspected for stains. A similar type of test using carbon black has been used to test the corners of paper packs (Thompson, 1969).

Microbiological tests may be carried out by immersing the packs in a bacterial suspension or tumbling them in a closed vessel containing a bacterial aerosol; after disinfection of the exterior surfaces, the pack is opened aseptically and the contents are cultured.

MAINTENANCE OF STERILITY

The contents of sterilized packs may become recontaminated during transport, storage or removal for use. Causes of recontamination include damage to the packaging material, broken seals, unclean storage conditions and unsatisfactory methods of opening the packs.

Transport

Commercial products may be transported over short distances by the manufacturer but public transport by land, sea or air must be used for distribution to country, interstate or international destinations. Hazards that could lead to contamination include rough handling, accidental dropping and gross soiling of the containers.

Within hospitals, trolleys, service lifts, passenger lifts or ducted systems may be used for distribution of sterile supplies to the departments where they are used. Closed trolleys or sterilized boxes

should be used unless the articles are contained in shelf storage cartons or plastic dust covers.

Storage

Packs from steam sterilizers should be cooled on open mesh shelves to prevent wetting of porous wrapping material by condensate. Equipment that has been sterilized in the hospital is transferred directly to a special store that is free from dust, draughts and dampness. Sudden temperature changes, which cause air movement that could carry microorganisms through porous material, should be avoided. The packs should be handled, as little as possible, by staff with clean, dry hands. Commercially sterilized supplies may be kept in the same store after they have been removed from the outer transport containers in a nonsterile area.

Storage facilities in operating rooms, wards and diagnostic departments should conform to the same standard of hygiene as is practised in the central store. Cupboards are superior to open shelves, as shown in Table 3.2. Packs which are placed in drawers may be damaged. Shelf storage cartons or plastic dust covers should be retained until the articles are taken to the place where they will be opened for use.

Duration of sterility

Hospital staff enquire frequently about the duration of shelf life for sterile articles. There is no

Table 3.2 Storage life of dressing packs (Standard et al, 1971, 1973)

Types of wrappings	Storage conditions	Duration of sterility (days)
Single cotton fabric[1]	Open shelves	3–14
	Closed shelves	14–21
Double cotton fabric	Open shelves	28–56
	Closed shelves	56–77
Single creped paper	Open shelves	28–49; >63
	Closed shelves	>63; >91
Single cotton cloth plus single paper	Open shelves	77–98
Single cotton cloth with polyethylene bag	Open shelves	>9 months

[1] A single wrapper of cotton fabric consisted of two layers stitched together at the edges

simple answer to this question because efficiency of packaging and conditions of transport and storage are more important than is the time that has elapsed since sterilization (Allen et al, 1965). Studies on the maintenance of sterility under normal storage conditions are time consuming and involve testing a large number of packs. However, the studies by Standard et al (1971, 1973), summarized in Table 3.2, show that one layer of crepe paper provides the same duration of sterility as do two layers of cloth, and that storage life may be prolonged indefinitely if an impervious dust cover is used. Although prediction of a meaningful shelf life for packaged equipment is not feasible, it is good hospital practice to avoid prolonged storage by ensuring rotational use. This may be achieved by organizing the distribution of supplies to prevent unnecessary hoarding. A small number of packs, containing emergency equipment that is rarely required but must always be available, may be kept for several months if they are placed in impervious dust covers after sterilization.

REFERENCES

Alder V G, Gingell J C, Mitchell J P 1971 Disinfection of crystoscopes by subatmospheric steam and steam and formaldehyde at 80°C. British Medical Journal 3:677–680

Allen S M et al 1965 Central sterile supply. Lancet ii: 1343

Barbeito M S, Gremillion G G 1968 Microbiological safety evaluation of an industrial refuse incinerator. Applied Microbiology 16: 291–295

Barrie J D 1974 'Make-safe' processing of theatre instruments Part II. Journal of the Association of Sterile Supply Administrators 3 (2): 6–7

Bennett P J, Cope D H P, Thompson R E M 1968 Decontamination of anaesthetic equipment. A 'one step' washing machine for processing anaesthetic equipment and tubing. Anaesthesia 23: 670–675

Cowtan R P 1974 Surgical instrument washing process Part III. Journal of the Association of Sterile Supply Administrators 3 (2): 8

Daley D, Kereluk K, Lloyd R S 1971 Microbiological aspects of the hospital environment: bacteriological effectiveness of a utensil washer-sanitizer. Health Laboratory Science 8: 21–28

Darmady E M, Hughes K E A, Drewett S E, Prince D, Tuke W, Verdon P 1965 The cleaning of instruments and syringes. Journal of Clinical Pathology 18: 6–12

Darmady E M, Hughes K E A, Tuke W 1957 Sterilization of syringes by infra-red radiation. Journal of Clinical Pathology 10: 291–298

Duncan M H 1972 Double-wrapping — is it really necessary? Part VI. Journal of the Association of Sterile Supply Administrators 1 (2): 12–14

Ernst R R 1973 Ethylene oxide gaseous sterilization for industrial applications. In: Phillips G B, Miller W S (eds) Industrial sterilization. Duke University Press, Durham, ch 12, p 181

Gamble D R, Bullin C H 1969 Bacteria and the washing machine. British Hospital Journal and Social Service Review 79: 492–494

Goddard B A 1967 Ultrasonic cleaning. British Hospital Journal and Social Service Review 77: 1735–1743

Hughes K E A, Drewett S E, Darmady E M 1967 The risk of contamination of sterile dressings packed in paper bags. British Hospital Journal and Social Service Review 77: 764–765, 781

Keall A A 1980 Washing machines. Sterile World 2(5): 2–3

Kelsey J C, Wagg R E 1969 The disinfection of textiles in laundering in hospitals. British Launderers' Research Association Bulletin 9: 231–236; 16: 239–246

Lewis C 1972 Double-wrapping — is it really necessary? Part V. Journal of the Association of Sterile Supply Administrators 1 (2): 9–12

Marotta C 1981a Tyvek: 'wonder' material of sterile packaging. Medical Device & Diagnostic Industry 3 (5): 18–20

Marotta C 1981b Vented flexible packaging. Medical Device & Diagnostic Industry 3 (9): 33–34

Marotta C 1982a High-barrier packaging for wet devices. Medical Device & Diagnostic Industry 4 (1): 21–22

Marotta C 1982b Tamper-evident packaging. Medical Device & Diagnostic Industry 4 (7): 18, 54

Marotta C D 1983 Particulate contamination in packaging materials. Medical Device & Diagnostic Industry 5 (1): 20, 22–23

Maurer I M 1972 The management of laboratory discard jars. In: Shapton D A, Board R G (eds) Safety in microbiology. Academic Press, London, p 53

McGuinness W J 1977 Introducing solvent drying of surgical instruments. Journal of the Association of Sterile Supply Administrators 6 (1): 4–5, 11

Meredith H G 1977 Corrosion of surgical instruments. Journal of the Association of Sterile Supply Administrators 6 (1): 6–8, 10–11

Mitchell E 1974 Merits or otherwise of sterilising theatre and other instruments prior to handling by staff of CSSD/TSSU, Part I. Journal of the Association of Sterile Supply Administrators 3 (2): 5–6

Nuffield Provincial Hospitals Trust 1963 Cleaning, drying and packaging. In: Central sterile supply. Principles and practice. Oxford University Press, London, ch 4, p 31

Nyström B 1973 Handling sterile products in the hospital. In: Phillips G B, Miller W S (eds) Industrial sterilization. Duke University Press, Durham, ch 20, p 359

O'Grady F, Thompson R E M 1962 Container for central sterile supply of instruments. Lancet i: 516

Perkins J J 1969 Principles and methods of sterilisation in health sciences, 2nd edn. Charles C. Thomas, Springfield, ch 10, p 239

Pressley T A, Morris F P 1962 Wool blankets in hospitals. Medical Journal of Australia 1: 43–44

Powell D B 1973 Packaging of sterile medical products. In: Phillips G B, Miller W S (eds) Industrial sterilization. Duke Unviersity Press, Durham, ch 5, p 79

Rogers K B, Slater N A J 1961 The disposal of infected linen. Lancet ii: 592–593

Rutter B 1972 Double-wrapping — is it really necessary? Part IV. Journal of the Association of Sterile Supply Administrators 1 (2): 6, 8–9

Schneider P M 1980 Microbiological evaluation of package and packaging-material integrity. Medical Device &

Diagnostic Industry 2 (5): 29–37

Speers R Jr, Shooter R A 1966 The use of double-wrapped packs to reduce contamination of the sterile contents during extraction. Lancet ii: 469–470

Standard P G, Mackel D C, Mallison G F 1971 Microbial penetration of muslin- and paper- wrapped sterile packs stored on open shelves and in closed cabinets. Applied Microbiology 22: 432–437

Standard P G, Mallison G F, Mackel D C 1973 Microbial penetration through three types of double wrappers for sterile packs. Applied Microbiology 26: 59–62

Standards Association of Australia 1962 Laundering of Shrink-resistant Wool Blankets. Australian Standard No.

CL2–1962

Talbot J M 1974 Disinfection of anaesthetic equipment. British Hospital Journal and Social Service Review 84: 2296

Thompson R E M 1969 Testing the seals of paper packs. British Hospital Journal and Social Service Review 79: 1397–1398

Thompson R E M, O'Grady F W 1959 An improved box for the sterilisation of dressings. Lancet ii: 445–446

Weymes C 1971 Sterilisation of water for topical use in plastic bags. British Hospital Journal and Social Service Review 81: 1553, 1555, 1557

Weymes C 1973 The Scottish scene and the present position of sterile supply in the United Kingdom. Journal of the Association of Sterile Supply Administrators 2 (2): 26–27

4

Principles of heat sterilization

Heat is generally regarded as the most reliable, readily available and economical method of sterilization for materials that are stable to temperatures above 121°C in wet conditions or above 160°C in dry conditions. The time required for sterilization decreases as the temperature is raised and many different combinations of temperature and time are equivalent in lethality. A set of parameters can be selected, therefore, that will achieve sterilization with minimum damage to heat-sensitive materials.

This chapter deals with the following topics:

Moist and dry heat
Mechanisms of biocidal action
Heat resistance of microorganisms
Factors influencing heat resistance
Design of heat sterilization processes.

MOIST AND DRY HEAT

The terms moist heat and dry heat, as applied to sterilization processes, refer to the moisture levels in the heating environment and the microbial cells. Moisture level is not identical with water content; it refers to the free, available water in a gaseous or liquid system. Moisture levels in air, steam or other gaseous environments are defined by relative humidity (RH). This is the water vapour content at a given temperature, expressed as per cent of the maximum content at that temperature. The RH scale ranges from zero to 100 per cent.

$$\% \text{ RH} = \frac{\text{actual water vapour content}}{\text{maximum at existing temperature}} \times 100$$

The moisture level of aqueous liquids is expressed as water activity (a_w):

$$a_w = \frac{\text{vapour pressure of solution}}{\text{vapour pressure of pure water}}$$

A_w values are always less than unity because the vapour pressure of solutions is less than that of pure water. If a_w values are multiplied by 100, they correspond to relative humidity; thus water activities of 0.2, 0.4 and 1.0 are equivalent to relative humidities of 20, 40 and 100 per cent respectively. Microbial protoplasm is a concentrated solution of organic and inorganic substances. The water activity within living cells cannot be measured directly but is assumed to be equivalent to that of the liquid in which the microorganisms are suspended or the relative humidity of air or other gases in their immediate gaseous environment.

The term moist heat is restricted to the condition of moisture saturation in the microorganisms and the heating environment. This exists when the organisms are in equilibrium with pure water or saturated steam. The term dry heat implies the absence of free water from the heating environment; it may refer to any moisture level from zero to just below saturation.

MECHANISMS OF BIOCIDAL ACTION

All types of microorganisms can be killed by moist or dry heat at a temperature appropriate to their level of resistance. This broad spectrum of biocidal action suggests that death is the result of physical or chemical changes that result in denaturation of major cell constituents, such as proteins or nucleic acids. Denaturation of proteins involves the rupture of bonds that maintain their coiled polypeptide chains in the configuration which is essential for specific functions, such as enzyme activity. Denaturation may lead to coagulation or precipitation.

Evidence for coagulation of proteins as the major cause of thermal death in microorganisms has been obtained by comparing the influence of moisture on the temperature required for protein denaturation and enzyme inactivation in vitro with its influence on the temperature required for biocidal action. Lewith (1890) observed that the temperature at which egg albumin coagulated increased from 56°C in excess water to 74–80°C, 145°C and 160–170°C as the water content was reduced to 25 per cent, 6 per cent and finally zero. The protection of a purified enzyme (luciferase) against inactivation by heat was demonstrated by Chappelle et al (1967), who found that it retained 40 per cent of its activity when heated to 135°C for 36 hours in a gel under conditions of low moisture and oxygen content. These effects are similar to the influence of moisture on the biocidal action of heat. Bacterial spores are killed rapidly at 121°C in saturated steam but the temperature must be increased to 160°C for a comparable death rate in dry conditions. Additional support for protein denaturation as the major mechanism of thermal death is provided by the similarity of the activation energies of the two processes (Rosenberg et al, 1971). Nucleic acids are also denatured by moist heat (Brannen, 1970) but coagulation of cytoplasmic proteins and the resulting inactivation of enzymes is probably sufficient to account for thermal death in the presence of moisture. At extremely low moisture levels, coagulation is replaced by other processes including oxidative destruction.

Most of the information about the biocidal action of heat has come from studies on bacterial spores at rapidly lethal temperatures. The primary cellular target cannot be determined in these conditions, but Allwood & Russell (1967) demonstrated initial damage to the cell membrane during sublethal heat treatment of *Staphylococcus aureus* in water at 50–60°C. Impairment of the essential function of the membrane as a semipermeable barrier resulted in the leakage of amino acids, nucleic acid constituents and other essential metabolites from the cells. This eventually resulted in death of the bacteria from loss of vital constituents but they recovered if they were transferred to favourable growth conditions before the loss was too great. Studies on cells of *Bacillus cereus* (Silva & Sousa, 1972) with the aid of electron microscopy confirmed that sublethal heat treatment affected the structure of the cell membrane. When the temperature was raised above 60°C, coagulation occurred throughout the cytoplasm and the action was biocidal. The production of single-strand breaks in the DNA of *Streptococcus faecalis* by sublethal heat treatment (Andrew & Greaves, 1979) and of bacterial spores by lethal heat treatment (Grecz & Bruszer, 1981) has been described.

HEAT RESISTANCE OF MICROORGANISMS

Vegetative microorganisms

Vegetative bacteria, including *Mycobacterium tuberculosis*, are killed rapidly in hot water (65–100°C). *Streptococcus faecalis* has the highest resistance among the common species but a Gram-negative bacterium, *Thermus aquaticus*, grows in thermal springs at 70°C (Brock & Freeze, 1969). Similar heat-tolerant non-sporing bacteria have been isolated from hospital hot water supplies (Pask-Hughes & Williams, 1975). *Salmonella senftenberg*, strain 775W, has unusually high resistance for the species when it is heated in food. Most viruses and fungi are killed in the same temperature range as are non-sporing bacteria but boiling may be required for viruses (e.g. hepatitis B virus) in association with blood or tissue. Fungal spores are susceptible to boiling water treatment but ascospores of *Byssochlamys fulva*, which can cause spoilage of canned berry fruits, may survive the canning process if the temperature fails to reach 98°C (Olliver & Rendle, 1934; Bayne & Michener, 1979).

Bacterial spores

Temperatures exceeding 100°C are usually required to kill bacterial spores but the level of heat resistance varies widely according to the species. Spores of *Clostridium botulinum* type E, *Bacillus anthracis* and *Clostridium perfringens* are relatively sensitive. Most pathogenic species, including *Clostridium tetani*, produce more resistant spores. The highest resistance occurs in thermophilic species, such as *Bacillus stearothermophilus* and *Clostridium thermosaccharolyticum*. They are not pathogenic but *B. stearothermophilus* is used as a biological indicator for testing the efficiency of steam sterilizers because it is more resistant than

the pathogens. Some common microorganisms are grouped in Table 4.1 according to their relative resistance to moist heat.

It is difficult to make valid comparisons for dry heat resistance from published reports because the moisture level at which the tests were carried out has not always been known. However, Bond & Favero (1975) obtained D values of 2.5 hours at 150°C and 139 hours at 125°C for spores of an extremely resistant *Bacillus* sp. (ATCC 27380) isolated from soil.

Mechanisms of heat resistance

The mechanisms underlying the high resistance of bacterial spores to heat and other biocidal agents have been the subject of speculation and experimental studies since they were discovered a century ago. The refractility of mature spores provided an early indication that their resistance to heat and lack of metabolic activity might be associated with a low water content. Measure-

Table 4.1 Resistance of microorganisms to moist heat

Grades of resistance	Types of microorganisms (examples)
Extremely susceptible	Non-sporing bacteria (including *M. tuberculosis*)
	Viruses (not protected by biological material)
	Moulds and yeasts (vegetative growth stages)
Moderately susceptible	Viruses (with blood or tissue)
	Mould spores
	Group D streptococci (e.g. *S. faecalis*)
Slightly resistant	Spores of: *B. anthracis* *B. megaterium* *C. botulinum* type E *C. perfringens*
Moderately resistant	Spores of: *B. subtilis* *C. botulinum* type A *C. tetani*
Highly resistant	Spores of: *B. stearothermophilus* *C. thermosaccharolyticum*

ments based on refractility are consistent with a water content of about 20 per cent in the spore core and a water activity of about 0.7 (Ross & Billing, 1957). A water activity of 0.73 has been found to provide extracted spore enzymes with the same degree of protection against heat inactivation that exists in the intact spore (Warth, 1981). However, the total quantity of water in spores ranges from 42 per cent to more than 90 per cent, depending on the water activity or relative humidity of their immediate environment; this led to the conclusion that water is distributed unequally among the different spore structures. The nature of the mechanism that controls water distribution within the spore is still a matter of theory rather than established fact. The following summary of current views on this important and interesting subject includes a brief account of the structure and chemical composition of spores and certain aspects of their development. Figure 4.1 is a simplified diagram of a mature spore.

Exosporium

An exosporium is not present in all species. It may be loose-fitting or closely adherent to the underlying spore coats and consists mainly of protein. Its presence is not required for heat resistance and no other function has been assigned to it.

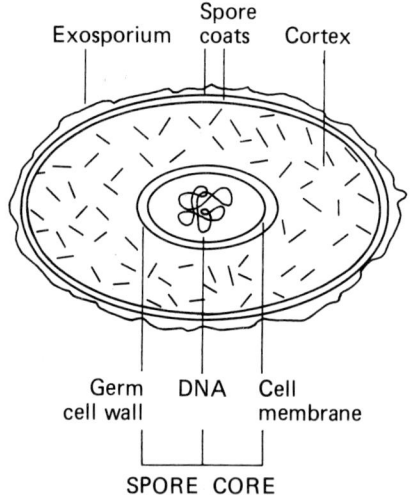

Fig. 4.1 Structure of a bacterial spore.

Spore coats

Electron microscopy reveals a complex structure of at least three layers, with a striated pattern in the centre. The coats consist mainly of proteins, with smaller amounts of carbohydrates, lipids and phosphorus-containing material. They are resistant to proteolytic enzymes and might protect the cortex against enzymic destruction by lysozyme but damage to the coats or their complete removal has no effect on heat resistance.

Cortex

The cortex is the most prominent of the layers that surround the spore core, occupying a wide zone between the coats and the germ cell wall. The electron microscope does not reveal any structure when the spore is intact but a network of fine fibres is revealed by a special staining method when the cortex swells during germination or as a result of artificial disruption of the spore. Swelling does not cause outward expansion of the cortex but the inner surface, adjacent to the germ cell wall, becomes densely folded. The principal component of the cortex is a peptidoglycan polymer which differs from that in the germ cell wall in having fewer cross links between the linear glycan chains. The porous cortex is assumed to contain most of the spore water. The lytic enzymes that break down the peptidoglycan during spore germination may be the only proteins in the cortex. The cortex is essential for heat resistance, which does not develop until its formation is at least 90 per cent complete.

Spore core

The central region of the spore is the germ cell, or protoplast, which contains a full complement of the macromolecular constituents of the living cell; that is, nucleic acids, ribosomes, enzymes and lipids. These make up 50–60 per cent of the dry weight of the core. The other core components are substances of low molecular weight that are markedly different in types and quantities from those in vegetative cells. All of the dipicolinic acid (DPA), a compound that is unique to the bacterial spore, is located in the core (Leanz & Gilvarg,

1973) and is accompanied by smaller amounts of glutamic acid, sulpholactic acid and phosphoglyceric acid. The DPA and other dicarboxylic acids are complexed with divalent ions, particularly calcium. As already mentioned, the spore core is severely dehydrated. Fifty per cent of the water that is normally present in bacterial cytoplasm is lost from the forespore before synthesis of the cortex or of DPA commences. It is possible that most of the remaining water is displaced by dipicolinic acid, which constitutes up to 15 per cent of the spore dry weight. The result of the severe dehydration is likely to be an amorphous, immobile matrix in which the concentrated macromolecules and the low molecular weight components are tightly packed together with a small amount of 'structured' water but complete absence of liquid water. The immobility would make the vital core resistant to physical or chemical alteration. Recent knowledge of the structure and chemistry of the spore core and its relation to heat resistance has been reviewed by Murrell (1981).

Regulatory mechanisms

The significance of DPA in the establishment or maintenance of heat resistance has received much attention. A consistent relationship between the amount of DPA in the spore and the degree of resistance has not been found; different species, or different types within a species, may contain similar amounts of DPA but vary widely in heat resistance (Murrell & Warth, 1965). Different strains of *C. botulinum* exhibit a thousandfold difference in resistance (Murrell, 1955). Studies of mutant spores have also given equivocal results; a strain of *B. cereus* which lacked DPA was resistant although the resistance was readily lost (Hanson et al, 1972) whereas a strain of *Bacillus subtilis* which also lacked DPA was not heat resistant (Balassa et al, 1979). DPA is thought to be necessary for the maintenance of heat resistance but not the level of resistance.

Heat resistance is most closely associated with the cortex, which contains no DPA (Leanz & Gilvarg, 1973). The main role of the cortex appears to be the maintenance of the heat resistance after it has been established in the spore core. There is agreement that the cortex exerts its influence by a physical pressure but the nature and source of this pressure have been the subject of at least three different theories.

The first theory involving a contractile cortex (Lewis et al, 1960) was abandoned when the expanded, water-filled structure of the peptidoglycan polymer was established. A similar fate has overtaken the proposal of Gould & Dring (1975) that a high osmotic pressure in the cortex, attributed to a surplus of electronegative groups on the peptidoglycan polymer and the mobile potassium ions that counterbalance them, might draw water away from the core, which is assumed to have a low osmotic pressure. Osmotic pressure has been ruled out as a major control mechanism firstly, because the swelling pressure caused by osmosis would be exerted inwards towards the spore core only if the coats were intact and secondly, because the calculated osmotic pressure in the cortex would only reduce the water activity in the core to about 0.97 — far short of the level of 0.73 that is required in vitro to stabilize the spore enzymes to the heat treatment which they withstand in the intact spore (Warth, 1981).

The physicochemical structure of the peptidoglycan polymer in the cortex is the focus of a theory proposed by Warth (1978), which is based on experimental evidence that the spore coats are not required for heat resistance and that the cortex does not expand outwards when the spore is disrupted. The concept of a pressure exerted in a particular direction was presented by Alderton & Snell (1963). It is now suggested that outward expansion may be restricted by orientation of the glycan chains parallel to the plane of the surface of the cortex, thus directing the pressure towards the inner zone where dense folding has been observed.

Difficulty in formulating a single, completely acceptable theory lies in the probability that all of the mechanisms that have been proposed make some contribution to the extraordinarily high heat resistance of bacterial spores.

Methods of determining heat resistance

Heat resistance is usually expressed as a D value, which is the time at a specified temperature that effects a tenfold reduction of the viable cells in a microbial population. Thermal death times (TDT), referring to some other level of reduction, may be used but the degree of reduction must be specified. In tests for heat resistance, all conditions that may influence heat resistance must be controlled before and during the heat treatment. The culture medium and conditions of incubation that are used to detect or enumerate survivors also influences the result. In the test, heating and cooling times must be reduced to a minimum, ideally to zero, so that the lethal action of heat is restricted to the temperature of the test. D values and thermal death times are read from a death rate curve, prepared by plotting viable counts on samples taken after increasing times of heat treatment.

Moist heat resistance

Resistance to moist heat at temperatures above 100°C may be investigated by exposure of the test organism for short time periods in a tubular flow reactor that has been heated to the temperature at which the test is to be performed (Wang et al, 1964). Alternatively, small volumes of a suspension containing a known number of organisms are injected into a buffer solution in screw-capped, thin-walled tubes which are heated in a glycerol bath. A neoprene liner in the caps allows the suspension to be injected without the atmosphere of the headspace losing its positive pressure. A thermocouple may be sealed into the side of the tube. The tubes are transferred to iced water after set time periods (Kooiman & Geers, 1975). Stumbo's resistometer (Stumbo, 1973) is a mechanical device for transferring tubes from ice water to the heating medium and returning them to the ice bath for rapid cooling. Miniature cans are used for determining the heat resistance of microorganisms in viscous liquids or in foods that contain solid particles.

Dry heat resistance

In tests for dry heat resistance, the microorganisms must be preconditioned to a specified moisture level and maintained at that level during the heat treatment. The microorganisms may be preadjusted by placing them in a tightly closed vessel, such as a desiccator, above a salt solution with the appropriate vapour pressure. For the heat treatment, they may be sealed into tubes with the correct amount of water for maintenance of the moisture level. The tubes are heated in a water or oil bath. Alternatively, the test organisms may be dried on metal strips or glass coverslips in small open cans where they will be severely desiccated during heat treatment on a thermostatically controlled hot plate or beneath an infrared heater. The time required to kill spores in flowing air may be determined by injecting them into a stream of preheated air and sampling in the range of 200–350°C at intervals of less than one second.

Recovering survivors

A culture medium that is normally adequate for the species of microorganism might contain substances that inhibit heat-damaged survivors (Roberts, 1970). Inhibitory substances can sometimes be removed or inactivated by the addition of powdered starch or finely divided charcoal to the medium (Stumbo, 1973; Labbe, 1979). Reducing the incubation temperature from 37°C to 32°C for mesophils, or from 50°C to 45°C for thermophils, also increases the number of survivors recovered. Sometimes it is necessary to stimulate the germination of surviving spores by adding calcium dipicolinate (Ca DPA) to the recovery medium (Riemann & Ordal, 1961).

FACTORS INFLUENCING HEAT RESISTANCE

The biocidal action of moist and dry heat is influenced by a variety of conditions that may alter the resistance of the microorganisms or protect them from effective contact with the lethal agent. The conditions that are used to grow vegetative cells or produce spores exert their effects prior to heating but the major influences operate during the heat treatment.

Conditions of growth or sporulation

It is generally accepted that differences in the physiological age of vegetative microorganisms and in the composition of the growth medium influence resistance. However, the reports indicate variation in the direction as well as the extent of the changes. The temperature at which spores are produced has a more predictable effect. Thermophils and most mesophils produce their most resistant spores in the upper part of the growth temperature range but the resistance of *Clostridium* spores may be enhanced when they are produced below the optimum growth temperature.

Temperature

The time required to kill microorganisms decreases as the temperature is raised. The influence of temperature is described by a temperature coefficient, such as the z value. The z value is equal to the change in temperature that brings about a tenfold change in the D value or a thermal death time. It is usually read from a linear thermal death time curve, as in Figure 4.2. The range and generally accepted averages of z values for bacterial spores in moist and dry heat are given in Table 4.2. A low z value corresponds to a large influence of temperature, and vice versa.

Moisture

The water activity of bacterial protoplasm is equivalent to that of the liquid in which the microorganisms are suspended or to relative humidity if the environment is gaseous. The relationship

Table 4.2 z values for bacterial spores in moist and dry heat (Molin, 1982)

z Value	Moist heat	Dry heat
Range	7–24°C	10–60°C
Average[1]	10°C	21°C

[1] Widely accepted values

between the moisture level and heat resistance of bacterial spores was demonstrated by Murrell & Scott (1966) and their findings are represented by the curves in Figure 4.3.

The different species used in the study varied widely in their resistance at 100 per cent moisture saturation (a_w 1.0). Curve A is typical of species which are relatively susceptible to moist heat and curve B represents more resistant species. As the moisture level was reduced, all of the species increased in resistance to reach a maximum between a_w 0.2 and a_w 0.4. There was little difference between species at this intermediate water activity because the resistance of the ones that were less resistant at the highest moisture level increased to a greater extent. As the moisture level

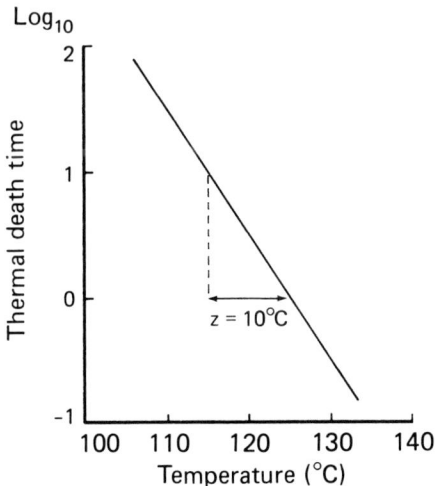

Fig. 4.2 Influence of temperature on the time required for sporicidal action (thermal death time curve).

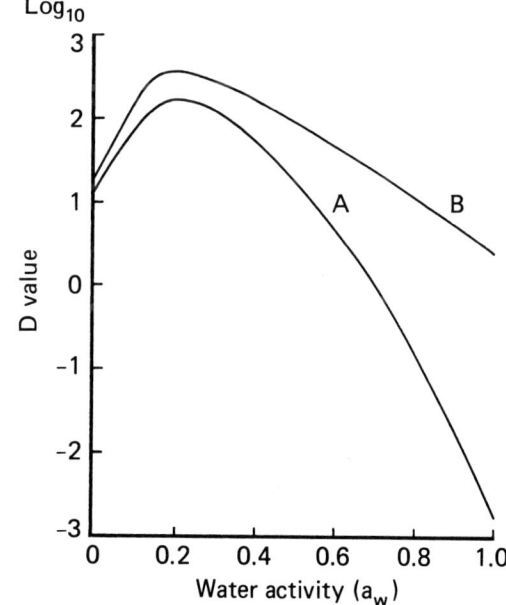

Fig. 4.3 Influence of water activity on the heat resistance of bacterial spores
  Curve A: a species relatively susceptible to moist heat
  Curve B: a species highly resistant to moist heat.

decreased below 0.2 a_w (20 per cent saturation), the resistance of the spores declined but it remained above the level associated with full saturation. The relative resistance of different species is occasionally reversed during the transition from the intermediate moisture level to severe desiccation. This occurs with B. stearothermophilus and B. subtilis, the former being more resistant to moist heat and the latter more resistant to dry heat. This is of practical importance in the selection of these species for use as biological indicators of sterilization efficiency. The findings of Murrell & Scott (1966) were confirmed by Angelotti et al (1968), who determined D values for spores of B. subtilis var. niger which were preconditioned to various water activities and then embedded in water-impermeable plastic blocks for heat treatment. Angelotti's results are shown in Table 4.3.

The heat resistance of non-sporing bacteria and yeasts is influenced by water activity in a similar manner. The effects are highly significant in the heat treatment of foods and other materials that have a low water activity because they contain a high concentration of sugar or salt.

Hydrogen ion concentration (pH)

Spores that are highly resistant to moist heat at pH 7 may be killed rapidly in an acid medium. In food canning, products are divided into groups according to the degree of acidity. Non-acid foods (pH >4.5), such as meat and vegetables, are processed at 121°C to ensure that the chance of a spore of C. botulinum surviving the treatment is reduced to 10^{-12}. However, acid products (pH 4.5 or below), such as tomatoes, could be processed at 100°C

Table 4.3 Influence of water activity on the heat resistance of B. subtilis var. niger spores embedded in impermeable methylmethacrylate polymer (Angelotti et al, 1968)

Water activity prior to embedding (a_w)	D value, 135°C (min)
0.1	59.5
0.2	73.5
0.4	88.7
0.6	67.4
0.8	36.0
0.9	10.9

with similar assurance of sterility.

Alderton & Snell (1963) demonstrated a reversible change in the resistance to moist heat of spores produced by B. stearothermophilus and Bacillus megaterium that depends on interchange between hydrogen ions and calcium ions in the spore integuments prior to heating. In a subsequent study (Alderton et al, 1964), spores of B. megaterium were converted to the more sensitive hydrogen form by immersion in mineral acid (pH 4) at 25°C for 4–5 hours. Reversion to the resistant state occurred when they were transferred to an alkaline solution containing calcium. The transition required several days at ambient temperature in the calcium-containing solution but occurred in 1–2 hours at 50–60°C. The determinations of heat resistance were carried out in a neutral, calcium-free medium. Similar results have been reported by Ando & Tsuzuki (1983) for C. perfringens type A.

Associated materials

Microorganisms may be associated with many different materials in their natural environments. These include blood, tissue, food, sugars, salts, lipids, crystalline deposits and garden soil. The protection of microorganisms by associated material may be caused by delay in heat penetration but is usually attributable to the influence of the material on the moisture level. High concentrations of sugar or salt affect the resistance of vegetative bacteria, spores and yeasts by lowering the water activity of the suspending medium. La Rock (1975) compared the heat resistance of spores in an anhydrous oil to their resistance in the same oil after incorporation of 0.02 and 0.1 per cent water. The death rate curves obtained in the anhydrous oil had a broad shoulder which was reduced in width by 0.02 per cent and abolished by 0.1 per cent water content. The results showed that a decrease in resistance occurred as the amount of water increased. Molin & Snygg (1967) also showed that addition of water to oils decreased the resistance of bacterial spores and found that the type of oil influenced resistance in a way that could not be entirely explained by reduced heat conductivity of lipids or their water content.

Sodium nitrate, sodium nitrite and sodium chloride, which are used as curing salts, appear to exert their main effect subsequent to heat treatment by inhibiting the germination of surviving spores. Briggs & Yazdany (1970) showed that aerobic spore-formers are increasingly sensitized to sodium chloride in the recovery medium by increasing heat damage. They proposed that the increase in salt sensitivity contributes to the stability of canned foods containing sodium chloride.

DESIGN OF HEAT STERILIZATION PROCESSES

Different temperature-time combinations which are equivalent in lethality may differ in their effects on the materials to be treated. These differences should be investigated when a process is designed for articles or solutions containing heat-sensitive ingredients. The first decision to be taken is whether steam sterilization or some form of dry heat treatment is appropriate. Secondly, a favourable temperature-time combination should be selected. Finally, a choice between maintaining the whole of the material at the selected temperature for a specified time, or calculating the lethality of the heating and cooling stages and subtracting this from the holding time at a fixed temperature may be made.

Heat-stable materials

The sterilization time for articles or liquids that withstand the usual moist or dry heat sterilization processes is the sum of the penetration time and the holding time. The penetration time is variable, depending on the nature and the bulk of the material. The holding time, for which the whole of the material must be held at the sterilizing temperature, depends on the temperature of the process. The relationship between sterilization time, penetration time and holding time for a textile pack in a steam sterilization process is shown by the temperature profiles in Figure 4.4.

Heat-sensitive materials

Rubber, synthetic polymers and many types of solutions deteriorate when they are subjected to conventional sterilization processes because they suffer unnecessary damage or deterioration during

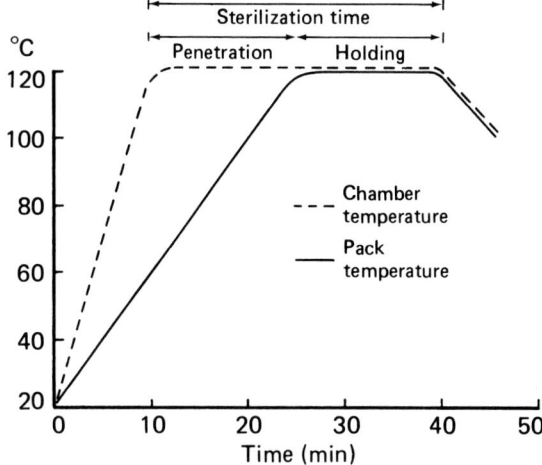

Fig. 4.4 Sterilization, penetration and holding times in heat sterilization.

prolonged heating and cooling periods. Solutions for injection or intravenous administration, microbiological culture media and canned foods contain ingredients that may lose biological activity, nutrient quality or palatability. The heat-sensitive substances include drugs, antibiotics, sugars, proteins and vitamins.

Deterioration can sometimes be reduced or prevented by better management of the sterilization cycle. Many rubber articles withstand sterilization at 134°C in a prevacuum steam sterilizer because air is removed before the chamber and load are heated to the sterilizing temperature, whereas they deteriorate after treatment at 121°C in a downward displacement jacketed sterilizer because air removal is not completed before the load becomes hot. Some pharmaceuticals can be stabilized against oxidation by removal of headspace air from the containers before they are sealed. Caramelization of sugars in intravenous solutions is reduced or prevented by rapid spray cooling.

The principal method of minimizing deterioration of heat-sensitive material involves the determination of a suitable processing temperature and calculation of the total lethality of the heating, holding and cooling stages of the process.

Processing temperature

Selection of the most favourable temperature requires knowledge of the different temperature coefficients for sporicidal action and for deterioration of a critically heat-sensitive component of the material to be treated. Curve A in Figure 4.5 describes the effect of increasing temperature on the D value of bacterial spores with a z value of 10°C and curve B represents a heat-sensitive substance with a z value of 30°C. In this example, the margin between achievement of sterility and the occurrence of deterioration increases as the temperature is raised because the rate of sporicidal action is accelerated more than is the rate of deterioration. The opposite situation would exist if the z value for the biocidal action were higher than that for the adverse reaction.

Practical application of this approach is limited by the difficulty of isolating and identifying the critically heat-sensitive ingredient of complex materials, such as microbiological culture media and foods. Further, the potential benefit of a high temperature-short time treatment might not be realized in a batch sterilization process because extended heat penetration and cooling times could outweigh the advantage of a decrease in holding time. An increase in the holding time is also required when the parameters of a batch process are translated to large scale operation. A heat treatment of increased severity is required because an increase in the volume of liquid is accompanied by a corresponding increase in the number of micro-bial contaminants to be killed. For example, if the volume, and the number, were increased by 1000, extra time equivalent to 3 times the D value would be required to match the level of sterility assurance for which the small scale operation was designed.

The deterioration of heat-sensitive liquids that is caused by prolonged heating and cooling times and extended holding times is greatly reduced if a continuous heat treatment process can be used. This is only practicable in a large scale operation, where a homogeneous, non-viscous liquid is rapidly heated and cooled by a heat-exchange system; in these circumstances full advantage can be taken of using the combination of temperature and time that provides the widest margin between the rates of sporicidal action and product deterioration. The difference between the heating profiles of a batch and a continuous process is shown in Figure 4.6.

Method of integrated lethality

The heat treatment of canned foods is designated by the symbol F, which represents the time at a specified temperature that will achieve the required levels of microbiological safety and keeping quality (Stumbo, 1973). If the recommended treatment (F) for non-acid canned foods is 4 minutes at 121°C, the time for which the product must be held at this temperature may be reduced by converting all temperature-time combinations

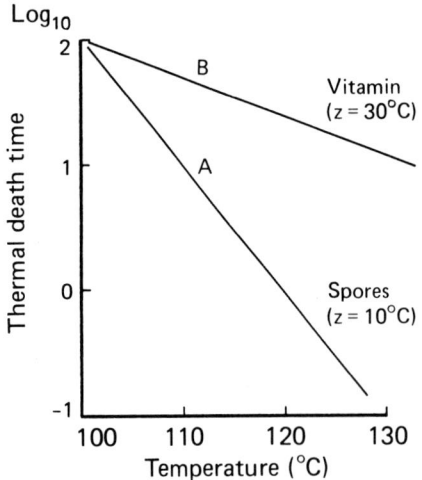

Fig. 4.5 Influence of temperature on the death rate of bacterial spores with a z value of 10°C and on the rate of deterioration of a heat-sensitive food constituent with a z value of 30°C.

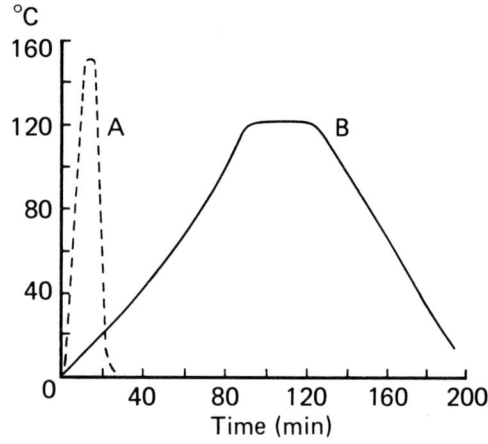

Fig. 4.6 Comparison of heating profiles of aqueous liquids in (A) a continuous process operated at 150°C and (B) a batch process at 121°C.

during the heating and cooling stages to equivalent time at 121°C. The total is then subtracted from the holding time of 4 minutes at the maximum temperature.

The lethality of a process is calculated from the heating profile of the product, which has been obtained by placing a thermocouple at the centre of a can at the slowest heating site in the sterilizer and recording the temperature continuously throughout the heat treatment. A hypothetical heating profile is shown in Figure 4.7, where it has been divided into separate segments, each representing a temperature that is assumed to have been maintained for 1 minute.

Different mathematical methods are used for converting the lethality of the heating and cooling times to equivalent times at the reference temperature of 121°C. The simplest method is the use of a Lethal Rate Table (Stumbo, 1973), which permits 1 minute at each temperature to be converted directly to a fraction of a minute at 121°C. The hypothetical data contained in Figure 4.7 have been subjected to this procedure and the result shows that the recommended holding time of 4 minutes at 121°C can be reduced by 3.74 minutes if the lethality of the heating and cooling stages is taken into account (Table 4.4).

The symbol F_0 refers to a process which is based on 121°C as the reference temperature and 10°C as

Table 4.4 Use of Lethal Rate Table to calculate total heat treatment

	1 min at °C	Equivalent time at 121°C (min)
Heating	100	0.001
	104	0.002
	107	0.007
	110	0.022
	113	0.062
	116	0.168
	118	0.348
	119	0.486
	120	0.683
	120.5	0.824
Cooling	120	0.683
	118	0.348
	114	0.087
	109	0.014
	104	0.002
	100	0.001
		Total 3.74

the z value for bacterial spores. The custom of designating a heat treatment in this way is now being extended to processes other than food canning. A recommendation for an F_0 value of 20 minutes at 121°C for a culture medium to be used in a sterility test allows the treatment to be delivered in the manner that is least detrimental to its growth-promoting quality. The decision may be influenced by the heat sensitivity of the material or the size of the containers and volume of material in each. Modern electronically controlled sterilizers provide evidence that a given load has received heat treatment equivalent to the F_0 value desired (Industrial Pharmacists Group, 1980).

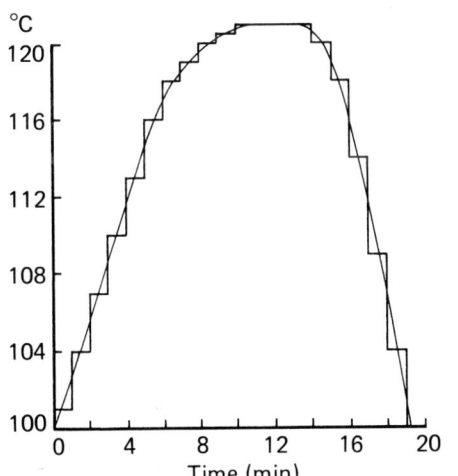

Fig. 4.7 Hypothetical temperature profile of a canned food, divided into 1 minute intervals for calculating the lethality of all temperature-time combinations (F_0 value)

REFERENCES

Alderton G, Snell N 1963 Base exchange and heat resistance in bacterial spores. Biochemical and Biophysical Research Communications 10: 139–143
Alderton G, Thompson P A, Snell N 1964 Heat adaptation and ion exchange in *Bacillus megaterium* spores. Science 143: 141–143
Allwood M C, Russell A D 1967 Mechanism of thermal injury in *Staphylococcus aureus* 1. Relationship between viability and leakage. Applied Microbiology 15: 1266–1269
Ando Y, Tsuzuki T 1983 Mechanism of chemical manipulation of the heat resistance of *Clostridium perfringens* spores. Journal of Applied Bacteriology 54: 197–202

Andrew M H E, Greaves J P 1979 Production of single strand breaks in the DNA of *Streptococcus faecalis* after mild heating. Journal of General Microbiology 111: 239–242

Angelotti R, Maryanski J H, Butler T F, Peeler J T, Campbell J E 1968 Influence of spore moisture content on the dry-heat resistance of *Bacillus subtilis* var. *niger*. Applied Microbiology 16: 735–745

Balassa G, Milhaud P, Raulet E, Silva M T, Sousa J C F 1979 A *Bacillus subtilis* mutant requiring dipicolinic acid for the development of heat-resistant spores. Journal of General Microbiology 110: 365–379

Bayne H G, Michener H D 1979 Heat resistance of *Byssochlamys* ascospores. Applied and Environmental Microbiology 37: 449–453

Bond W W, Favero M S 1975 Thermal profile of a *Bacillus* species (ATCC 27380) extremely resistant to dry heat. Applied Microbiology 29: 859–860

Brannen J P 1970 On the role of DNA in wet heat sterilization of micro-organisms. Journal of Theoretical Biology 27: 425–432

Briggs A, Yazdany S 1970 Effect of sodium chloride on the heat and radiation resistance and on the recovery of heated or irradiated spores of the genus *Bacillus*. Journal of Applied Bacteriology 33: 621–632

Brock T D, Freeze H 1969 *Thermus aquaticus* gen. n. and sp. n., a nonsporulating extreme thermophile. Journal of Bacteriology 98: 289–297

Chappelle E W, Rich E Jr, MacLeod N H 1967 Prevention of protein denaturation during exposure to sterilization temperatures. Science 155: 1287–1288

Gould G W, Dring G J 1975 Heat resistance of bacterial endospores and concept of an expanded osmoregulatory cortex. Nature 258: 402–405

Grecz N, Bruszer G 1981 Lethal heat induces single strand breaks in the DNA of bacterial spores. Biochemical and Biophysical Research Communications 98: 191–196

Hanson R S, Curry M V, Garner J V, Halvorson H O 1972 Mutants of *Bacillus cereus* strain T that produce thermoresistant spores lacking dipicolinate and have low levels of calcium. Canadian Journal of Microbiology 18: 1139–1143

Industrial Pharmacists Group 1980 Sterilisation: need for a new approach. Pharmaceutical Journal 224: 41–43

Kooiman W J, Geers J M 1975 Simple and accurate technique for the determination of heat resistance of bacterial spores. Journal of Applied Bacteriology 38: 185–189

Labbe R G 1979 Recovery of spores of *Bacillus stearothermophilus* from thermal injury. Journal of Applied Bacteriology 47: 457–462

LaRock P A 1975 Effect of water on the thermal death of a hydrocarbon bacterium in a nonaqueous fluid. Applied Microbiology 29: 112–114

Leanz G, Gilvarg C 1973 Dipicolinic acid location in intact spores of *Bacillus megaterium*. Journal of Bacteriology 114: 455–456

Lewis J C, Snell N S, Burr H K 1960 Water permeability of bacterial spores and the concept of a contractile cortex. Science 132: 544–545

Lewith S 1890 Ueber die Ursache der Widerstandsfähigkeit der Sporen gegen hohe Temperaturen. Ein Beitrag zur Theorie der Desinfektion. Archiv für Experimentelle Pathologie und Pharmakologie 26: 341–354

Molin G 1982 Destruction of bacterial spores by thermal methods. In: Russell A D, Hugo W B, Ayliffe G A J (eds) Principles and practice of disinfection, preservation and sterilization. Blackwell, Oxford, ch 13B, p 454

Molin N, Snygg B G 1967 Effect of lipid materials on heat resistance of bacterial spores. Applied Microbiology 15: 1422–1426

Murrell W G 1955 The bacterial endospore. Monograph published by the University of Sydney, Australia. (Quoted by Grecz N, Tang T 1970 Relation of dipicolinic acid to heat resistance of bacterial spores. Journal of General Microbiology 63: 303–310)

Murrell W G 1981 Biophysical studies on the molecular mechanisms of spore heat resistance and dormancy. In: Levinson H S, Sonenshein A L, Tipper D J (eds) Sporulation and germination. American Society for Microbiology, Washington, p 64–77

Murrell W G, Scott W J 1966 The heat resistance of bacterial spores at various water activities. Journal of General Microbiology 43: 411–425

Murrell W G, Warth A D 1965 Composition and heat resistance of bacterial spores. In: Campbell L L, Halvorson H O (eds) Spores III. American Society for Microbiology, Ann Arbor, p 1–24

Olliver M, Rendle T 1934 A new problem in fruit preservation. Studies on *Byssochlamys fulva* and its effect on tissues of processed fruit. Journal of the Society of Chemical Industry 53: 166T–172T

Pask-Hughes R, Williams R A D 1975 Extremely thermophilic Gram-negative bacteria from hot tap water. Journal of General Microbiology 88: 321–328

Riemann H, Ordal Z J 1961 Germination of bacterial endospores with calcium and dipicolinic acid. Science 133: 1703–1704

Roberts T A 1970 Recovering spores damaged by heat, ionizing radiations or ethylene oxide. Journal of Applied Bacteriology 33: 74–94

Rosenberg B, Kemeny G, Switzer R C, Hamilton T C 1971 Quantitative evidence for protein denaturation as the cause of thermal death. Nature 232: 471–473

Ross K F A, Billing E 1957 The water and solid content of living bacterial spores and vegetative cells as indicated by refractive index measurements. Journal of General Microbiology 16: 418–425

Silva M T, Sousa J C F 1972 Ultrastructural alterations induced by moist heat in *Bacillus cereus*. Applied Microbiology 24: 463–476

Stumbo C R 1973 Thermobacteriology in food processing, 2nd edn. Academic Press, New York

Wang D I-C, Scharer J, Humphrey A E 1964 Kinetics of death of bacterial spores at elevated temperatures. Applied Microbiology 12: 451–454

Warth A D 1978 Molecular structure of the bacterial spore. In: Rose A H, Morris J G (eds) Advances in microbial physiology 17: 1–45

Warth A D 1981 Stabilization of spore enzymes to heat by reduction in water activity. In: Levinson H S, Sonenshein A L, Tipper D J (eds) Sporulation and germination. American Society for Microbiology, Washington, p 249–252

5

Sterilization by dry heat

Dry heat sterilization refers to a variety of methods, in which the only common factor is the absence of liquid water from the heating environment. The dry condition actually embraces a wide range of moisture levels, from just above complete dryness to just below full saturation. The relationship between moisture levels, expressed as the relative humidity of a gaseous heating environment, or the corresponding water activity of the microbial cells, and heat resistance has been explained in Chapter 4 (Fig. 4.3). Dry heat sterilization is usually carried out towards the lower limit of the humidity scale, where the resistance of bacterial spores is about 100 times less than that at the peak level which occurs at 20–40 per cent saturation. More severe treatments are required if the organisms are at an unfavourable moisture level and cannot gain or lose water during the heating process.

The need for dry heat sterilization in hospitals declined sharply with the introduction of single-use syringes and needles that are sterilized commercially by radiation or ethylene oxide. However, the method is required for sterilization of reusable glass syringes, needles, delicate cutting instruments, surgical drills, articles made from non-stainless steel, and oily materials. Dry heat sterilization is used extensively in microbiological laboratories for routine production of dry sterile glassware.

The following sources of dry heat will be discussed in this chapter but most attention will be paid to hot air sterilization:

Hot air
Radiant heat
Conducted heat
Direct flaming
Incineration.

SUSCEPTIBILITY OF MICROORGANISMS

Species of sporing bacteria differ in their resistance to dry heat to a lesser extent than they do to moist heat. Reported D values and thermal death times vary widely because, although the importance of specifying the moisture level is now appreciated, it was not always known or controlled during the tests. D values of 0.35 minutes for *Bacillus stearothermophilus* and 1.8 minutes for *Bacillus subtilis* var. *niger* at 160°C have been reported (Bruch et al, 1963). This explains their selection for use as biological indicators for moist and dry heat respectively.

The resistance of non-sporing microorganisms at water activities in the upper part of the humidity scale (e.g. 0.9–0.95) is of considerable importance in food canning and food preservation but is not particularly relevant to the sterilization of medical and laboratory equipment by dry heat.

Heat resistance tests that were carried out in connection with research on dry heat sterilization of spacecraft components containing electronic elements revealed a range of D values from less than 5 minutes to 58 minutes at 125°C (Bond et al, 1971); D values up to 5 hours have been reported in closed heating systems (Pflug, 1970) and a particularly resistant species of *Bacillus* had a D value at 125°C of 139 hours (Bond et al, 1973).

FACTORS INFLUENCING EFFICIENCY OF STERILIZATION

Temperature

The time required for sterilization varies inversely with temperature, as in moist heat sterilization. However, dry heat sterilization is conducted in a higher temperature range as the rate at which spores are killed accelerates markedly in the range 160–180°C.

Temperature coefficients (z values) for spores range from 14°C at high environmental humidity to 55.5°C in a hot dry gas at a high flow rate (Fox & Pflug, 1968); values are usually between 15–30°C and an accepted average for bacterial spores within the temperature range of 105–135°C is 21°C (Pflug & Holcomb, 1983).

Moisture levels

The efficiency of dry heat sterilization depends on the initial moisture level of the microbial cells and the direction and extent of changes that may occur during the heat treatment by exchange of water between the microorganisms and the heating environment. Heating systems may be characterized as open or closed.

Open systems

An open system is one in which there is no limit to water transfer between the microorganisms and their environment. When the organisms are directly exposed to hot dry air in a large oven, they will lose intracellular water and reach a very low moisture level. The water activity in an open system is not constant and its adjustment may be hindered if the contaminated articles are enclosed in material that is not fully permeable to water vapour.

Closed systems

In closed systems, the microorganisms are isolated from the main heating environment by material that is impermeable to water vapour. They may be in a partly closed situation, represented by a small, impervious container or a closely wrapped film of aluminium foil. They may also be trapped in an air bubble within an impervious solid. In these situations, the microorganisms exchange moisture with the limited space around them until the levels are equalized. The final level depends on the initial levels in the cells and the air space and on the volume of the space. It may be predicted by calculation if this information is available.

The less common situation of a completely closed system occurs when microorganisms are embedded in direct contact with an impervious solid, with no surrounding space available for transfer of water. The resistance of the microorganisms is therefore determined by their initial moisture level, which is maintained during the heat treatment, and it will be very high if this happens to be in the region of 20–40 per cent saturation. Encapsulation of spores of *B. subtilis* var. *niger* in crystals of calcium carbonate was associated with a ninefold increase in their resistance to dry heat at 121°C (Doyle & Ernst, 1967). Closed systems are encountered when dry heat is used to sterilize impervious solids or anhydrous oils in depth.

D values in closed systems are about 10 times those that apply to open systems (Pflug, 1970). Microorganisms that are trapped between closely mated surfaces, which are common in space exploration vehicles, are in a partly closed system but their resistance is closer to levels encountered in open systems than to those associated with completely closed systems (Pflug, 1970; Simko et al, 1971).

Gaseous atmosphere

Experiments conducted in open systems at 160°C have revealed no significant differences between air, oxygen, carbon dioxide, nitrogen and helium (Pheil et al, 1967). D values for spores of *B. subtilis* 5230 at 160°C fell within the range 1.4–1.7 minutes and minor variations were attributed to differences in the humidity of the gases obtained from the cylinders. Fox & Pflug (1968) obtained a similar result and commented that the failure of nitrogen to increase resistance to dry heat is at variance with the view that oxidation has a major role in the lethal action.

APPLICATIONS OF DRY HEAT STERILIZATION

The main advantage of dry heat sterilization is its ability to penetrate solids, nonaqueous liquids and closed cavities. Lack of corrosion is also important in the sterilization of non-stainless metals and instruments with fine cutting edges. Disadvantages are the high temperature and the long time required for sterilization.

Glassware and metalware for which dry heat is the preferred method of sterilization include non-stainless and fine cutting instruments, syringes, hollow needles, test tubes and pipettes. Dry heat provides the only method of sterilization for heat-

stable powders (e.g. drugs), waxes and nonaqueous liquids. Nonaqueous liquids include Vaseline (petrolatum), paraffin, Vaseline or paraffin gauze dressings, eye ointment bases, oily injections, silicone lubricant and pure glycerol.

Rubber, plastics and substances that will vaporize or ignite at the sterilizing temperature do not withstand dry heat sterilization. Glycerol containing water should not be sterilized in a hot air oven because there is a risk of explosion.

HOT AIR STERILIZATION

Dry heat (hot air) sterilization is carried out in electrically heated ovens with mechanical air convection. Gas-heated ovens are no longer used because temperature distribution within the chamber may vary by as much as 60°C (Darmady & Brock, 1954). The same authors reported that electrically heated ovens in which temperature distribution depends only on gravity convection are also unsatisfactory because variations of 9–28°C were observed. Detailed specifications for sterilizing ovens with mechanical convection and automatic controls are provided by the Department of Health and Social Security (1980) in Health Technical Memorandum No. 10.

Design of sterilizing ovens

The non-pressurized chamber should be insulated against heat loss, and provision for the entry of 12 thermocouples is required. There may be one door at the front, or a door at each end to permit removal of the sterilized load into the appropriate storage area. The chamber should be fitted with shelves for separating the layers of packs or containers. An interconnected electrical heater and fan unit circulates hot air between the shelves.

The controls include an overheat cutout (manually resettable) and a sterilizing stage timer that returns to zero if power is disconnected. It should not re-start automatically because a decision must be made on whether to continue the process or start again from the beginning. Door operation is subject to controls that prevent a cycle being started if the door is not locked and prevent the door from being opened while a cycle is in progress.

The recommended indicators include an indicating thermometer and chart recorder. The separate sensing elements should be placed where they will not interfere with loading but be close enough to give similar readings of temperature. Indicator lights should show when the power is switched on, the electrical system is operating and when the process had been completed. In the event of a faulty cycle, the door should remain locked until it is attended to by a designated responsible person. While ovens equipped for an automatic cycle are now recommended, manual operation is acceptable; the door may be locked by a key and access should be restricted to the person in charge of the process.

Packing and loading

A single layer of wrapping material should be used. Kraft paper bags are acceptable for individually wrapped pipettes in laboratories but aluminium foil and aluminium containers are recommended for hospital use. Aluminium tubes and oval canisters closed with crimped foil caps have been designed for glass syringes (Darmady et al, 1957) and small instruments (Darmady et al, 1963) respectively. Syringes should be assembled and forceps may be closed. Heavy instruments should be supported in a metal cradle to facilitate heating by conduction. Delicate instruments, such as cataract knives, should also be supported to guard against physical damage.

Canisters are widely used in laboratories for sterilizing unwrapped pipettes. Foil caps and lids may admit airborne contaminants during cooling. However, the insertion of cotton wool plugs may be undesirable because they generate fibres.

Sterilization process

The oven may be preheated to the sterilizing temperature before loading, or it may be loaded when cold. Loading into a heated oven reduces the time taken for the chamber to reach the sterilizing temperature because heat is not absorbed by the walls and fittings. The sterilization cycle includes the following stages:

1. Heating the chamber to the selected sterilizing temperature
2. Sterilizing the load
3. Cooling the load.

The oven and its heating system should be designed to reach the sterilizing temperature in the range 160–180°C within a specified time. The sterilizing stage starts when this has been achieved and the sterilization time is the sum of:

a. Heat penetration time
b. Holding time.

The duration of the sterilization cycle is governed mainly by the penetration and holding times. The penetration time varies widely with the type of material, ranging from 15 minutes for small instruments or syringes, individually packed, to 4 hours or more for a canister filled with glass pipettes. Powders and oils have particularly long penetration times because they are poor conductors of heat. Some heating times for different quantities of powder and Vaseline, adapted from Perkins (1969), are shown in Table 5.1.

Table 5.1 Times required for powders and oils to heat from room temperature to 160°C in a hot air oven (Perkins, 1969)

Material	Quantity	Time (min)
Powder	28 g (1 oz)	80
	112 g (4 oz)	115
Vaseline	28 g (1 oz)	110
	112 g (4 oz)	165

Holding times recommended in the United Kingdom are shorter than those recommended in the United States, as shown in Table 5.2. The British Pharmacopoeia (1980) permits pharmaceuticals to be sterilized for a holding time of

Table 5.2 Holding times in dry heat sterilization

Temperature °C	Authority	
	DHSS[1], 1980 (min)	Perkins, 1969 (min)
150	—	150
160	60	120
170	40	60
180	20	30

[1] Department of Health and Social Security

60 minutes at 150°C but the United States Pharmacopeia (1980) recommends a temperature of 160°C for not less than 2 hours if the material is sufficiently stable.

Testing efficiency of sterilization

The methods that are described here are recommended by the Department of Health and Social Security (1980). The tests required when a new sterilizing oven is purchased are of two types: a basic performance test that is carried out by the manufacturer and repeated when necessary, and a production load test to validate methods of preparation, packaging and loading of the materials for which the sterilizer will be used.

Twelve thermocouples are required for each test. Two are placed close to the sensors for the indicating thermometer and the chart recorder. In the basic performance test, the remaining leads are distributed at strategic positions in a standard load of jars containing a nonflammable, non-toxic silicone fluid. In a production load test, they are placed in packs or containers that represent the 'worst case' load for which the oven will be used. The purpose of the thermocouples in the chamber is to determine temperature overshoot that may occur before a steady state temperature has been reached in the chamber; temperature drift, which is the variation in temperature over a prolonged recording period; reproducibility of the chamber temperature in two independent cycles; and temperature variation between the indicating thermometer and the chart recorder. The thermocouples placed in various load units measure the temperature reached, its uniformity throughout the load, and the time required for the whole of the load to reach the sterilizing temperature after it has been reached in the chamber (i.e. the heat penetration time).

If the sterilizer has passed the basic performance test but the production load is unsatisfactory, the methods of packing and loading must be examined and adjusted to conform to the capability of the oven. In between annual full scale tests, a half-yearly test may be carried out using three thermocouples.

Biological indicators prepared from spores of *B. subtilis* var. *niger* are available for hot air ovens but their use for validation or routine control is generally considered unnecessary. Chemical indicators of appropriate type may be useful for demonstrating that the packages have been processed.

STERILIZATION BY RADIANT HEAT

Infrared and microwave radiations are characterized by long wavelengths and very low levels of radiant energy. Their minor role in sterilization depends entirely on the conversion of the radiant energy to heat when it is absorbed by solids or liquids. Microwave ovens are unsuitable for dry heat sterilization although they can be used for decontamination of moist bacterial cultures (Latimer & Matsen, 1977). Infrared heaters may be used in sterilizing ovens where they transmit radiant energy directly to the exposed surfaces of articles to be sterilized, eliminating the slow process of conduction by air in the chamber. However, the heat that is produced on the surface of the load can only penetrate to the interior by conduction. Two types of infrared ovens, each designed for a special purpose and now mainly of historical interest, will be described briefly.

Conveyor oven

An infrared conveyor oven was developed by Darmady et al (1957) for use in a regional service supplying sterile glass syringes to a group of British hospitals. The syringes were packed individually in aluminium tubes with crimped foil caps. Tubes with a dull black anodized surface were used for the larger syringes and a dull aluminium surface for the smaller ones so uniform heating was obtained. The tunnel-shaped oven, about 2 m in length and closed by flaps at each end, contained four infrared heaters and a moving belt. The syringes were heated to 180°C with the assistance of a forced draught and the throughput time of 22 minutes included a holding time of 7.5 minutes. The efficacy of the system was confirmed by Russell & Abdurahman (1960) but the use of conveyor ovens declined when commercial production of single-use syringes, made from heat-sensitive materials, commenced.

High-vacuum oven

A prototype sterilizer was designed for rapid dry heat sterilization of instruments in situations where a steam supply might not be available for sterilization and the cost of a special installation would be prohibitive (Darmady et al, 1961). The oven was evacuated rapidly to a very low level and then heated to 280°C by infrared heaters. The sterilization cycle of 15 minutes included a holding time of 7 minutes and the load was cooled with nitrogen to prevent damage by oxidation. However, portable, electrically heated steam sterilizers are now readily available for the sterilization of instruments.

STERILIZATION BY CONDUCTED HEAT

Small metal or glass articles may be heated rapidly if they are placed in direct contact with a metal block on a thermostatically controlled hot plate (Darmady et al, 1958). Cavities bored in the block accommodate syringes; instruments are placed in a shallow covered tray recessed into the top. When the hot plate was preheated to 190°C, the syringes reached 180°C in 10 minutes and the instruments in 23 minutes. A holding time of 7.5 minutes was added to these penetration times.

Conducted heat, in the form of oil baths, has been used in dental surgeries for disinfection of conventional handpieces, and crucibles containing heated glass beads are sometimes used for chairside disinfection of the small reamers and broaches that are used for debridement of root canals. However, these techniques are inconvenient and unsatisfactory and sterilization in a hot air oven is recommended.

STERILIZATION BY FLAMING

Sterilization by direct flaming is limited to wire loops that are used for inoculating bacterial cultures. The loop is held in the flame of a bunsen burner until it becomes red hot. Precautions must be taken to avoid spattering of unsterilized material from the loop as it is heated. Darlow (1959) designed a metal tubular device to be mounted over the burner. Electrically heated loop incinerators are now commonly used; they are especially suitable for use in safety cabinets or enclosures where anaerobic conditions are maintained. A support for the handle of the loop has been described by Gordon & Davenport (1973), who advise that handles should be insulated to guard against the possibility of electric shock if the loop comes in contact with the heating element.

The practice of flaming transfer forceps, glass rods, the outer surface of sterilized pipettes, and the mouths of culture tubes or bottles does not guarantee sterilization or protection against airborne contaminants because the temperature is too low and the time is too short. These limitations apply also to the method of dipping forceps, hypodermic needles or glass spreaders in alcohol and burning it off. Evaporative cooling lowers the temperature at the surface of the instrument to 118°C although the air temperature a short distance away may be 204°C (Doyle & Ernst, 1969). The suspicion of many microbiologists that flaming of test tubes and bottles when opening them to transfer cultures is a waste of time receives support from an investigation by Brunker & Fernandez (1972), who found no significant difference in contamination rates between containers that were flamed and those that were not flamed.

INCINERATION

Combustible waste

Much of the waste material that is generated in hospitals and microbiological laboratories is contaminated with large numbers of microorganisms, including recognized and opportunistic pathogens. Hospital waste and certain types of laboratory waste materials, such as those from animal units, are incinerated but the efficacy of incineration cannot be taken for granted. Vegetative and sporing bacteria have been found in solid residues and gaseous effluents from incinerators. An investigation by Barbeito & Gremillion (1968) showed that a temperature of 371°C in the firebox and 196°C in the brick lining were required to kill spores of *B. subtilis* var. *niger* when they were mixed with dry animal bedding.

Air incinerators

The effluent from safety cabinets or chambers where aerosols are generated for investigational purposes must be made safe for discharge to the outside environment. High-efficiency filters are commonly used but methods of heat sterilization have also been studied. Decker et al (1954) reported that exposure times of 3 seconds at 300°C, 5 seconds at 275°C and 10 seconds at 245°C sterilized bacterial spores suspended in an air stream. Mullican et al (1971) obtained a much shorter time of 0.02 second at 260°C for aerosolised spores of *B. subtilis* var. *niger*. They used an experimental system that reduced the heating time of the bacterial aerosol almost to zero and calculated that their findings were in accord with the resistance to dry heat of bacteria on solid surfaces if allowance was made for the heating time of the supporting material.

REFERENCES

Barbeito M S, Gremillion G G 1968 Microbiological safety evaluation of an industrial refuse incinerator. Applied Microbiology 16: 291–295

Bond W W, Favero M S, Korber M R 1973 *Bacillus* sp. ATCC 27380: a spore with extreme resistance to dry heat. Applied Microbiology 26: 614–616

Bond W W, Favero M S, Petersen N J, Marshall J H 1971 Relative frequency distribution of D_{125C} values for spore isolates from the Mariner-Mars 1969 spacecraft. Applied Microbiology 21: 832–836

British Pharmacopoeia 1980 HMSO, London 2: A196

Bruch C W, Koesterer M G, Bruch M K 1963 Dry-heat sterilization: its development and application to components of exobiological space probes. Developments in Industrial Microbiology 4: 334–342

Brunker T, Fernandez B 1972 Effect of flaming cotton-plugged tubes upon the contamination of media during culture transfers. Applied Microbiology 23: 441–443

Darlow H M 1959 A device for flaming platinum loops. Lancet ii: 651

Darmady E M, Brock R B 1954 Temperature levels in hot-air ovens. Journal of Clinical Pathology 7: 290–299

Darmady E M, Hughes K E A, Tuke W 1957 Sterilization of syringes by infra-red radiation. Journal of Clinical Pathology 10: 291–298

Darmady E M, Hughes K E A, Tuke W 1963 Instrument container for dry-heat sterilisation. Lancet ii: 498–499

Darmady E M, Hughes K E A, Jones J, Tuke W 1958 Sterilisation by conducted heat. Lancet ii: 769–770

Darmady E M, Hughes K E A, Jones J D, Prince D, Tuke W 1961 Sterilization by dry heat. Journal of Clinical Pathology 14: 38–44

Decker H M, Citek F J, Harstad J B, Gross N H, Piper F J 1954 Time temperature studies of spore penetration through an electric air sterilizer. Applied Microbiology 2: 33–36

Department of Health and Social Security 1980 Sterilizers Health Technical Memorandum 10. HMSO, London

Doyle J E, Ernst R R 1967 Resistance of *Bacillus subtilis* var. *niger* spores occluded in water-insoluble crystals to three sterilization agents. Applied Microbiology 15: 726–730

Doyle J E, Ernst R R 1969 Alcohol flaming — a possible source of contamination in sterility testing. American Journal of Clinical Pathology 51: 407–408

Fox K, Pflug I J 1968 Effect of temperature and gas velocity on the dry-heat destruction rate of bacterial spores. Applied Microbiology 16: 343–348

Gordon R C, Davenport C V 1973 Simple modification to improve usefulness of the Bacti-cinerator. Applied Microbiology 26: 423

Latimer J M, Matsen J M 1977 Microwave oven irradiation as a method for bacterial decontamination in a clinical microbiology laboratory. Journal of Clinical Microbiology 6: 340–342

Mullican C L, Buchanan L M, Hoffman R K 1971 Thermal inactivation of aerosolized *Bacillus subtilis* var. *niger* spores. Applied Microbiology 22: 557–559

Perkins J J 1969 Principles and methods of sterilization in health sciences, 2nd edn. Charles C. Thomas, Springfield, ch 12, p 289; 295

Pflug I J 1970 Dry heat destruction rate for micro-organisms on open surfaces, in mated surface areas and encapsulated in solids of spacecraft hardware. Life Sciences and Space Research 8: 131–141

Pflug I J, Holcomb R G 1983 Principles of thermal destruction of microorganisms. In: Block S S (ed) Disinfection, sterilization, and preservation, 3rd edn. Lea & Febiger, Philadelphia, ch 38, p 770

Pheil C G, Pflug I J, Nicholas R C, Augustin J A L 1967 Effect of various gas atmospheres on destruction of microorganisms in dry heat. Applied Microbiology 15: 120–124

Russell F, Abdurahman R 1960 Sterilization of syringes by an infra-red conveyor oven. Scottish Medical Journal 5: 213–218

Simko G J, Devlin J D, Wardle M D 1971 Dry-heat resistance of *Bacillus subtilis* var. *niger* spores on mated surfaces. Applied Microbiology 22: 491–495

United States Pharmacopeia 1980 20th rev. Mack Publishing Company, Easton, p 1037

6

Sterilization by steam at increased pressure

Sterilization by moist heat depends on the use of steam above 100°C, usually at a temperature in the range 121–134°C. Minimum holding times for the sterilization of medical equipment are 15 minutes at 121°C, 10 minutes at 126°C and 3 minutes at 134°C (Working Party on Pressure-Steam Sterilizers, 1959). The slightly shorter times recommended by Perkins (1969) may be adequate for aqueous liquids if they are cooled slowly. Steam can be heated to temperatures above 100°C only by increasing the pressure above that of a normal atmosphere at sea level.

As the International System (SI) of measurement might not yet be used on the gauges and recorders of all pressure steam sterilizers, some relevant conversions are given in Table 6.1. Two pressure scales may be used: absolute pressure and gauge pressure. On the absolute pressure scale, zero represents a complete vacuum and all values are positive. The gauge pressure scale, in which zero represents standard atmospheric pressure at sea level, is more commonly used in steam sterilization. Values above atmospheric pressure are positive and values below zero are negative, representing degrees of vacuum. Gauge pressure measurements are subject to variation with the prevailing weather.

PROPERTIES AND QUALITY OF STEAM

Saturated steam

Saturated steam is water vapour, free from any other gases, which is in equilibrium with water.

Table 6.1 Temperature and pressure measurements in steam sterilization[1]

Temperature[2]		Gauge pressure[3]	
°C	°F	kPa	lb.f/in²
100	212	0	0
116	240	69	10
121	250	101	15
126	260	138	20
132	270	185	27
134	273	203	30
150	302	380	55

[1]Some measurements are approximate for simplicity
[2]Temperature conversion   1°C = 1.8°F
                                1°F = 0.56°C
[3]Pressure conversion   1 kPa = 10 mbar
                                1 kPa = 0.145 lb.f/in²
                                1 lb.f/in² = 6.9 kPa

On the boundary between the liquid and vapour phases of water, evaporation and condensation occur at equal rates and the relative humidity of the vapour is at the maximum value of 100 per cent.

The temperature of steam corresponds to that of the boiling water that gives rise to it. The boiling point, which is 100°C at standard atmospheric pressure at sea level, rises when the pressure is increased. When steam is generated within, or piped under pressure into, a closed vessel from which air has been removed, the temperature rises in a fixed relationship to the pressure, as shown in Figure 6.1, where the phase boundary has been drawn by joining separate temperature-pressure combinations. Any point on the line represents saturated steam.

The biocidal efficiency of saturated steam depends on:

1. Moisture content
2. Heat content
3. Penetration.

Moisture content

Saturated steam has a relative humidity of 100 per cent; as explained in Chapter 4, this is the condition in which bacterial spores are least resistant to heat. When steam condenses on the articles to be sterilized, it deposits a film of water on all accessible surfaces, ensuring that the microbial contaminants will be killed rapidly.

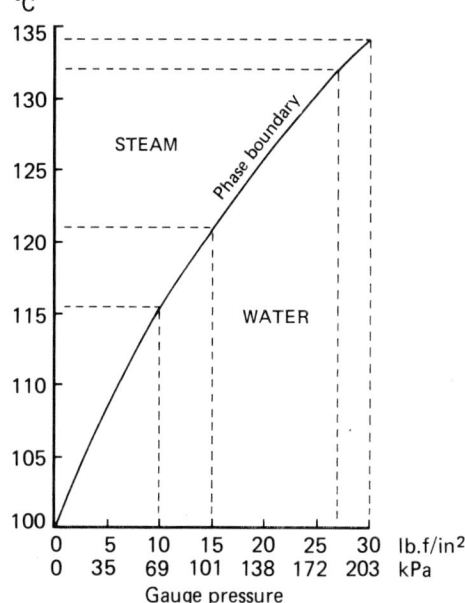

Fig. 6.1 Temperature and pressure relationships in saturated steam.

Heat content

Steam has a greater heat content than does water at the same temperature, as shown by the figures in Table 6.2.

The sensible heat is the quantity of heat that is required to raise the temperature of water to the boiling point. The latent heat is the additional heat that is absorbed when boiling water is converted to steam at the same temperature. This heat is converted to energy of motion (kinetic energy) as the water molecules are released from the cohesive forces of the liquid state and acquire the rapid motion that is characteristic of gases. When steam condenses on cooler objects in the sterilizing chamber, the latent heat is released but the sensible heat is retained and the condensate remains at the same temperature. The large amount of latent heat that is released is communicated directly to the surfaces of the load in the sterilizer, heating them rapidly to the temperature selected for sterilization.

Penetration

Penetration of steam through porous paper and

Table 6.2 Heat content of water and steam

Phase of water	Temperature °C	Heat content (kJ/kg) Sensible heat	Latent heat	Total heat
Liquid	100	419	0	419
Vapour	100	419	2257	2676
Vapour	121	509	2199	2708
Vapour	135	567	2160	2727

cloth wrapping materials to the interior of large textile packs and into partly enclosed cavities of glass or metal equipment is essential for sterilization. Effective penetration depends mainly on removal of air from the chamber and load, but is assisted by the large decrease in volume (e.g. 1600 ml to 1 ml) that accompanies condensation. This is of special importance in the sterilization of textiles.

Superheated steam

Steam is in a superheated state when the temperature is above that corresponding to the phase boundary at the existing pressure; that is, above the phase boundary line in Figure 6.1. In this condition, the relative humidity is less than 100 per cent and condensation does not occur unless the steam is cooled to the phase boundary temperature. Thus, deposition of moisture and release of latent heat are delayed, and the resistance of the microbial contaminants is increased (see Ch. 4, Fig 4.3). The degree of superheat is expressed by the difference between the actual temperature of the steam and the expected phase boundary temperature. If the temperature is 130°C and the pressure is 100 kPa (which corresponds to 121°C in saturated steam), the steam has 9°C superheat. The maximum acceptable degree of superheat in steam sterilization is 5°C (Working Party on Pressure-Steam Sterilizers, 1959).

The steam in a sterilizing chamber may become superheated from a variety of causes:

1. Overheated steam jacket
2. Pressure reduction in supply line
3. Dehydration of textiles.

Overheating in the steam jacket should be prevented by correct design of the sterilizer. It was formerly common in downward displacement porous load sterilizers with separate supply lines to the jacket and chamber but is now avoided by passing steam through the jacket to the chamber. This type of superheat may occur in prevacuum porous load sterilizers as the steam enters the evacuated chamber but the duration is too short to cause dehydration of the load, especially when steam is introduced in the prevacuum stage of the cycle to assist the removal of air.

Excessive pressure reduction in the supply line before the high-pressure steam from the boiler reaches the chamber causes water droplets in the steam to evaporate. The appropriate degree of reduction ensures that the steam in the chamber will be 'just dry' (i.e. close to the phase boundary) but excessive reduction causes superheat. The degree of reduction required depends on the amount of water in the steam supply.

A less obvious, but quite common cause of superheat is dehydration of textile packs prior to sterilization. This may occur if packs are placed in a hot, steam-jacketed sterilizer and left for some time before loading is completed and the sterilization cycle started. If the moisture content of cotton materials is reduced below the normal level of 5 per cent, they will absorb more steam to satisfy their affinity for moisture than is required to heat them to the sterilizing temperature and the excess latent heat raises the temperature of the steam (Henry, 1959). The relationship between dehydration of cotton and superheat is shown in Table 6.3.

Table 6.3 Relation between dehydration and superheating of cotton fabrics (Henry, 1959)

Moisture content of cotton goods (%)	Degree of superheat °C
8	0
5 — normal level (45% RH)	1–2
1	4
0 — completely dehydrated	9

Wet steam

'Wet' steam carries a fog of small droplets of water, usually resulting from condensation in long supply lines that are not adequately insulated. Droplets may also be entrained from an overfilled boiler. Wet steam is undesirable because it soaks porous material, creates a barrier to air removal and delays or prevents drying after sterilization. Excess moisture may be prevented by installation of a steam separator in the supply line after the pressure reducing valve. The dryness fraction of steam is expressed as the weight of pure, saturated steam divided by the weight of steam plus entrained water. The steam supply to sterilizers should have a dryness fraction of at least 0.95 when it enters the chamber (Working Party on Pressure-Steam Sterilizers, 1959). The resolution of problems caused by wet steam depends on correct management of the boiler and adequate insulation of the supply lines. The steam supply to the sterilizer should be tapped from the top of the main line, which should slope downward towards the separator and steam trap adjacent to the sterilizer. The degree of reduction is critical, depending on quality and pressure of the steam supply; a dryness fraction of 0.9 in the mains and a reduction of pressure in the ratio 2:1 have been recommended (Department of Health and Social Security 1980).

Chemical impurities

The absence of toxic residues is one of the advantages of steam sterilization. However, it has been common practice in the past to add volatile amines (e.g. octadecylamine, cyclohexylamine, morpholine) to the water in the boiler to prevent corrosion. Although traces of these substances in the steam may also reduce corrosion of carbon steel instruments (Holmlund, 1965), their use in boilers that supply steam for sterilization should be avoided as far as possible (Department of Health and Social Security, 1980) because they may be toxic to patients if they gain access to intravenous solutions or infant feeds. Their presence in tissue culture media is also detrimental to the laboratory culture of viruses (Robbins & Jones, 1971).

Steam and air mixtures

The temperature-pressure relationships of saturated steam shown in Figure 6.1 apply only to pure steam. If air is mixed with steam, it registers as a partial pressure but does not influence the temperature of the steam. If only half of the air in a sterilizing chamber is removed and the pressure is raised to 100 kPa above atmospheric pressure, the vapour in the chamber will contain 25 per cent air and the temperature will reach only 112°C instead of 121°C, as expected for pure steam at that pressure (Perkins, 1969). The problem cannot be solved by increasing the total pressure until the desired temperature is reached because residual air interferes with penetration and condensation. It is also likely that the total pressure will exceed the design pressure of the sterilizing chamber.

PRESSURE STEAM STERILIZERS

A steam sterilizer is a metal chamber, constructed to withstand the pressure that is required to raise the temperature of steam to the level required for sterilization. Early models were termed 'autoclaves' because they were fitted with a self-closing door of a type that is still used in domestic pressure cookers. The internally fitted lid was sealed to the rim of the vertical chamber by the pressure of steam that was generated within the chamber.

Present-day sterilizers are usually horizontal chambers with a door at the front for convenience in loading. An additional door may be provided at the opposite end for unloading into a storage area for sterile supplies. Although the term 'autoclave' is not appropriate for modern steam sterilizers and is not officially recognized, its continued use as a verb (to autoclave) or adjective (autoclavable) may be justified by the convenient brevity and long-established familiarity. Detailed, highly technical descriptions of the design, construction and controls of steam sterilizers are contained in Standards that are officially recognized in the particular country. These documents are prepared for the guidance of sterilizer manufacturers but persons who are responsible for purchasing or operating the sterilizers should also be familiar with them. A brief account of general design features will suffice, in this chapter, as an introduction to the specially designed sterilizers that are used for processing porous loads, instruments and utensils, or solutions.

General design

Chamber and fittings

The chamber is usually constructed from stainless steel or from mild steel clad with a specified thickness of stainless steel. Nickel cladding is recommended for bottled liquid sterilizers because it is more resistant to corrosion. Small chambers may be cylindrical but larger models are usually rectangular to allow better utilization of the space available for loading. The floor of the chamber slopes downwards to an outlet near the front of the chamber for discharge of air and condensate. When a jacket is required, it is an outer shell that surrounds the chamber on all sides, enclosing a space that can be filled with steam under pressure. The sterilizer is insulated externally to prevent heat loss. Fittings inside the chamber include a baffle plate in front of the steam inlet to protect the load from direct contact with condensate, and ledges or rails for baskets containing the load. Pressure gauges are fitted to the jacket and chamber and a safety valve is set to release pressure if it exceeds the maximum for which the chamber is designed.

Doors

Doors are constructed from material similar to that used in the chamber and insulated to ensure that parts which may present a hazard to the operator are maintained at a safe temperature. The door closure is sealed by a replaceable gasket of heat-resistant material that is fitted to the rim of the chamber. Hinged doors may be closed manually or mechanically; alternatively, mechanically operated sliding doors may be used.

Pipework and valves

The steam supply line is fitted with a pressure-reducing valve and steam separator just before the entrance to the chamber or jacket. If air is removed

by mechanical evacuation, as in prevacuum porous load sterilizers, air and condensate are discharged separately. Air and the steam which is introduced into the chamber in the prevacuum stage are evacuated by a water ring-seal vacuum pump or by powerful steam ejectors. Separate discharge lines from the jacket and chamber discharge into a sanitary sewer; backflow of condensate in the line is prevented by a non-return valve and backflow from the sewer by a compulsory air break and tundish.

All discharge lines for condensate and those which discharge air and condensate together, as in conventional downward displacement sterilizers, slope downwards and are fitted with a balanced pressure thermostatic steam trap or other approved valve. The balanced pressure trap is illustrated in Figure 6.2. The bellows element contains a small volume of volatile liquid, which causes it to expand and close the valve when it is surrounded by saturated steam. An air-steam mixture, which has a lower temperature than that of pure steam, brings about contraction of the bellows and the valve opens to discharge it. The unit should open automatically in response to a decrease of 1°C in the temperature of the effluent.

When the sterilization cycle terminates with a vacuum in the chamber, air must be admitted through a bacterial filter until atmospheric pressure is restored before the chamber can be opened. The filter should have a retention efficiency of 99.997 per cent for particles with a diameter of 0.3 μm. A non-return valve in the air line prevents wetting of the filter material. If a prefilter is used, the high-efficiency filter should have a working life of one year (Working Party on Pressure-Steam Sterilizers, 1960). The air flow rate into the chamber

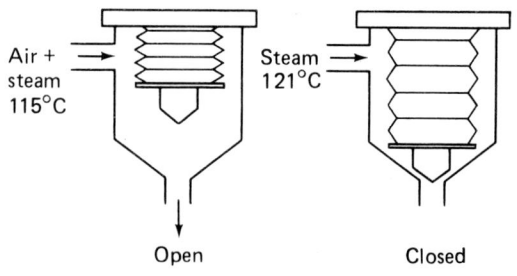

Fig. 6.2 Balanced pressure thermostatic steam trap.

should restore it to atmospheric pressure within 3 minutes.

Indicators and controls

Hospital sterilizers are designed to operate an automatic sterilization cycle, which may include the following sequence of stages:

1. Removal of air and heating of the chamber
2. Sterilization of the load
3. Removal of steam, followed by drying of textiles or cooling of liquids
4. Restoration of the chamber to atmospheric pressure.

Each stage is controlled by a timer that is activated by temperature, positive pressure or vacuum, as appropriate to the particular cycle.

The first stage is initiated by switching on the electric power and the steam supply to the unit. The second stage is controlled by a temperature-sensing device in the opening of the chamber drain, where residual air is most likely to accumulate. Independently of the control system, the temperature in the drain, together with pressure and vacuum readings, is indicated by gauges and recorded on a chart, all located on the instrument panel on the front of the sterilizer casing.

The second stage must be continued, under thermostatic control, until the whole of the load has reached the selected sterilizing temperature and is thereafter maintained at the temperature for a holding time that is sufficient to kill all the microbial contaminants. At the end of the preset sterilization time, the steam is exhausted from the chamber. The pressure is reduced slowly to atmospheric pressure for bottled liquids, more rapidly for a load of instruments and utensils, and porous loads are dried by drawing a low or high vacuum for an appropriate time while the chamber is kept hot by the steam jacket.

Indicator lights on the instrument panel show which stage in the cycle has been reached and when the cycle has been completed. If the sterilizer has a door at the opposite end for removal of the sterilized load, appropriate indicators are also required at this end. In the event of failure to achieve the specified sterilizing conditions, the cycle may be terminated prematurely or it may be completed with visual and audible signals. The door remains locked until it is released by an authorized person who can initiate investigation of the fault. Other controls for the operation of the door ensure that the cycle cannot be started until the door or doors have been locked and that they cannot be reopened until the cycle has been completed and the chamber restored to atmospheric pressure. The door of a sterilizer containing bottled liquids should not be released for opening until the temperature in the bottles has been reduced to 80°C. When the sterilizer has a door at each end, means are provided to ensure that both cannot be open at the same time. A counter that records the number of cycles performed by the sterilizer is useful for maintenance purposes.

Installation and maintenance

The intended location of the sterilizer, whether it is to be built-in or free standing, and the adequacy of steam, water and compressed air supplies should be examined and discussed with the manufacturer before placing an order for purchase. Relevant Standards should be consulted for further details.

The engineer who is responsible for preventive maintenance of the sterilizer and for carrying out minor repairs is usually a member of the hospital staff, who has received the necessary instruction. Some problems might require the advice or assistance of a specialist engineer who is employed by a regional health authority or by the sterilizer manufacturer (Department of Health and Social Security, 1980). Routine engineering tasks that are included in a planned preventive maintenance (PPM) programme are checking chart records and the performance of the operator's daily tasks, observance of an automatic cycle in operation, and inspection of working parts of the sterilizer. The latter includes inspection of the chamber (for signs of corrosion) and the condensate discharge lines (for blockage), the door gasket, door safety interlocks, steam traps, valve seals, drains, air filters, gauges and recorders. The engineer is responsible for the quality and pressure of steam supplied to the sterilizer and ensuring that the pressure settings of steam control valves and safety valves are correct. The involvement of the engineer in tests for efficiency of sterilization has been outlined in Chapter 2 and will be mentioned again in the appropriate sections of this chapter.

Methods of air removal

Steam sterilizers are divided into downward displacement or mechanically evacuated (prevacuum) types according to the method that is used for the removal of air in the first stage of the sterilization cycle.

The downward displacement system relies on gravity for the displacement of cool, relatively heavy air by the steam. When the steam enters the upper region of the chamber it moves downwards gradually, displacing the air from the free space in the chamber towards the outlet at the lowest point in the floor. Displacement of air from the load occurs more slowly and is critically dependent on methods of packing and loading that ensure minimum resistance to the movement of steam and air.

The downward displacement system is appropriate for sterilization of unwrapped instruments, utensils and liquids but has now been replaced in porous load sterilizers by mechanical evacuation, using high-vacuum pumps or steam ejectors and condensers that can reduce the partial pressure of air within the chamber to less than 133 Pa (1 mm Hg) above absolute zero (Knox & Pickerill, 1964). When steam is admitted to the evacuated chamber, it penetrates the entire load within a minute; thus the load heats at the same rate as the chamber and the heat penetration component of the sterilization time is eliminated. The complete removal of air before the load becomes hot reduces damage to cotton fabric (Henry, 1964) and rubber articles which can be sterilized at 134°C for 3 minutes. The overall advantages of prevacuum sterilizers are the certainty of steam penetration into the most difficult loads and reduction of the processing time to 30 minutes or less. The methods of air removal that are used in different types of steam sterilizers are listed in Table 6.4.

Porous load sterilizers (prevacuum type)

Applications

Mechanically evacuated sterilizers were developed for use in British hospitals after the report of a survey on sterilization practice (Nuffield Provincial Hospitals Trust, 1958) had revealed serious defects in the design and operation of old style downward displacement 'dressing' sterilizers. Special attention was given to errors in packing and loading which resulted in failure of steam penetration into packaged materials and equipment. Prevacuum sterilizers were also used in Germany but their adoption in the United States occurred later because the downward displacement type was more highly developed and the importance of factors that influence the efficiency of sterilization was more widely appreciated (Perkins, 1969).

Special design features

The earliest models were appropriately termed 'high prevacuum' sterilizers (Bowie, 1958) because the chamber was evacuated to at least 98.8 kPa below atmospheric pressure (corresponding to

Table 6.4 Types of steam sterilizers

Method of air removal	Type of load	Steam jacket	Sterilizing temperature °C	Drying or cooling
Mechanical evacuation	Wrapped articles (porous loads)	Present	134–138	Mechanical evacuation
Downward displacement	Wrapped articles (porous loads)	Present	121–126	Partial evacuation by steam ejector
Downward displacement	Unwrapped instruments and utensils	Absent	132–134	Fast steam exhaust
Downward displacement	Bottled aqueous liquids	Absent	115–121	Slow steam exhaust (unsealed containers) Rapid spray cooling (hermetically sealed containers)

2.5 kPa, or 20 mm Hg absolute pressure) by means of a water ring-seal pump to remove air from the chamber and load. However, prolonged evacuation (up to 8 minutes) was necessary and it proved difficult to prevent air from leaking into the chamber. An unexpected problem was discovered by Harris & Allison (1961) and confirmed by Henry & Scott (1963); when a test pack was placed in an otherwise empty chamber, thermocouples indicated that sterilizing temperatures were not reached or were not sustained sufficiently in certain parts of the pack, and biological indicators gave erratic results. The 'small load effect' was explained by entrainment of residual air (up to 2 per cent of the amount originally present) by the incoming steam, so that it was all carried into the solitary pack. When the chamber was filled with packs, this residual air was immobile and it was evenly distributed among the packs so that the amount in each pack was not sufficient to interfere with sterilization.

The problems caused by air leaks and small loads have both been solved by introducing a small quantity of steam into the chamber during the evacuation process. A continuous flow of steam was effective in removing all of the air from the chamber. However a further modification, involving a rapid succession of pressure-vacuum pulses, improved the efficiency of extracting air from textile packs. Both methods overcome the need to reduce the pressure in the chamber to an extremely low level. The partial pressure of air in the chamber can be reduced to less than 0.5 mm Hg absolute without the use of high vacuum (Knox & Pickerill, 1964). It has also been suggested that the risk of air leakage can be reduced further if steam pulsing is performed above atmospheric pressure (Knox & Pickerill, 1967). The basic features of a prevacuum porous load sterilizer are shown in Figure 6.3.

An air detection device is an essential component of a prevacuum sterilizer. In its simplest form, an air detector is a short metal tube, closed at one end, which communicates with the chamber and therefore competes with the load for residual air in the chamber. Thus the sample of chamber gas which collects in the air detector reflects the amount of air that would be available to accumulate in the packs (Pickerill et al, 1971). The design varies with the brand of sterilizer but the presence

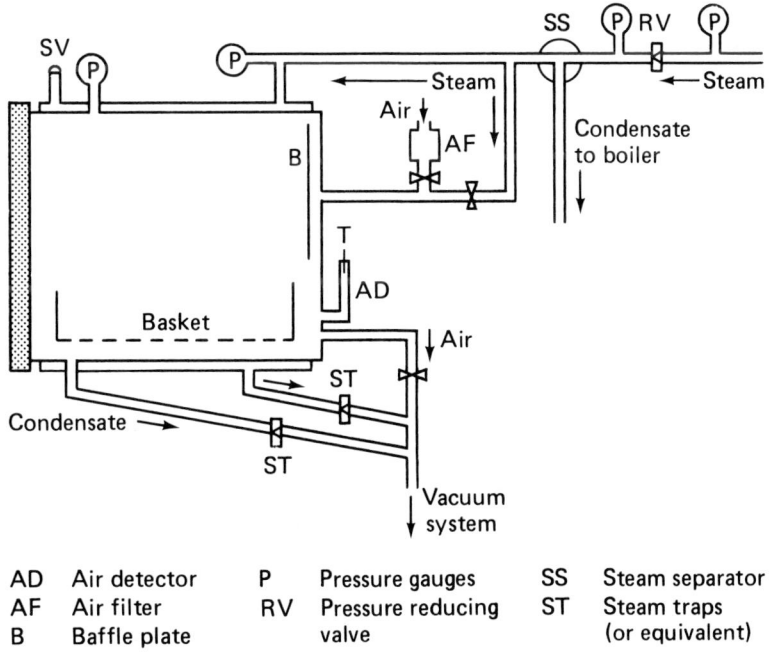

AD	Air detector	P	Pressure gauges	SS	Steam separator
AF	Air filter	RV	Pressure reducing	ST	Steam traps
B	Baffle plate		valve		(or equivalent)

Fig. 6.3 Schematic diagram of a prevacuum porous load steam sterilizer.

of air in the detector can be determined by measurement of temperature. If no air is present, the temperature of the sensing device rises to that of saturated steam at the appropriate pressure; but, if air is present, then a lower temperature will be reached at the same pressure. Some devices operate by measurement of the pressure that remains after the steam has been condensed by cooling. The temperature in the sterilizing stage of the sterilization cycle is controlled by the sensing device in the air detector, which also signals failure to achieve sterilizing conditions. The signal may be activated at the conclusion of the air removal stage or in the sterilizing stage of the cycle.

The development of the prevacuum system, which is also used in gas sterilization processes using ethylene oxide or formaldehyde, has led to the production of dual purpose sterilizers by some manufacturers. These are disapproved strongly by British regulatory authorities because their complexity results in frequent breakdowns and delays for maintenance and repair. Human error, which could result in a load of heat-sensitive equipment, such as endoscopic instruments, being subjected to the high-temperature steam sterilization process cannot be ruled out.

Packing and loading

Double layers of cloth or paper are used for primary packaging. Textile packs may be supported in cardboard boxes, previously autoclaved to kill bacterial spores. Special perforated metal caskets, incorporating bacterial filters, have been designed for use in Bowie-Dick tests, where the density of packing is specified. However, there is danger in using any type of metal container for hospital linen packs unless overpacking is prevented. Textiles and instruments may be combined in the same pack, or they may be packed separately. In the 'Edinburgh tray' system (Bowie et al, 1963) the instruments are placed in a heavy gauge, heat-retaining aluminium tray; the cloth wrapper is used to line the deep tray and is fastened by cord to the flange. The drapes and surgical dressings required for the same operation are laid on top of the instruments and the wrapping material is folded to enclose them. The tray itself remains outside the wrappings.

Although different articles or materials can be sterilized in the same load, the inclusion of metalware (e.g. bowls) frequently causes wetness of wrappings and textile packs (Rowe & Kusay, 1961; Department of Health and Social Security, 1980). The drying process may be extended to a limit imposed by a maximum sterilization cycle time of 30 minutes, but this might not be sufficient. The problem is caused by deposition of excess condensate on the cool metal surfaces. The condensate coalesces and migrates from the site where its latent heat content was liberated to a new location where this heat is not available to revaporize it. If the problem cannot be overcome by adjusting the proportion of textiles and metalware in the load, absorbent material, additional to the normal wrappings, should be placed within packs containing metal.

The method of loading packs into the sterilizer is not critical, provided that those containing metal are not placed in contact with textile packs. The size of textile packs is limited to 30 × 30 × 50 cm but they may be loaded in more than one layer. It is not necessary, although it may be advisable, to place the fabric layers vertically.

Sterilization process

The sterilization cycle includes the following sequence of stages:

1. Evacuation of air from the chamber and load, assisted by a small quantity of steam
2. Sterilization of the load for 3 minutes at a minimum temperature of 134°C, with a maximum time of 6 minutes
3. Removal of steam and drying of the load by mechanical evacuation
4. Admission of filtered air to restore atmospheric pressure.

The prevacuum stage may be managed by the continuous passage of steam through the chamber or by a rapid succession of pressure-vacuum pulses, carried out below or slightly above atmospheric pressure but not reaching the temperature or pressure of the sterilizing stage. Finally, the chamber is evacuated and steam is admitted rapidly to penetrate the entire load in less than 1 minute.

The drying stage may be adjusted to suit the load but the sterilization cycle must be completed within 30 minutes. A cycle that is representative of a steam pulsing prevacuum sterilizer is shown as a pressure-time chart in Figure 6.4, alongside the corresponding chart for a downward displacement sterilizer.

Downward displacement jacketed sterilizers

Applications

Failure to replace this type of porous load sterilizer by the more reliable prevacuum type may be justified only by lack of accessible skilled maintenance services or by the constraints of hospital finance.

Special design features

A steam jacket is essential; in addition to keeping the chamber hot between sterilization cycles, it assists drying of the wrapped articles and textile packs. A steam ejector (venturi) is also required to exhaust steam from the chamber and draw a partial vacuum in the drying stage of the cycle. This relatively inefficient vacuum system should not be used for removal of air from the chamber because the remaining air mixes slowly with the steam and repeated low-order vacua merely produce a 'breathing' motion of the same air within the packs (Working Party on Pressure-Steam Sterilizers, 1959).

The balanced pressure thermostatic steam trap in the air and condensate discharge line from the chamber may be described as the 'heart' of a downward displacement sterilizer. If it malfunctions by sticking in the closed position, or if the line is blocked by solids through negligent maintenance or by condensate because of incorrect installation, air is trapped in the chamber and the sterilizing temperature will not be reached. The bellows element must re-open during sterilization to expel air that accumulates from the load.

Packing and loading

All of the packaged articles and textiles must be positioned in the sterilizer so that air can flow out in a downward direction. Textiles should be packed loosely within cloth and paper wrappings; the layers should be parallel within the pack, and vertically oriented in the sterilizer. The large differ-

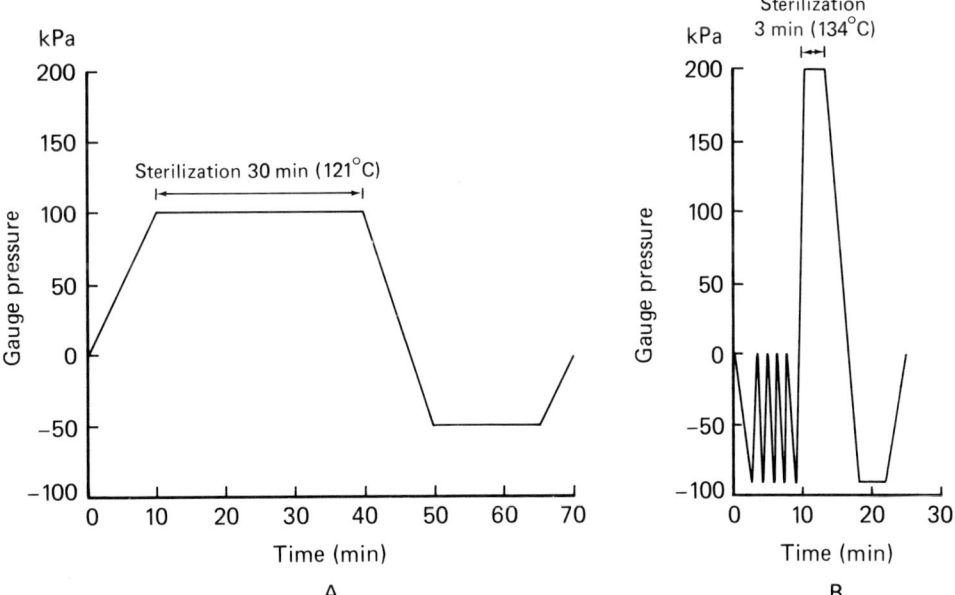

Fig. 6.4 Sterilization cycles in (A) an old-fashioned downward displacement jacketed sterilizer and (B) a modern prevacuum porous load sterilizer.

ence between the heat penetration times for similar packs which have been placed vertically and horizontally in a downward displacement sterilizer is shown in Figure 6.5.

Bowls and other empty containers should be placed on edge, or inverted; lids, if present, should be loosened. If metalware is sterilized in the same load as textiles, it must be placed so that condensate does not drain on to packs underneath. Instruments should be opened and set out on a perforated tray. If rubber sheeting is sterilized the folded layers must be separated by inserts of permeable material. Glass syringes must be disassembled, and the barrel and plunger placed in the same bag. Tubing should be wetted internally and drained, and should not be tightly coiled. Additional details, with illustrations, are provided by Perkins (1969).

Sterilization process

The sterilization cycle consists of the following stages:

1. Displacement of air by incoming steam while the chamber is heated to the selected sterilizing temperature
2. Sterilization of the textile packs for the recommended minimum sterilization time of 15 mi-

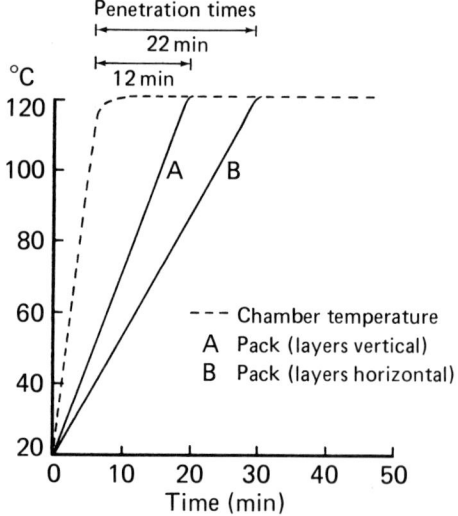

Fig. 6.5 Heat penetration times for identical textile packs in a downward displacement steam sterilizer with parallel layers of fabric positioned (A) vertically and (B) horizontally.

nutes heat penetration time and 15 minutes holding time at 121°C
3. Drying of the load to its original condition by a partial vacuum, assisted by heat from the jacket
4. Restoration of the chamber to atmospheric pressure by admission of filtered air.

A pressure recording from a sterilization cycle in a downward displacement porous load sterilizer, together with one from a prevacuum sterilizer, is shown in Figure 6.4. The presence of residual air while the load is being heated causes cumulative damage to cotton textiles. Rubber is also damaged by prolonged exposure to the conditions that are used in the sterilization of large textile packs. Mixed loads should therefore be avoided to prevent damage to the smaller or more heat-sensitive articles. The use of a sterilizing temperature above 121°C in a downward displacement porous load sterilizer is not recommended because prolongation of the heat penetration time is likely to counterbalance the shorter holding time at the higher temperature and harmful effects may be increased (Perkins, 1969). The drying stage may be the slowest part of the sterilization cycle. Packs that have absorbed surplus condensate from a wet steam supply or by drainage from bowls cannot be dried to the condition that existed before sterilization.

Instrument and utensil sterilizers

This type of downward displacement sterilizer is designed to sterilize only unwrapped articles that may be used immediately or articles that require decontamination after use. Provision may be made for drying the surface of solid articles but porous material cannot be dried by this system.

Special design features

The non-jacketed chamber is relatively small and usually cylindrical. Air is removed by downward displacement. Piped steam may be connected or steam may be produced within the chamber from distilled or demineralized water that is boiled by an immersion heater or by elements fixed to the outside of the chamber. These bench models are described as portable, electrically heated steam sterilizers. The heaters are programmed to switch off if the water boils dry. The air outlet cannot be placed at the bottom of the chamber but the opening of the discharge line should be as close to the water level as possible. The discharge line should be fitted with a balanced pressure steam trap, or other approved valve, and a safety valve. If the sterilizer is designed for surface drying, an independent external heating element is provided. A tank mounted above the sterilizing chamber serves as a water reservoir and also as a condenser when steam is exhausted from the chamber. Figure 6.6 is a diagram of a manually operated, portable, electrically heated sterilizer that is suitable for use in microbiological laboratories.

Loading

The load-carrying basket or perforated tray should not be overloaded and each article should be positioned so that air can flow out by gravity; bowls should be placed on edge and hinged instruments opened.

Sterilization process

The following stages in the sterilization cycle may be carried out under manual or automatic control:

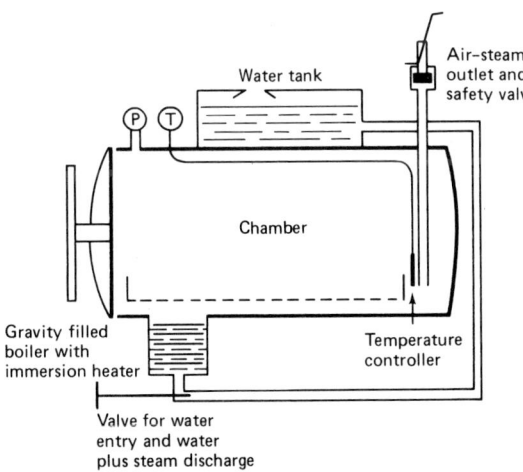

Fig. 6.6 A portable, electrically heated sterilizer, of a manually operated type, for unwrapped instruments and utensils.

1. Removal of air and heating of the chamber to the sterilizing temperature
2. Sterilization for 4 minutes at 132°C or 3 minutes at 134°C
3. Restoration of the chamber to atmospheric pressure by rapid exhaustion of steam.

The chamber should be vented and opened immediately after atmospheric pressure has been reached. Delay increases the wetness of the load and a vacuum in the chamber causes an inrush of unsterile air. The cycle should be completed in 10 minutes unless the sterilizer is initially cold. The sterilizing stage must be temperature-controlled and accurately timed. The rapid removal of air from the chamber permits rubber tubing (e.g. corrugated breathing tubes from an anaesthetic circuit) to be processed in an instrument sterilizer. Ultra-rapid 'flash' sterilizers, in which the chamber is brought to 150°C, after a come-up time of not less than 60 seconds, and immediately exhausted have been described and reported to be satisfactory (Lane et al, 1964; Phillips & Taylor, 1965).

Bottled fluid sterilizers

The term 'liquid' is more appropriate than 'fluid' because fluid includes gases. The types of aqueous liquids that are sterilized by steam under pressure include water, irrigating solutions, injections, intravenous solutions, dilute disinfectants (e.g. chlorhexidine) and microbiological culture media. Most of the pharmaceuticals are sterilized commercially but sterile water and simple solutions for surgical use may be produced in hospital pharmacies or sterilizing departments.

Special design features

The non-jacketed chamber may be constructed from stainless steel or from mild steel clad with nickel, which is more resistant to corrosion by salt solutions. Sterilizers for use in microbiological laboratories or other places where liquids are sterilized in unsealed containers (closed with cotton wool plugs or screw caps) must be programmed for slow exhaustion of steam from the chamber. A rapid spray-cooling system is required when large scale production of sterile water or solutions in hermetically sealed containers is carried out in hospital pharmacies or commercial operations. Although the load can be cooled by means of a cold water spray with a mean droplet size of 80 μm (Wilkinson et al, 1960), cooling with heated condensate, which has been collected in a separate steam-heated tank during sterilization, is more successful. The temperature of the spray is initially close to that of the bottles and is gradually reduced. Compressed air may be admitted to the chamber during cooling to guard against breakage of bottles or bursting of plastic bags. The use of heated condensate for cooling and the filtration of air that is admitted to the chamber after sterilization reduce the possibility of microbial contaminants entering bottles through faulty closures. The sterilization cycle for bottled liquids may be controlled by a temperature sensor in a load simulator, such as a bottle of water or a metal block with similar heating characteristics. The simulator must be cooled or replaced between cycles.

Packing and loading

Glass bottles, plastic containers, flexible plastic pouches, flasks or test tubes containing water or solutions must be supported in a container from which air can be removed by downward displacement. Wire baskets should be coated with heat-resistant plastic to prevent staining when the liquid is in flexible pouches (Weymes, 1971). The use of a double wrapping for plastic pouches necessitates the introduction of a small volume of water between the two layers to provide steam for sterilization of the adjacent surfaces which are not accessible to steam in the chamber. A problem that is associated with the need to use leak-proof containers for discarded cultures of microorganisms will be discussed later.

Sterilization process

There are three stages in a sterilization cycle for bottled liquids:

1. Removal of air and heating of the chamber to the selected sterilizing temperature
2. Sterilization of the liquid

3. Cooling the liquid.

It is not necessary for steam to enter the bottles because steam is produced from the contained liquid when it reaches the sterilizing temperature. Heat is transmitted from steam in the chamber to the liquid in the bottles by the release of latent heat on the outer surface and conduction through the wall of the container. Convection assists the uniformity of temperature within the container as heated liquid rises and cooler liquid flows down to replace it. As most of the steam entering a chamber that is filled with a large load of bottles condenses on the surfaces until they have reached 100°C, air displacement does not commence until the later part of the first stage. The mechanisms of heating are illustrated in Figure 6.7.

Sterilization of water and heat-stable solutions is carried out at 121°C; the recommended holding time is 15 minutes but 12 minutes might be adequate for unsealed containers which are cooled slowly. A temperature of 115°C and holding time of 30 minutes may be adequate for solutions containing heat-sensitive ingredients (Department of Health and Social Security, 1980) but the liquid must be dispensed in small volumes because this temperature-time combination is not equivalent in lethality to 12 minutes at 121°C.

The sterilization time for liquids varies widely because the heat penetration time is influenced by the following factors:

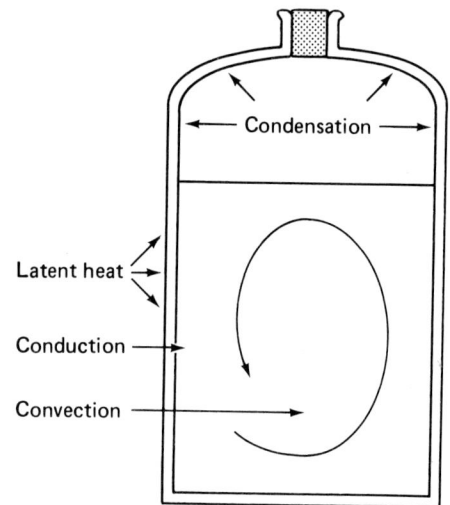

Fig. 6.7 Mechanisms of heat transfer in a bottle of aqueous liquid in a steam sterilizer.

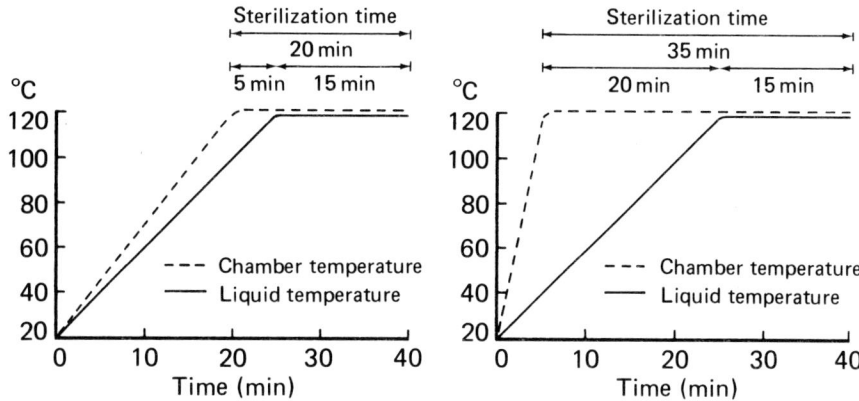

Fig. 6.8 Effect of rate of heating of the sterilizing chamber on the heat penetration time and the sterilization time of bottled liquids.

1. *Rate of heating of the chamber.* There is little variation in the time required to heat a given volume of liquid from ambient temperature to 121°C. However, the rate at which steam is admitted to the chamber affects the heat penetration time because this depends on the difference in temperature between the steam and the liquid at the moment when the sterilizing temperature is reached in the chamber. The penetration time, and therefore the sterilization time, is extended when the chamber is heated quickly, as shown in Figure 6.8.

2. *Type of container.* As glass is a poor conductor of heat, a liquid in a thick-walled bottle has a longer heat penetration time than does the same volume in thin-walled laboratory glassware.

3. *Viscosity of the liquid.* Agar-containing culture media which have been allowed to solidify before sterilization take 5–10 minutes longer to reach the sterilizing temperature than do media that do not contain agar or are above the setting temperature of 42°C when they are sterilized. Canned foods, which may also be regarded as aqueous liquids, may be viscous or contain suspended particles that delay heat penetration.

4. *Volume of liquid.* The influence of the size of the container and volume of liquid may be seen by examination of the temperature charts in Figure 6.9.

5. *Trapped air.* The headspace air in vessels containing aqueous liquid does not interfere with sterilization because the upper surfaces are flushed

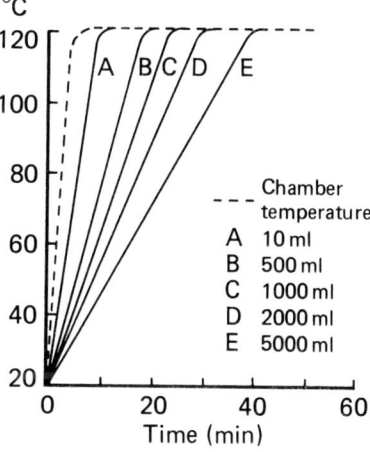

Fig. 6.9 Influence of volume on the heat penetration time of aqueous liquids in a batch sterilization process.

liberally with condensate. However, the large amount of air that is trapped in bins or plastic bags which are used for the collection, transportation and sterilization of clinical specimens and discarded cultures of microorganisms causes long delays in heat penetration. The difference in penetration times when a single 100 ml bottle is placed in an impervious container or a wire basket in the chamber is shown in Figure 6.10.

Perforated containers cannot be used for discarded cultures and the penetration time is inevitably long, a fact that is not always realized by those who are responsible for sterilizing them. The depth of bins should not be greater than 20–25 cm

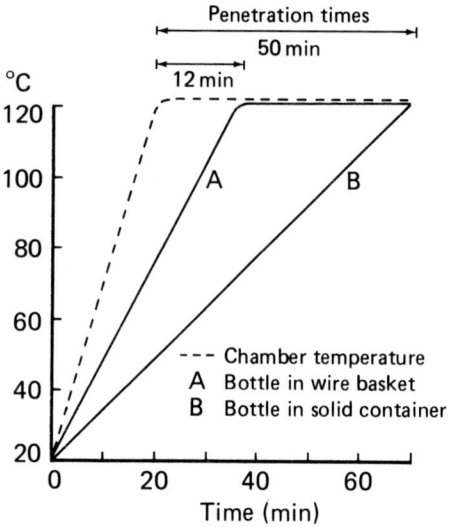

Fig. 6.10 Effect of air trapped in a deep metal container on the heat penetration time of a bottle of aqueous liquid.

to 17 minutes in a large one (Wilkinson et al, 1960). Rapid cooling also prevents the caramelization of sugars in intravenous solutions.

Slow cooling is mandatory when the liquid is in unsealed containers because the liquid becomes superheated and boils violently if the pressure is reduced rapidly. However, the rate should be controlled so that the decrease in pressure keeps pace with the temperature. The chamber should be vented when it has been restored to atmospheric pressure to avoid the entrance of contaminated air into containers with unfiltered closures, such as screw caps, when a terminal vacuum is released.

Whichever method of cooling is used, the door of the chamber should not be opened to remove the load until the temperature has fallen to a safe level to prevent breakage; 80°C is recommended for glass bottles (Department of Health and Social Security, 1980).

and bags should not be more than half full. The contents of a metal bin heat more rapidly than those in a polypropylene bin (Lauer et al, 1982). The addition of water to the container does not result in a dramatic improvement. A method of injecting steam into the containers through tubes with inverted funnel-shaped openings has been described (Everall et al, 1978) but may be difficult to implement on a large scale. Some penetration times which have been measured by thermocouple recordings in metal or plastic bins and in plastic bags are listed in Table 6.5.

The cooling stage of the sterilization cycle for liquids is important for reasons that include shortening the cycle, minimizing deterioration of heat-labile ingredients and avoiding the danger of breakage or spillage. In spray-cooling sterilizers, the cooling time may be reduced from 3 hours to 10 minutes in a small sterilizer and from 22 hours

TESTS FOR EFFICIENCY OF STEAM STERILIZERS

The principles and methods of testing the mechanical performance of sterilizers and the achievement of sterilizing conditions in the chamber and throughout the load have been explained in Chapter 2. The appropriate tests that are required to qualify each type of steam sterilizer for its intended purpose and to monitor its continued efficiency in routine operation will be listed here, with some discussion of important details that govern the validity of particular tests. All of the tests should be carried out according to the specifications of the Department of Health and Social Security (1980).

The mechanical performance test will be described first because it is similar for all types of steam sterilizers. A sterilization cycle is performed under automatic control and the times for separate

Table 6.5 Heat penetration times in containers for discarded cultures[1]

Type of container	Contents	Penetration time (min)
Metal bin	Bijoux bottles (full load)	45–50
Polypropylene bin	Bijoux bottles (full load)	60
Plastic bag	Plastic petri dishes	
	Half-filled	30
	Filled	55–60

[1]Data provided by Gorry J P, Department of Microbiology, University of Melbourne.

stages and the complete cycle are checked. During the cycle, readings of temperature, pressure and vacuum gauges are noted at all stages, including at least three sets of readings at intervals during the sterilizing stage. Record charts should be examined carefully at the end of the cycle, labelled and kept until all tests have been completed, when one from a cycle that passed all tests is preserved as a master temperature record (MTR) to serve as a standard of comparison for future qualifying tests on the same sterilizer.

Tests for prevacuum porous load sterilizers

Performance test

The performance test should be carried out weekly by the operator or engineer. A temperature of 134^{+4}_{-0} °C must be maintained in the chamber for at least 3 minutes and not more than 6 minutes in Stage 2. The cycle should be completed within 30 minutes. If a test pack is included, the towels should be close to the normal air-dry condition.

Leak rate test

The sterilizer controls are switched to an automatic leak test position or to manual operation if it has not been provided. A preliminary warming up cycle is required if the test is carried out in the air removal stage but this may be avoided by deferring it to the drying stage. A vacuum is drawn to 80–90 kPa below atmospheric pressure and then the valves are closed and the vacuum system disconnected. After the reading on the absolute pressure gauge has stabilized, it is observed for 10 minutes. The pressure should not increase by more than 133 Pa (1.3 mbar or 1 mm Hg) per minute.

Thermocouple test

This is a time-at-temperature test. Two thermocouples are placed in a standard Bowie-Dick test pack (see below) and one in the chamber drain. The test should be carried out with the pack alone in the chamber and, if the result is successful, repeated with a full load of similar packs. The temperature recorded in the pack should be identical with that in the chamber drain for the last 2 minutes of the

prescribed 3 minute holding time. The thermocouple test should be repeated at three-monthly intervals.

Bowie-Dick autoclave tape test

The test was designed for convenience in daily performance because complex equipment is required for the thermocouple test. However, the tape test does not measure time-at-temperature and therefore it does not confirm that sterilizing conditions have been achieved in the test pack. It is a test for air removal and uniformity of steam penetration.

The test pack, described in detail in Health Technical Memorandum No. 10 (Department of Health and Social Security, 1980) is prepared from cotton towels of a specified quality, which are folded and stacked to correspond to a density of 160 kg/m³ of chamber space and to dimensions of 300 × 225 mm cross section and 279 mm height. It may be wrapped in fabric or paper or placed in a perforated metal casket designed for the purpose (British Standards Institution, 1960). The towels should be washed before the first use and then once a week; they must be unfolded and aired for at least 1 hour between tests.

The indicator is a paper sheet of the same area as the pack on which a St Andrew's cross has been prepared with specified brands of autoclave tape (DRG 2538 or 3M 1222). It is placed at the centre of the stacked towels. To perform the test, the pack is placed with its layers horizontal, alone in the chamber and 100 mm from the base and the door. A preliminary warming up cycle is required to ensure that a satisfactory cycle is not failed. The sterilization cycle must be modified for the test so that the temperature of the pack is not held at 134°C for more than 3.5 minutes.

When the cycle is completed, the pack is opened and the autoclave tape cross is examined carefully to detect non-uniformity of the colour change. Any paler area indicates retention of air and that the sterilizer has failed the test.

The Bowie-Dick test must be performed at the start of each working day. It is the principal routine test, in conjunction with the weekly leak test, for efficiency of prevacuum sterilizers. The result is invalid if the specified towels are not used or the sterilizing stage is not limited to 3.5 minutes. Batch variations in the indicator tape have been shown not to affect the result of the test (Bowie & Dick, 1969; Bowie, 1974) and the test is still valid in steam-pulsing sterilizers because the colour of the tape is not significantly changed by the temperature reached or the time for which it is maintained (Department of Health and Social Security, 1980).

Air detector tests

The function of the air detector is to pass or fail the sterilization cycle according to the amount of air in the chamber. An air detector function test must be carried out if the Bowie-Dick test has failed or the leak test is unsatisfactory and a cause has not been detected. It is necessary to induce air leaks into the chamber to demonstrate that the detector passes the cycle if the leak rate is 3 mm Hg/minute or less but will fail it at a leak rate of 6 mm Hg/minute.

If the air detector function test is unsatisfactory, an air detector performance test must be carried out. A Bowie-Dick test pack containing a thermocouple is placed in the chamber and a predetermined quantity of air is admitted to cause the temperature in the pack to fall 2°C below that in the chamber drain for the last 3 minutes of the 6 minute sterilizing stage of the cycle. The air detector should then fail the cycle.

Biological and chemical indicators

Biological indicator tests with *Bacillus stearothermophilus* spore papers, and chemical indicators which are known to respond accurately to specified conditions of temperature and time may be included in a qualifying test programme but their routine use is unnecessary and is not recommended.

Downward displacement jacketed sterilizers

As this type is no longer officially recognized as a porous load sterilizer, tests for efficiency of sterilization are not standardized. The Bowie-Dick tape test is not applicable because the colour change is likely to occur during the prolonged heating time although air is still present in the pack.

Performance test

This is carried out in the usual way with close attention to correspondence of temperature and pressure, clearance of the discharge line and correct functioning of the balanced pressure steam trap.

Thermocouple test

Thermocouple tests are essential to determine the heat penetration time and the temperature reached in the chamber and load. The test pack should be similar in size and weight to the largest and densest packs for which the sterilizer will be used. It should be placed near the air outlet, with fabric layers vertical, and accompanied by a full load; the small load effect does not occur in downward displacement sterilizers. When thermocouples are placed in packs, care must be taken to ensure that steam cannot enter along the path of the leads. A reference thermocouple is also placed in the chamber drain.

Biological and chemical indicators

A reliable chemical indicator may be placed in selected packs from time to time to provide warning of sterilization failure caused by a change in materials or packing methods. Routine use of biological indicators is unnecessary if temperature measurements are carried out; they should not be used frequently.

Instrument and utensil sterilizers

The usual sterilizer performance test is carried out, with particular attention to accuracy of timing in the sterilizing stage. A thermocouple test should be performed with two leads in the chamber, one close to the air outlet and one fixed to the surface of an article in the full load. Regular observation of the temperature and pressure gauges is sufficient for routine testing. Biological and chemical indicators are not required in these sterilizers.

Bottled fluid sterilizers

Performance test

The need for special attention to the correct operation of the balanced pressure steam trap was high-lighted in 1972 when failure to investigate a discrepancy between the temperature and pressure readings was responsible for the death of several patients who received intravenous infusions that were contaminated with Gram-negative bacteria (Clothier, 1972). The control mechanism that prevents opening of the door of the sterilizer until the liquid has cooled to a safe temperature must also be checked.

Thermocouple test

Thermocouple tests are essential for the determination of the sterilization parameters for a particular liquid, in particular containers, to be sterilized in a particular sterilizer. Penetration times determined in one set of circumstances do not apply in another situation.

As a result of the deaths from contaminated intravenous solutions, a rigorous thermocouple test was introduced. Eleven leads are required for commissioning a new sterilizer and for annual tests. Eight are placed in test bottles at the corners of a multilayered load and the nineth is placed in a bottle at the centre of the bottom row. The others are placed in the chamber drain and another at some other site in the chamber. The test bottles should be filled to a maximum of 80 per cent of capacity and all should be at the same temperature at the start of the test. A modified test, requiring only three thermocouples is required at 3 monthly intervals. The breakage rate of glass bottles should not exceed 1 per cent of the load.

REFERENCES

Bowie J H 1958 Requirements for an automatically controlled, high pre-vacuum steriliser. Health Bulletin (Edinburgh) 16: 36–40

Bowie J H 1974 Bowie and Dick test. Lancet i: 1233

Bowie J H, Dick J 1969 Autoclave tape test. British Hospital Journal and Social Service Review 79: 868

Bowie J H, Campbell I D, Gillingham F J, Gordon A R 1963 Hospital sterile supplies: Edinburgh pre-set tray system. British Medical Journal 2: 1322–1327

British Standards Institution 1960 Specification for Rectangular Metal Boxes for Use in High Vacuum Steam Sterilizers. British Standard 381: 1960

Clothier C M (Chairman) 1972 Report of the Committee appointed to inquire into the circumstances, including the production, which led to the use of contaminated infusion fluids in the Devonport Section of Plymouth General Hospital. HMSO, London

Department of Health and Social Security 1980 Sterilizers Health Technical Memorandum 10. HMSO, London

Everall P H, Morris C A, Yarnell R 1978 Sterilisation in the laboratory autoclave using direct air displacement by steam. Journal of Clinical Pathology 31: 144–147

Harris H F, Allison V D 1961 Steam sterilisation. Lancet ii: 603–604

Henry P S H 1959 Physical aspects of sterilizing cotton articles by steam. Journal of Applied Bacteriology 22: 159–173

Henry P S H 1964 The effect on cotton of steam sterilization with pre-vacuum. Journal of Applied Bacteriology 27: 413–421

Henry P S H, Scott E 1963 Residual air in the steam sterilization of textiles with pre-vacuum. Journal of Applied Bacteriology 26: 234–245

Holmlund L G 1965 Steam corrosion and steam corrosion inhibition in autoclave sterilization of dental and surgical steel materials. Biotechnology and Bioengineering 7: 177–198

Knox R, Pickerill J K 1964 Efficient air removal from steam sterilisers without the use of high vacuum. Lancet i: 1318–1321

Knox R, Pickerill J K 1967 Steam sterilisation: a pre-sterilising stage combining a flush-aided pre-vacuum with bursts of steam above atmospheric pressure. British Hospital Journal and Social Service Review 77: 2377, 2379–2380, 2382

Lane C R, Cook G T, Kelsey J C, Beeby M M 1964 High-temperature sterilisation for surgical instruments. Lancet i: 358–360

Lauer J L, Battles D R, Vesley D 1982 Decontaminating infectious laboratory waste by autoclaving. Applied and Environmental Microbiology 44: 690–694

Nuffield Provincial Hospitals Trust 1958 Studies of sterile supply arrangements for hospitals. Present sterilizing practice in six hospitals. The Nuffield Provincial Hospitals Trust, London

Perkins J J 1969 Principles and methods of sterilization in health sciences, 2nd edn. Charles C. Thomas, Springfield, ch 7, p 154; ch 9, p 193

Phillips I, Taylor T A 1965 Sterilisation of surgical instruments in a 'flash' autoclave. Lancet ii: 840–842

Pickerill J K, Perera R, Knox R 1971 Air detection in dressings steam sterilizers. Laboratory Practice 20: 406–413

Robbins J H, Jones G A 1971 Autoclave which sterilises with highly purified steam for tissue-culture laboratories. Lancet ii: 1236–1237

Rowe T W G, Kusay R 1961 Steam sterilisation. Lancet ii: 604–605

Weymes C 1971 Sterilization of water for topical use in plastic bags. British Hospital Journal and Social Service Review 81: 1553, 1555, 1557

Wilkinson G R, Peacock F G, Robins E L 1960 A shorter sterilising cycle for solutions heated in an autoclave. Journal of Pharmacy and Pharmacology Supplement 12: 197T–202T

Working Party on Pressure-Steam Sterilisers 1959 Sterilisation by steam under increased pressure. A report to the Medical Research Council. Lancet i: 425–435

Working Party on Pressure-Steam Sterilisers 1960 Sterilisation by steam under increased pressure. A report to the Medical Research Council. Lancet ii: 1243–1244

FURTHER READING

Alder V G, Simpson R A 1982 Sterilisation by heat methods. In: Russell A D, Hugo W B, Ayliffe G A J (eds) Principles and practice of disinfection, preservation and sterilisation. Blackwell, Oxford, ch 13, p 433

Joslyn L J 1983 Sterilization by heat. In: Block S S (ed) Disinfection, sterilization, and preservation, 3rd edn. Lea & Febiger, Philadelphia, ch 1, p 3

7

Sterilization by gaseous chemicals

The past three decades have seen the development and production of an increasing amount and variety of medical equipment which cannot withstand sterilization at high temperatures. The equipment may be separated into two categories:

1. Relatively simple devices that are produced and sterilized commercially; they are usually intended to be used once only and then discarded
2. Complex surgical or diagnostic equipment which is reusable and is sterilized on the hospital premises if a suitable process is available.

Commercial producers of sterile devices may choose between ethylene oxide at a temperature within the range 30–55°C and ionizing radiation at ambient temperature by gamma rays or electron beam. The decision is based on the nature of the equipment to be sterilized, the availability of an irradiation facility and the relative costs of installing and operating the two processes. Radiation sterilization is not available in hospitals but there is a choice between two processes in which a chemical vapour is used at a relatively low temperature. Ethylene oxide is used in the temperature range 45–60°C, whereas the alternative low-temperature steam and formaldehyde process is operated at 70–75°C. Some diagnostic instruments and electronic devices might not withstand the higher temperature of the formaldehyde process. The choice of sterilizing agent must be made before ordering a gas sterilizer because the same machine cannot be used for both processes.

Gas sterilization should not be used for equipment or materials that withstand steam or dry heat sterilization. The low-temperature processes are slower, more expensive to operate, and may leave toxic residues which necessitate aeration of the sterilized products before they can be released for use. The steam and formaldehyde process, which was developed in the United Kingdom as an alternative to ethylene oxide, is quite distinct from older methods in which formaldehyde vapour is used as a disinfectant in rooms and cabinets where control of concentration, temperature and humidity is usually lacking.

The following explanation of mechanisms of biocidal action applies to ethylene oxide and formaldehyde; thereafter, the processes will be described separately.

BIOCIDAL ACTION OF ALKYLATING AGENTS

Ethylene oxide (C_2H_4O) and formaldehyde (H.CHO) are alkylating agents. Alkylation involves the addition of certain saturated hydrocarbon groups to reactive amino (NH_2), sulphydryl (SH), hydroxyl (OH) or carboxyl (COOH) groups on protein molecules and to imino (NH) groups which are part of the ring structure of nucleic acid bases.

Typical alkylation reactions with reactive groups on proteins or nucleic acids are:

$$— NH_2 \ + \ C_2H_4O \ \rightarrow \ — NH(C_2H_4OH)$$

$$— SH \ + \ H.CHO \ \rightarrow \ — S(H.CHOH)$$

$$> NH \ + \ C_2H_4O \ \rightarrow \ > N(C_2H_4OH)$$

The biocidal activity of ethylene oxide parallels its alkylating power and depends on an unstable three-membered ring structure, as shown in Table 7.1. Cyclopropane, with a non-reactive ring structure, has neither alkylating power nor biocidal activity. At the other extreme, ethylene imine is so reactive that it is unsuitable for sterilization. The substitution of a hydrogen atom in ethylene oxide by a carbon-containing side chain, as in propylene oxide, reduces activity.

Alkylation of nucleic acids by ethylene oxide has been proposed as the principal mechanism of biocidal action (Gunther, 1980) because these vit-

Table 7.1 Biocidal activity of alkylating agents

Agent	Formula	Biocidal activity
Ethylene imine	$H_2C \longrightarrow CH_2$ with NH	Very high
Ethylene oxide	$H_2C \longrightarrow CH_2$ with O	High
Propylene oxide	$H_2C \longrightarrow CH.CH_3$ with O	Moderate
Cyclopropane	$H_2C \longrightarrow CH_2$ with CH_2	None

al cell components control protein synthesis. The ring nitrogen atoms of purine and pyrimidine bases are critical sites (Bruch, 1973). The direct alkylation of reactive groups in proteins and their amino acid or peptide components is considered less important. Formaldehyde has been found to react with DNA during the replication process, when the double-stranded helix is unwinding (Vologodskii & Frank-Kamenetskii, 1975; Shikama & Miura, 1976).

Chemical alkylating agents resemble ionizing radiation in their potentiality for toxicity, mutagenicity and carcinogenicity. They also share with ionizing radiation a broad spectrum of biocidal action, with a less than tenfold difference between the resistance of bacterial spores and the vegetative cells. This contrasts with a very large difference, up to 5 factors of 10, in the heat resistance of bacteria and their spores.

ETHYLENE OXIDE

PROPERTIES OF ETHYLENE OXIDE

Physical and chemical properties

Ethylene oxide, which boils at 10.7°C at ambient temperature and pressure, is liquefied at a relatively low pressure in storage cylinders. The pure gas is 1.5 times as heavy as air and usually diffuses downwards if it escapes into the atmosphere. However, upward movement has been demonstrated when small amounts are released, together with warm air, from a sterilizing chamber (Samuels & Corn, 1979). Ethylene oxide is highly diffusible, moving through air pockets and dissolving in rubbers, plastics, silicones and oils. The vapour is freely soluble in water, with which it reacts to form ethylene glycol. Reaction with sodium chloride in solutions or materials that have absorbed ethylene oxide yields non-volatile ethylene chlorohydrin (2-chloro-ethanol).

Flammability

Ethylene oxide is flammable and highly explosive at all concentrations above 3.6 per cent by volume in air; the explosive force is 50 times as great as would be expected for a purely oxidative reaction. The pure gas may be used below atmospheric pressure in sterilization chambers from which air has been removed by evacuation. Mixtures containing 12 per cent by weight of ethylene oxide and 88 per cent fluorocarbon–12 (CCl_2F_2) or 10 per cent in carbon dioxide are nonflammable. The 12%/88% (m/m) mixture with fluorocarbon produces a much lower pressure in the storage cylinders and sterilizing chambers than does the carbon dioxide mixture. The latter also has the disadvantage of varying in composition as the cylinder empties (Ernst & Doyle, 1968). Ethylene oxide is the sole sterilizing agent in the nonflammable gas mixtures; the diluent gases have no biocidal activity. The mixture with fluorocarbon–12 is more expensive than pure ethylene oxide and the carbon dioxide mixture but is generally used in hospital ethylene oxide sterilizers. However, the economic factor must be considered in industrial sterilization processes.

Polymerization

Ethylene oxide tends to polymerize in storage cylinders, pipelines and sterilizing chambers. Rust, rough metal edges, constrictions in pipes and valves, and the polymer itself act as catalysts. Stainless steel should be used in the construction of sterilizing chambers and storage cylinders. The rate of polymerization is accelerated by a rise in temperature. The products may be solid, semi-solid or liquid and the colour may be white, yellow, green or brown. A white powder is formed in the sterilizing chamber at sites where water accumulates but a yellow liquid, which turns to gum, is formed in pipelines where the temperature

and pressure are highest (Ernst & Doyle, 1968). Accumulation can be prevented by the use of high quality gases and regular steam cleaning of empty storage cylinders. The cylinders should be protected from direct sunlight and from high storage temperatures. However, if the recommended precautions are taken, the sterilizing gases can be transported over long distances without deterioration.

Absorption by natural and synthetic materials

Natural rubber absorbs up to 35 000 p.p.m. and synthetic rubbers up to 20 000 p.p.m. ethylene oxide. Polyvinyl chloride (PVC) absorbs more than any other material because ethylene oxide reacts with the phthalic acid plasticizer. Polyethylene and polypropylene absorb smaller but significant amounts. Paper wrapping material absorbs up to 10 000 p.p.m. and cotton absorbs less than 5000 p.p.m. These figures have been taken from published reports (e.g. Bruch, 1973; McGunnigle et al, 1975). They are subject to wide variation because the amount of ethylene oxide absorbed varies with the concentration and time of exposure and may be affected by the diluent gas. Accurate estimation is difficult because the amounts of ethylene oxide are small and must be extracted quantitatively from the solid material before analysis by gas chromatography (Mogenhan et al, 1971; Spitz & Weinberger, 1971; Warren, 1971; McGunnigle et al, 1975).

Desorption

The rate at which ethylene oxide desorbs from various materials has been studied extensively to determine when sterilized articles are safe to use. The times required for natural desorption from packaged articles on open shelves at ambient temperature range from a few hours for those which contain only a small component of absorbing material to about 2 days for articles made from polyethylene and polypropylene and to 1–2 weeks for PVC and some types of rubber. Some silicones are reported to desorb rapidly (White & Bradley, 1973; McGunnigle et al, 1975). As desorption is an exponential process, most of the ethylene oxide is lost quickly but the final stages are very slow.

Aeration of sterilized products in ambient conditions is satisfactory in commercial production because sufficient time elapses between sterilization and use. Special aeration cabinets are required in hospitals, where the types of articles that are sterilized by ethylene oxide are often required for use on the following day. The gas is driven out of the material at 50–60°C and flowing air removes it from the cabinet. Aeration times range from 2–24 hours (Gunther, 1974; McGunnigle et al, 1975).

Toxicity

Inhalation

Inhalation of large or small amounts of ethylene oxide presents an occupational hazard to operators of the sterilization process and sometimes to persons who work in adjoining areas. Acute toxicity, which is manifested by irritation of eyes and respiratory tract, headache, nausea, dizziness and vomiting, is equivalent to that caused by ammonia. Moreover, ethylene oxide concentrations below 700 p.p.m. in air cannot be detected by smell, whereas levels down to 1 p.p.m. may be toxic.

The association of long-term occupational exposure to ethylene oxide with the carcinogenic, mutagenic and possibly reproductive effects which characterize alkylating agents is now recognized. However, statistical evidence has accumulated slowly and its significance is not always established. Increases in leukaemia (Hogstedt et al, 1979) and spontaneous abortions (Hemminki et al, 1982) in persons who have been occupationally exposed to ethylene oxide have been attributed to the vapour but the possibility of other causes has not always been ruled out. However, observation of an increased rate of sister chromatid exchange in the peripheral lymphocytes of persons who were exposed to ethylene oxide for as little as 3.6 minutes per day regularly over a period of months has provided evidence of DNA damage and may serve as a sensitive method of early detection (Yager et al, 1983). Threshold exposure levels, in terms of a time-weighted average, have not been firmly established but any detectable level of ethylene oxide is considered hazardous if it extends throughout working hours. Higher concentrations may be tolerated for short periods.

Contact

Harmful effects may result from contact of skin and tissues with materials containing absorbed ethylene oxide. Liquid ethylene oxide evaporates too quickly to burn or blister the skin, but contact with clothing, shoes, rubber gloves, anaesthetic face masks, endotracheal tubes and wound dressings which have not been adequately aerated after sterilization may cause dermatitis in hospital patients or staff. In a single episode, 19 patients were seriously burned by surgical drapes and gowns containing 3600–10 800 p.p.m. of residual ethylene oxide; healing took 3–6 weeks in some individuals (Biro et al, 1974). Synthetic materials, sterilized by ethylene oxide and used in cardiopulmonary bypass surgery, have been identified as the cause of severe toxic shock and some deaths in small children (Stanley et al, 1971). The degree of tissue toxicity depends on the concentration of ethylene oxide in the material and the duration of contact. Reyniers et al (1964) reported that multiple tumours developed on the skin of mice that were in contact with bedding material that had been treated with ethylene oxide, instead of gamma radiation as intended.

Ethylene chlorohydrin has less than 15 per cent of the toxicity of ethylene oxide (Gunther, 1974). A report that ethylene chlorohydrin may be present in toxic amounts in PVC if the material has been previously sterilized by gamma radiation (Cunliffe & Wesley, 1967) has been contradicted by subsequent investigations in which no significant amount of ethylene chlorohydrin was detected in irradiated or unirradiated PVC (Bogdansky & Lehn, 1974). However, the amount of chlorides in some pharmaceuticals and foods might result in the production of toxic levels of ethylene chlorohydrin, and ethylene oxide is not used for the sterilization of such materials, with the possible exception of spices or other additives that are used in small quantities (Wesley et al, 1965; Ragelis et al, 1968; Holmgren et al, 1969).

SUSCEPTIBILITY OF MICROORGANISMS

All types of microorganisms are susceptible to ethylene oxide if they are exposed to suitable conditions of concentration, temperature and relative humidity for an adequate time. The relatively small difference between the susceptibility of vegetative bacteria and spores is an advantageous feature of the biocidal action of ethylene oxide.

Dadd & Daley (1980) compared the resistance of different bacteria, spores and fungi with that of the spores of *Bacillus subtilis* var. *niger* (NCTC 10073), which are commonly used as a biological monitor of ethylene oxide sterilization. The vegetative bacteria, fungi, and the spores produced by *Bacillus stearothermophilus* and *Clostridium sporogenes* constituted a highly sensitive group. Strains of *Bacillus pumilus, Clostridium thermosaccharolyticum, Bacillus megaterium* and *Bacillus sphaericus* produced spores which were intermediate in resistance between the first group and *B. subtilis* var. *niger*. However, some species of *Bacillus* isolated from natural habitats produced spores of higher resistance. The spores of the reference strain of *B. subtilis* var. *niger* were only 8 times as resistant as the corresponding vegetative cells of this species. The virus that causes foot-and-mouth disease in domestic animals is susceptible to ethylene oxide (Tessler & Fellowes, 1961).

FACTORS INFLUENCING EFFICIENCY OF BIOCIDAL ACTION

The efficiency of ethylene oxide sterilization depends on achieving an adequate concentration of the chemical vapour at an appropriate temperature and relative humidity. Efficiency may be adversely affected if the microorganisms have previously been desiccated or are occluded within dried organic or crystalline material.

Concentration and temperature

The influences of concentration and temperature are interrelated (Ernst & Shull, 1962). If the concentration is above 450 mg/l, the temperature may be varied between 45°C and 60°C without affecting the time required for sterilization. Conversely, when the temperature is above 45°C, an increase in concentration above 450 mg/l has little effect on biocidal action. However, a concentration of 800–1200 mg/l is used in practice to over-

come penetration barriers and to allow for absorption by packaging material. If the concentration and relative humidity are constant, the rate of sporicidal action will double for every 10°C rise in temperature (Caputo & Rohn, 1982).

Moisture

Relative humidities below 30 per cent are consistently adverse to the biocidal action of ethylene oxide. Levels ranging from 50–100 per cent, depending on the nature and bulk of the materials to be sterilized, are generally used in hospital and industrial sterilization processes; 70 per cent is recommended for the hospital process which is operated at 55°C. The penetration of moisture is more likely to be the limiting factor in sterilization efficiency than is penetration of ethylene oxide gas.

The critical role of moisture was emphasized by Phillips & Kaye (1949) in their original investigation into the application of ethylene oxide to the sterilization of medical equipment. Working with a low concentration and at ambient temperature, Gilbert et al (1964) found that the optimum relative humidity for biocidal action was 33 per cent. A similar result has been obtained more recently by Caputo & Rohn (1982). At lower humidity levels, the death rate curves tailed sharply as a small proportion of spores survived despite an increase in the time or the concentration. Above 33 per cent, the curves were linear but the rate of killing decreased slightly. The resistant residue from the original desiccated population could be restored to sensitivity immediately by wetting or, more slowly, by exposure to a relative humidity above 75 per cent.

These phenomena are subject to alternative explanations, both of which are probably correct. Gunther (1980) has proposed that moisture is necessary for combination of ethylene oxide with reactive groups on the bacterial surface. A surface film of water would promote contact by dissolving ethylene oxide to form a concentrated solution and would also provide a medium for ionization of the reactive groups. The rate of reaction would be much slower if contact depended only on bombardment by molecules in the vapour.

The alternative explanation, proposed by Doyle

& Ernst (1967), is that moisture is necessary to dissolve organic or crystalline material which may protect some of the spores. This proposal was based on the observation that only about 1 per cent of desiccated spore populations survive and their sensitivity can be restored by moisture saturation. This was confirmed by demonstrating that the difference in the susceptibility of spores of *B. subtilis* var. *niger* on impervious and porous materials disappeared if the spores were thoroughly washed before inoculation on the carriers (Doyle & Ernst, 1968). The higher resistance on impervious material, such as metal foil or plastic, was explained by incrustation with material from the suspending fluid, whereas this was absorbed into the interstices of a porous material such as filter paper, leaving the bacteria in a cleaner condition on the surface. The decrease in susceptibility at high humidity which was found by Gilbert et al (1964) does not appear to apply to the conditions of higher ethylene oxide concentration and temperature that are used in the sterilization process.

Associated materials

Organic deposits do not confer complete protection on the microorganisms unless the material is very dry. However, occlusion in crystalline material confers complete protection unless the humidity in the sterilizer is high enough to dissolve it.

ETHYLENE OXIDE STERILIZATION IN HOSPITALS

The requirement for an ethylene oxide sterilization process and the availability of trained staff to operate it should be evaluated before a decision is made to install a sterilizer. The quantity of reusable medical, surgical and diagnostic equipment that cannot withstand heat sterilization should be assessed in order to ensure that the sterilizing capacity of the apparatus will be fully utilized. If the requirements of one hospital are insufficient to justify the cost involved, another might welcome an opportunity to share the facilities. The purchase of small, apparently simple, bench model sterilizers to meet a low level need cannot be recommended, because they rarely fulfil the conditions that are required to provide an adequate level of sterility assurance (Walter & Kundsin, 1959). They are also likely to be used by untrained staff. Lack of expertise in the supervision and operation of an ethylene oxide process is often a cause of sterilization failure.

The sterilizer and accompanying aeration cabinet should be installed in a central sterilizing department where the suitability of the process for different types of heat-sensitive equipment can be assessed and the proper preparation can be supervised. The advice of a microbiologist who has studied the ethylene oxide process should be readily available because regular biological tests are required for qualifying the sterilizer and monitoring it in routine operation. The services of a specially trained engineer are also required.

Applications of ethylene oxide sterilization

Low-temperature sterilization by ethylene oxide is required for articles that are made partly or entirely from heat-sensitive rubber or synthetic materials or contain electronic components, telescopes and lamps. Most of the articles withstand treatment at 50–60°C but a lower temperature (e.g. 48°C) may be required for some diagnostic equipment. The manufacturer's advice concerning the sterilization of complex equipment should be sought because components are changed from time to time. The ethylene oxide process is too slow for sterilization of instruments, such as endoscopes, between successive uses on the same day.

Ethylene oxide gas sterilization is not applicable to liquids or to articles in impervious packaging material. It is also unsuitable, because of possible toxic effects, for producing sterile diets for infection-susceptible patients or germfree animals. The availability of ethylene oxide sterilization in a hospital does not justify the resterilization of commercially sterilized devices which are intended for a single use only. Some types of hospital equipment for which an ethylene oxide process is required are listed in Table 7.2.

Table 7.2 Some articles that may be sterilized by ethylene oxide

Type of articles	Examples
Endoscopic instruments	Cystoscopes
	Laparoscopes
	Resectoscopes
Cardiac equipment	Cardiac catheters
	Heart-lung apparatus
	Transducers
Devices for implantation	Breast implants
	Cardiac pacemakers and leads
	Orthopaedic prostheses
Medical and dental equipment	Centrifuge bowls (for blood cell separation)
	Cryoprobes
	Dental handpieces (air rotor type), if not autoclavable
	Electrical[1], electronic equipment
	Mechanical ventilators
	Microsurgical accessories
	Nebulizers
	Oxygen tents
	Plastic bath linings

[1]Electrical equipment should be checked by an electrician before reuse

Preparation and packaging

Articles to be sterilized by ethylene oxide must be thoroughly cleaned. They should be dried at room temperature to avoid excessive dehydration and inspected for cleanliness and absence of water droplets. It may be difficult to check cavities in hollow instruments and it is impossible to verify the cleanliness of fine tubes such as cardiac catheters, which should not be reprocessed. Cleaned articles and packaging materials should be stored in a room at 40–60 per cent relative humidity.

Packaging materials recommended for hospital use are the same as those used for steam sterilization because permeability to air, steam and ethylene oxide vapour is essential. Bags made from paper or from paper and transparent plastic film (window pack) are most convenient for small articles but wrapping sheets of crepe paper or cotton fabric may be required for trays containing endoscopes or other large objects. Thin polyethylene film is permeable to ethylene oxide but packages made entirely from the film are impermeable to moisture and are likely to burst under vacuum because air cannot be removed. A porous paper-like material (Tyvek) made from spun-bonded polyethylene is ideal for ethylene oxide sterilization but its use for hospital packaging is limited by its high cost.

Design of sterilizers

A hospital ethylene oxide sterilizer is designed to perform an automatic cycle in which appropriate conditions of ethylene oxide concentration, temperature and relative humidity are produced in the chamber and maintained for a sufficient time to sterilize the load. A nonflammable mixture of ethylene oxide with fluorocarbon–12 or carbon dioxide may be used as the sterilant; the fluorocarbon diluent provides a suitable concentration of ethylene oxide below 100 kPa gauge pressure; the carbon dioxide mixture exerts a much higher pressure at a similar concentration. Pure ethylene oxide may be used in small sterilizers, providing concentrations of up to 1200 mg/l at subatmospheric pressure. The risk of leakage or explosion is very low as the sterilant is released from a small cartridge in the closed chamber after the air has been removed, but an explosion-proof chamber is required. Features of the design, construction and control systems of hospital ethylene oxide sterilizers are described by the Standards Association of Australia (1975) and the Canadian Standards Association (1977). These documents are intended for the guidance of manufacturers and hospital personnel who are responsible for the purchase, installation, operation and maintenance of the sterilizer.

Chamber and connections

The steel chamber is built to withstand degrees of vacuum and positive pressure appropriate to the particular process. The chamber may have a single door or a door at each end, the mechanisms and controls being similar to those for pressure steam sterilizers. If pure ethylene oxide is used, the explosion-proof chamber should have a spring-loaded door. A jacket in which hot water is circulated from a thermostatically controlled tank, is more likely to provide a uniform temperature in the chamber than external heating elements on the wall. The principal connections to the chamber are supply lines for steam, vaporized sterilant and filtered air. Outlets are required for removal of air, ethylene oxide and water vapour by mechanical evacuation and for drainage of condensate. Safety valves should be fitted with bursting devices which operate in the event of blockage by ethylene oxide polymer.

Indicators and controls

The sterilization cycle may be controlled by an electromechanical system with recording charts or by microprocessor technology with computer printouts. Coloured lights indicate the stage of the cycle. When a cycle has been completed but has failed to fulfil the conditions for sterilization, the door should remain locked until it is opened by a responsible supervisor or engineer. Alternatively, sterilizers may be provided with a means of terminating an unsatisfactory cycle before it has been completed. The source of heat should be cut off automatically if the chamber temperature rises more than 5°C above that for which the process is set. A humidity sensor/controller should be installed in the chamber; however, this requirement is not always met because contact with ethylene oxide is deleterious to electronic devices, which have a short working life.

Aeration cabinets

An aeration cabinet is a metal chamber in which

sterilized packs are exposed to flowing heated air at 50–60°C for times ranging from 2–24 hours. The heating system should cut out if the temperature rises more than 5°C above that selected for operation. The flow rate should provide at least two air changes per minute. All air drawn through the chamber must pass through a bacterial filter.

Sterilization cycle

The sterilization cycle comprises the following stages, which are illustrated in Figure 7.1, for a process using an ethylene oxide/fluorocarbon–12 mixture:

1. Removal of air from the chamber followed by humidification and heating of the load
2. Sterilization of the load
3. Removal of gases from the chamber.

Stage 1. Air must be evacuated to 90 kPa below atmospheric pressure to ensure deep penetration of moisture and to permit the introduction of sufficient sterilizing gas mixture to provide the ethylene oxide concentration required in stage 2.

Humidification of the load in the sterilizing chamber is necessary because a moisture level that has been established at room temperature decreases when the chamber is heated to 45–50°C for sterilization. Humidification is carried out by passing steam through the chamber which is maintained at 90 kPa below atmospheric pressure. The preconditioning process must be completed before

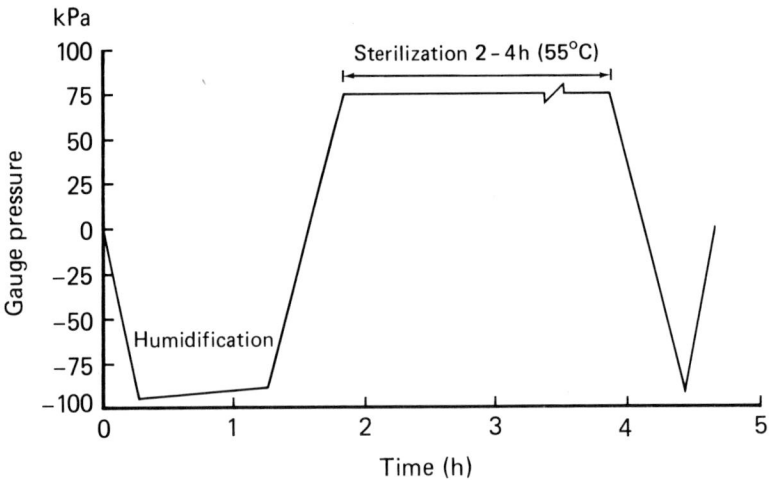

Fig. 7.1 An ethylene oxide sterilization cycle (original McDonald process) at 55°C

ethylene oxide is admitted to the chamber. The duration of the preconditioning stage is 30–60 minutes.

Stage 2. The sterilizing gas mixture must be vaporized and heated before it is admitted to the evacuated, humidified chamber. The entry of liquid sterilant would cause depletion of moisture by freezing and temperature stratification in the chamber could cause separation of flammable ethylene oxide from the diluent (Ernst & Doyle, 1968). An effective combination of sterilization parameters may be selected within the following range:

Ethylene oxide concentration	— 700–1000 mg/litre
Temperature	— 45–60°C
Relative humidity	— 70 per cent
Sterilization time	— 4 hours

The concentration of ethylene oxide in the chamber is regulated by pressure of the gas mixture. Gauge pressures of 56.3 kPa and 123.7 kPa correspond to 700 mg/l and 1000 mg/l when a 12%/88% ethylene oxide/fluorocarbon–12 mixture is used at 55°C. The sterilant is replenished as it is absorbed by the load.

Stage 3. The gases are removed from the chamber and exhausted to a suitable vent. This may be done by the following methods:

1. The chamber is evacuated and then restored to atmospheric pressure by admission of filtered air. The vacuum/air cycle may be repeated once. This is sufficient to remove the gases from the chamber; additional evacuations do not reduce the amount of ethylene oxide in the load or the rate at which it elutes (Roberts & Rendell-Baker, 1972).

2. After initial evacuation, the chamber may be purged with filtered air for 15 minutes, or until the chamber is opened. This stage may be extended, if necessary, to deliver a dry load. Materials, such as polypropylene and polycarbonate, which are poor conductors of heat, may attract a large amount of condensate which absorbs ethylene oxide and the solution may damage the material. This problem, which has been encountered in the sterilization of blood cell centrifuge bowls, may be avoided

by reducing the temperature of the process (e.g. to 30°C) and extending the sterilization time.

The door of the sterilizer should be opened immediately on completion of the cycle to avoid hazard to the operator resulting from build-up of ethylene oxide as it is released from the load. If the chamber cannot be opened immediately, it should be purged with air until it is opened. The load should be transferred immediately to an adjoining aeration cabinet.

Aeration of sterilized packs

An aeration cabinet is an essential component of the apparatus for sterilization by ethylene oxide. The long and uncertain aeration times required for desorption of ethylene oxide at ambient temperature are unsatisfactory in hospitals where complex equipment is often required for use as quickly as possible. Articles composed of PVC require at least 12 hours at 50°C in the aeration cabinet, where the heat accelerates desorption and the flowing air removes it from the chamber. Articles that are made from metal and glass may be aerated in 2 hours. If air purging has been extended (for safety reasons) while the load remained in the sterilizer, this time may be deducted from that required in the aeration cabinet.

Safety precautions in the sterilizing department

Stringent safety precautions are necessary to protect the operator of an ethylene oxide process and persons who may be passively exposed because they work in the area. The recommendations refer to:

1. Venting of gases from the sterilizing chamber and aeration cabinet
2. Release of residual ethylene oxide from the chamber or load when the door is opened
3. Managing accidental leakage or spillage of ethylene oxide from the chamber or storage cylinders.

The concentration of ethylene oxide in the atmosphere should be reduced below 5 p.p.m. (as near to zero as possible) for the safety of persons who may be exposed throughout working hours. An infrared gas analyser, which is positioned at fixed sites, such as the breathing zone of the operator, provides the most accurate result but the equipment is expensive. Small glass tubes packed with activated charcoal are more versatile because they can be worn by individuals as they work. A sample of air is drawn through the tube by a small portable pump and sent to the laboratory for analysis (Samuels & Corn, 1980). The same diffusion principle may be used in badges that could be worn by workers at risk.

The gases exhausted from the sterilizer and aeration cabinet should be vented directly to the outside atmosphere or to an existing exhaust vent that is known to be working at the time. If they are discharged to a sanitary sewer, a gas-liquid separator must be installed at the air break to direct the gas to an exhaust vent. Water trays are not effective absorbers of ethylene oxide. The area in which sterilization and aeration are carried out should be well ventilated; 8–10 air changes per hour have been recommended. The ventilation system must not interfere with the operation of the aeration cabinet (Association for the Advancement of Medical Instrumentation, 1981).

The main risk to the operator occurs when the chamber is opened and the load is transferred to the aeration cabinet. The most reliable method of minimizing the risk at this stage is to instal an exhaust hood over the door or to purge the chamber with filtered air until it is opened (Samuels & Corn, 1979, 1980). In the absence of these precautions, the operator and other individuals who work in the vicinity should vacate the area for 15 minutes to allow residual gas to dissipate, but this is less satisfactory.

Unloading the sterilizer and transferring the articles to the aeration cabinet may also present a risk. Rubber or fabric gloves should be worn for handling packs and the operator should move ahead of the transfer basket or trolley to avoid exposure to the gas that trails behind (Samuels, 1978).

Leaks and spills should be dealt with by an organized team according to a written programme with which all relevant staff are familiar. In the event of personal contact with liquid ethylene oxide, clothing, shoes and any rubber materials should be removed promptly and washed or aerated; if necessary, the skin should be washed and the eyes flushed with water.

Gas cylinders should always be in an upright position and chained to a fixed support. Care is required when changing to a new cylinder because the pipelines are filled with liquid sterilant. Quantities of pure ethylene oxide exceeding 10 kg should be kept in a store for flammable liquids. If cartridges are used in a small sterilizer, the number kept in a hospital sterilizing department should be limited to that required for one day's supply.

Testing efficiency of sterilization

Sterilization parameters

The temperature at selected sites in the chamber and load may be measured by thermocouples, as in steam sterilization. Direct measurement of the ethylene oxide concentration in routine operation is not feasible. The concentration in the chamber may be calculated from the weight of sterilant taken from the storage cylinder during the cycle or it may be read from a chart that relates concentration, pressure and temperature for the particular sterilant. Electronic humidity sensors are sometimes installed in ethylene oxide sterilizers but their working life is shortened because they are affected by exposure to ethylene oxide. The relative humidity in the chamber can be deduced from the difference between the temperatures of the jacket and chamber drain. A temperature of 54°C in the chamber and 45°C in the drainline corresponds to 70 per cent relative humidity.

Biological indicators

Standardized spore preparations provide the best evidence for a successful combination of sterilization parameters in the chamber and load. Spores produced by *B. subtilis* var. *niger* ('*B. globigii*') are most widely used. *B. stearothermophilus* is unsuitable because these spores are not highly resistant to ethylene oxide. The United States Pharmacopeia (1980) prescribes D values of 3 minutes at 600 mg/l and 1.7 minute at 1200 mg/l at a temperature of 55°C and relative humidity of 50 per cent. The inclusion of polymeric substances in the spore suspension which is used to inoculate the filter paper strips enhances the resistance of the washed spores (Doyle, 1971). Biological indicators should be standardized at temperatures at or above 50°C and at 50 per cent relative humidity (Oxborrow et al, 1983).

When qualifying tests are being performed on a newly installed, repaired or modified sterilizer, it is advisable to include 5–10 spore papers in every cycle until the efficiency of the process has been established. Thereafter, two spore papers per cycle are sufficient for routine use as long as failures are not detected. Devices for implantation into tissues should not be released for use until the biological test has been completed. Although it may be necessary to release some instruments before the sterilization cycle has been validated, the spore tests should be conducted regularly to ensure that a failure is detected as early as possible.

Chemical indicators

Small polyethylene sachets containing an acidified solution of magnesium chloride and a pH indicator (Royce & Bowler, 1959) can be calibrated to provide an estimate of the quantity of ethylene oxide absorbed. A colour change occurs when reaction with ethylene oxide renders the solution alkaline.

Other chemical indicators are limited to paper strips impregnated with a dye that changes from yellow to blue and adhesive tapes that develop coloured stripes during sterilization. Neither type provides an assurance of sterilizing conditions but immediate indication of a gross deficiency in ethylene oxide concentration is important.

Test packs

Challenge test packs containing cotton towels and enclosing items of rubber and plastic equipment are described in Canadian Standard Z314.1–M1977. The person in charge of operating the sterilizer may devise a test pack which is representative of the types that are sterilized in the hospital process.

ETHYLENE OXIDE STERILIZATION IN INDUSTRY

Ethylene oxide is an alternative to ionizing radia-tion as a sterilizing agent for medical devices that are produced and sterilized commercially. The gaseous process may be chosen because it can be carried out more easily on the manufacturer's premises than radiation sterilization.

Packaging

Tyvek (see Ch. 3) and treated papers are ideal because they are permeable to ethylene oxide and water vapour. Polyethylene film (*ca* 0.076 mm thickness) is also permeable to ethylene oxide, and water vapour may be carried through with the gas if it has been previously concentrated on the outer surface of the pack (Ernst & Doyle, 1968). However, sealed packs made entirely from plastic film are likely to burst during sterilization unless they contain a segment of breathable material. Products which are sterilized industrially by ethylene oxide can be enclosed in the outer packaging before sterilization.

Preconditioning

If the sterilization process is operated at a high temperature (above 30°C), the packs must be heated and humidified in the sterilization cycle because the humidity level established at ambient temperature decreases when the temperature is raised. However, when sterilization takes place at 20–30°C, preconditioning outside the chamber may be more satisfactory (Gillis, 1982). The relative humidity should be at least 50 per cent and the temperature approximately 10°C below that selected for sterilization. The conditioning room should accommodate two sterilizer loads. The same conditions should be maintained during transfer to the sterilizer, especially if condensation occurs within the package because the contents have low thermal conductivity.

Sterilization

The severity of treatment that is required to sterilize articles in several layers of packaging material depends on the contamination level and the resistance of the microbial population. It is also influenced by capacity of the packaging materials to absorb ethylene oxide and moisture, thus reducing the amounts available for sterilization.

The sterilization cycle is based on the same principles as those which govern the hospital process but modifications may be required to prevent the breakage of product packages caused by retention of air. The development of a high vacuum and sudden pressure changes may be avoided by a process in which the level of vacuum is modified and the remaining air is displaced from the chamber by the incoming sterilant. Alternatively, the pressure changes may be carried out in a series of steps (Ernst, 1973).

Aeration

Ambient aeration is satisfactory because the packs are held until all monitoring tests have been completed. The period between sterilization and use of the articles is further extended by the time required for storage and distribution.

Testing efficiency of sterilization

The methods are the same as those used in the hospital process. Ten or more biological indicators should be distributed in the load (Christensen et al, 1969). In the United States, the requirements for product sterility tests are modified if the process has been tested by biological indicators. A method of monitoring the concentration of ethylene oxide continuously during the sterilizing stage of the cycle has been recommended (Solomon & Macdonald, 1981). It involves taking samples from the chamber at frequent intervals and analysing them by gas chromatography.

FORMALDEHYDE

The low-temperature steam and formaldehyde process (Alder et al, 1966) was designed primarily for sterilization or disinfection of cystoscopes and other heat-sensitive instruments. It is also applicable to a wide variety of equipment that withstands a temperature of 70–75°C but cannot be sterilized by steam above atmospheric pressure. The process requires a specially designed prevacuum sterilizer which operates at subatmospheric pressure and is

quite different from formaldehyde fumigation. Like the ethylene oxide process, the steam and formaldehyde process is too slow for resterilizing equipment that is reused on the same day but the sterilizer can be used for an alternative disinfection process that may be completed within 30 minutes.

PROPERTIES OF FORMALDEHYDE

Physical and chemical properties

Formaldehyde is not available as a pure gas or liquid. Formalin is an aqueous solution containing 37 per cent w/v formaldehyde, from which the vapour can be released by heating. Formaldehyde polymerizes gradually in the solution, depositing paraformaldehyde as a white powder. It also polymerizes from the vapour state at low temperature and high humidity but this does not occur at the temperature (above 70°C) of the steam and formaldehyde sterilization process. Formaldehyde vapour is nonflammable at the concentration used in this process.

Toxicity

The potential toxicity of formaldehyde is similar to that of ethylene oxide. However, exposure is more readily detected by the odour and irritant effects of the vapour at concentrations below 5 p.p.m. in air. Exposure to 2–5 p.p.m. causes immediate irritation of the respiratory tract and eyes, with the shedding of tears. Skin irritation or allergic contact dermatitis may result from contact with solutions containing formaldehyde. Effects on the respiratory tract and skin have been reviewed by Clark (1983) and Yodaikin (1981).

The effects of long-term exposure to formaldehyde are being studied but retrospective surveys of large numbers of persons who have been subjected to occupational exposure for many years, at higher concentrations than would now be permitted, have yielded only negative evidence of a causal association with human cancer (Editorial Lancet, 1983).

Absorption by natural and synthetic materials

Relatively high levels of residual formaldehyde

have been found in paper and cloth wrappings after treatment by the steam and formaldehyde process. However, the quantity absorbed by rubber and plastics is reported to be low (Gibson et al, 1968). In view of increased concern about formaldehyde toxicity, further investigation of the quantities absorbed and the rate of desorption are required.

SUSCEPTIBILITY OF MICROORGANISMS

Formaldehyde has a broad spectrum of biocidal action, similar to that of ethylene oxide. Sporicidal action is slow at room temperature, but is accelerated by combination with saturated steam at 70–75°C. Viruses, fungi and tubercle bacilli are susceptible.

FACTORS INFLUENCING EFFICIENCY OF BIOCIDAL ACTION

Concentration and temperature

An increase in the concentration of formaldehyde vapour increases the killing rate if the temperature and relative humidity are constant. The direct effect of temperature on the killing rate cannot be separated from its other effects of increasing the concentration of formaldehyde vapour, retarding polymerization and decreasing absorption, all of which assist penetration of the vapour to relatively inaccessible sites.

LOW-TEMPERATURE STEAM AND FORMALDEHYDE STERILIZATION

Applications

The types of materials and equipment treated by this process are generally similar to those which may be sterilized by ethylene oxide, but the minimum operating temperature of 70°C may be unsuitable for cardiac pacemakers, some pressure transducers and other electronic devices; these can be sterilized by ethylene oxide at 45–50°C. The formaldehyde process should not be used for equipment that withstands conventional sterilization.

Natural and synthetic rubbers and most plastics are stable to steam and formaldehyde at 70–75°C. Polyethylene, leather, wood and painted surfaces are seriously damaged. The lubricating systems of mechanical ventilators may become contaminated with water but electrical connections can be protected by maintaining slight superheat in the chamber. A list of articles that have been sterilized without adverse effects is given in Table 7.3.

Preparation and packaging

Articles should be clean and just dry, as for ethylene oxide sterilization. Paper and cotton fabric are suitable wrapping materials; polyethylene film and glassine paper are unsuitable, except as a transparent window in a paper pouch. Cysto-

Table 7.3 Some applications of low-temperature steam and formaldehyde sterilization

Types of equipment and materials	Examples
Surgical instruments	Airways
	Anaesthetic masks, tubing, bags
	Arthroscopes
	Cardiac catheters (Teflon, Dacron)
	Cuffed endotracheal tubes (rubber)
	Cystoscopes, with leads and lights (including fibre light system)
	Laparoscopes
Medical equipment	Blood oxygenators
	Catheters (gum elastic, latex rubber)
	Drainage sets
	Gloves (latex)
	Humidifiers
	Hyperbaric equipment parts
	Mechanical ventilators, with electric motors, switches and heaters
	Syringes (large polypropylene)
Electrical equipment	Capacitors
	Defibrillator electrodes
	Electrode implants for physiological experiments
	Leads, switches, bakelite plugs and bulbs
	Motors (water contaminates lubricating system)
	Potentiometers
	Transformers

scopes may be packed in light cardboard boxes, which should be sterilized in a prevacuum steam sterilizer at 134°C to kill spores and eliminate bituminous material before they are used. Tubing should be loosely packed to avoid retention of air and water droplets, which interfere with steam penetration. Formaldehyde does not diffuse through the wall of plastic tubing. Excessive quantities of porous packaging material may reduce the amounts of steam and formaldehyde reaching the articles to be sterilized.

Design of sterilizers

A low-temperature steam and formaldehyde sterilizer is similar to a prevacuum steam sterilizer, but is operated at negative pressure with subatmospheric steam at 70–75°C. The jacket is heated continuously by water which is circulated from a thermostatically controlled reservoir. The floor of the chamber must be sloped towards the drain to prevent accumulation of condensate and consequent wetting of the load. Steam and condensate are discharged to an evacuated condenser because the balanced pressure steam traps that are used in steam sterilizers do not operate at negative pressure. Formaldehyde vapour is generated by passing formalin into a steam-heated vaporizer. Air that is admitted to the chamber at the end of the sterilization cycle to remove formaldehyde from the chamber must pass through a bacterial filter. Automatic controls include a mechanism to cut out the heating system if the temperature exceeds that selected for the process by more than 2°C.

Dual purpose machines which operate alternative cycles using steam at 134°C or steam with formaldehyde at 73°C are manufactured but are generally disapproved by regulatory authorities. Besides the risk of human error in activating a high-temperature process when the chamber is loaded with heat-sensitive equipment, the engineering problems are greatly increased.

Sterilization cycle

The cycle is divided into four stages:

Stage 1. Air is removed from the chamber and load by evacuation to 90 kPa below atmospheric pressure. This is followed by steam pulses ranging from 60–95 kPa below atmospheric pressure to assist steam penetration into the load; the introduction of formaldehyde at this stage assists penetration into narrow tubes (Marcos & Wiseman, 1979).

Stage 2. Sterilization of the load requires 40 minutes to 2 hours at 70–75°C, depending on the types of articles and the method by which the sterilizing agents are introduced into the chamber. The concentration of formaldehye in the chamber should be at least 5 mg/ml.

Stage 3. Formaldehyde vapour is removed by pulsing repeatedly with pure steam.

Stage 4. The load is dried by a series of evacuations to 95 kPa below atmospheric pressure, alternating with admission of filtered air.

Aeration

Levels of formaldehyde residues in materials sterilized by the steam and formaldehyde process have not been established. However, it is generally recommended they receive the same treatment as for ethylene oxide.

TESTING EFFICIENCY OF STERILIZATION

Sterilization parameters

The quality of steam, which is near to complete saturation, may be monitored by the temperature and pressure gauge readings and recorded charts. A pressure of 68 kPa below atmospheric corresponds to 73°C. Thermocouples may be used to determine heating rates within the load and to verify the temperature and time of exposure.

Biological indicators

Routine monitoring of the steam and formaldehyde process with biological indicators is required because they provide the only method for confirming penetration of formaldehyde into packs and instruments with hollow tubes. Spores of *B. stearothermophilus* are used because they are not affected at 75°C in the absence of the chemical vapour. Two spore papers may be placed in a small glass tube with a cotton wool stopper. The small tube is placed in a bottle tightly closed by a cap to which a length of metal tubing that simulates a cystoscope (Alder et al, 1971) or a coiled cardiac catheter (Line & Pickerill, 1973; Gibson, 1977) is attached. If a test pack is used, it should be designed to present a challenge to steam and formaldehyde penetration.

Chemical indicator

Browne formaldehyde control indicator papers are available. The blue spot changes to green after sufficient exposure to formaldehyde.

REFERENCES

Alder V G, Brown A M, Gillespie W A 1966 Disinfection of heat-sensitive material by low-temperature steam and formaldehyde. Journal of Clinical Pathology 19: 83–89

Alder V G, Gingell J C, Mitchell J P 1971 Disinfection of cystoscopes by subatmospheric steam and steam and formaldehyde at 80°C. British Medical Journal 3: 677–680

Association for the Advancement of Medical Instrumentation 1981 Good hospital practice: ethylene oxide gas — ventilation recommendations and safe use. Association for the Advancement of Medical Instrumentation, Arlington, AAMI EO-VRSU 3/81

Biro L, Fisher A A, Price E 1974 Ethylene oxide burns. A hospital outbreak involving 19 women. Archives of Dermatology 110: 924–925

Bogdansky S, Lehn P J 1974 Effects of γ-irradiation on 2–chloroethanol formation in ethylene oxide-sterilized polyvinyl chloride. Journal of Pharmaceutical Sciences 63: 802–803.

Bruch C W 1973 Sterilization of plastics: toxicity of ethylene oxide residues. In: Phillips G B, Miller W S (eds) Industrial sterilization. Duke University Press, Durham, ch 4, p 49

Canadian Standards Association 1977 Ethylene Oxide Sterilizers for Hospitals. CSA Standard Z314.1–M1977

Caputo R A, Rohn K J 1982 The effects of EtO sterilization variables on B1 performance. Medical Device & Diagnostic Industry: 4(7). 37–41, 68–69

Clark R P 1983 Formaldehyde in pathology departments. Journal of Clinical Pathology 36: 839–846

Christensen E A, Kallings L O, Fystro D 1969 Microbiological control of sterilization procedures and standards for the sterilization of medical equipment. Ugeskrift for Laeger 131: 2123 (Translation p 1–15)

Cunliffe A C, Wesley F 1967 Hazards from plastics sterilized by ethylene oxide. British Medical Journal 2: 575–576

Dadd A H, Daley G M 1980 Resistance of micro-organisms to inactivation by gaseous ethylene oxide. Journal of Applied Bacteriology 49: 89–101

Doyle J E 1971 Sterility indicator with artificial resistance to ethylene oxide. Bulletin of the Parenteral Drug Association 25: 98–104

Doyle J E, Ernst R R 1967 Resistance of *Bacillus subtilis* var. *niger* spores occluded in water-insoluble crystals to three sterilization agents. Applied Microbiology 15: 726–730

Doyle J E, Ernst R R 1968 Influence of various pretreatments (carriers, desiccation, and relative cleanliness) on the destruction of *Bacillus subtilis* var. *niger* spores with gaseous ethylene oxide. Journal of Pharmaceutical Sciences 57: 433–436

Editorial 1983 Formaldehyde and cancer. Lancet ii: 26

Ernst R R 1973 Ethylene oxide gaseous sterilization for industrial applications. In: Phillips G B, Miller W S (eds) Industrial sterilization. Duke University Press, Durham, ch 12, p 181

Ernst R R, Doyle J E 1968 Sterilization with gaseous ethylene oxide: a review of chemical and physical factors. Biotechnology and Bioengineering 10: 1–31

Ernst R R, Shull J J 1962 Ethylene oxide gaseous sterilization 1. Concentration and temperature effects. Applied Microbiology 10: 337–341

Gibson G L 1977 Processing urinary endoscopes in a low-temperature steam and formaldehyde autoclave. Journal of Clinical Pathology 30: 269–274

Gibson G L, Johnston H P, Turkington V E 1968 Residual formaldehyde after low-temperature steam and formaldehyde sterilization. Journal of Clinical Pathology 21: 771–775

Gilbert G L, Gambill V M, Spiner D R, Hoffman R K, Phillips C R 1964 Effect of moisture on ethylene oxide sterilization. Applied Microbiology 12: 496–503

Gillis J 1982 Outside preconditioning in EtO sterilization. Medical Device & Diagnostic Industry 4(1): 24, 26–27

Gunther D A 1974 Safety of ethylene oxide residuals Part 2. American Journal of Hospital Pharmacy 31: 684–686

Gunther D A 1980 The chemistry and biology of EtO sterilization. Medical Device & Diagnostic Industry 2(12): 31–35

Hemminki K, Mutanen P, Saloniemi I, Niemi M-L, Vainio H 1982 Spontaneous abortions in hospital staff engaged in sterilising instruments with chemical agents. British Medical Journal 285: 1461–1463

Hogstedt C, Malmqvist N, Wadman B 1979 Leukemia in workers exposed to ethylene oxide. Journal of the American Medical Association 241: 1132–1133

Holmgren A, Diding N, Samuelsson G 1969 Ethylene oxide treatment of crude drugs Part V. Formation of ethylene chlorohydrin. Acta Pharmaceutica Suecica 6: 33–36

Line S J, Pickerill J K 1973 Testing a steam-formaldehyde sterilizer for gas penetration efficiency. Journal of Clinical Pathology 26: 716–720

Marcos D, Wiseman D 1979 Measurement of formaldehyde concentrations in a subatmospheric steam-formaldehyde autoclave. Journal of Clinical Pathology 32: 567–575

McGunnigle R G, Renner J A, Romano S J, Abodeely R A Jr 1975 Residual ethylene oxide: levels in medical grade tubing and effects on an in vitro biologic system. Journal of Biomedical Materials Research 9: 273–283

Mogenhan J A, Whitbourne J E, Ernst R R 1971 Determination of ethylene oxide in surgical materials by vacuum extraction and gas chromatography. Journal of Pharmaceutical Sciences 60: 222–224

Oxborrow G S, Placencia A M, Danielson J W 1983 Effects of temperature and relative humidity on biological indicators used for ethylene oxide sterilization. Applied and Environmental Microbiology 45: 546–549

Phillips C R, Kaye S 1949 The sterilizing action of gaseous ethylene oxide I. Review. American Journal of Hygiene 50: 270–279

Ragelis E P, Fisher B S, Klimeck B A, Johnson C 1968 Isolation and determination of chlorohydrins in foods fumigated with ethylene oxide or with propylene oxide. Journal of the Association of Official Analytical Chemists 51: 709–715

Reyniers J A, Sacksteder M R, Ashburn L L 1964 Multiple tumors in female germfree inbred albino mice exposed to bedding treated with ethylene oxide. Journal of the National Cancer Institute 32: 1045–1057

Roberts R B, Rendell-Baker L 1972 Aeration after ethylene oxide sterilisation. Failure of repeated vacuum cycles to influence aeration time after ethylene oxide sterilisation. Anaesthesia 27: 278–282

Royce A, Bowler C 1959 An indicator control device for ethylene oxide sterilisation. Journal of Pharmacy and Pharmacology Supplement 11: 294T–298T

Samuels T M 1978 Personnel exposures to ethylene oxide in a central service assembly and sterilization area. Hospital Topics 56: 27–33

Samuels T M, Corn R 1979 Modification of large, built-in, ethylene oxide sterilizers to reduce operator exposure to EO. Hospital Topics 57: 50–55

Samuels T M, Corn R 1980 Evaluation of a new generation ethylene oxide sterilizer relative to reduction in operator exposure to ETO. Hospital Topics 58: 31–35

Shikama K, Miura K-I 1976 Equilibrium studies on the formaldehyde reaction with native DNA. European Journal of Biochemistry 63: 39–46

Solomon D, Macdonald M M 1981 Continuous monitoring of EtO during sterilization. Medical Device & Diagnostic Industry 3(12): 65–66

Spitz H D, Weinberger J 1971 Determination of ethylene oxide, ethylene chlorohydrin, and ethylene glycol by gas chromatography. Journal of Pharmaceutical Sciences 60: 271–274

Standards Association of Australia 1975 Ethylene Oxide Sterilizers (Using Ethylene Oxide/Dichlorodifluoromethane 12%/88% m/m Sterilizing Gas Mixture). Australian Standard 1714–1975

Stanley P, Bertranou E, Forest F, Langevin L 1971 Toxicity of ethylene oxide sterilization of polyvinyl chloride in open-heart surgery. Journal of Thoracic and Cardiovascular Surgery 61: 309–314

Tessler J, Fellowes O N 1961 The effect of gaseous ethylene oxide on dried foot-and-mouth disease virus. American Journal of Veterinary Research 22: 779–782

United States Pharmacopeia 1980 20th rev. Mack Publishing Company, Easton, p 1039

Vologodskii A V, Frank-Kamenetskii M D 1975 Theoretical study of DNA unwinding under the action of formaldehyde. Journal of Theoretical Biology 55: 153–166

Walter C W, Kundsin R B 1959 Faulty function of table model ethylene oxide sterilizer. Journal of the American Medical Association 170: 1543–1544

Warren B 1971 The determination of residual ethylene oxide and halogenated hydrocarbon propellants in sterilized plastics. Journal of Pharmacy and Pharmacology Supplement 23: 170S–175S

Wesley F, Rourke B, Darbishire O 1965 The formation of persistent toxic chlorohydrins in foodstuffs by fumigation with ethylene oxide and with propylene oxide. Journal of Food Science 30: 1037–1042

White J D, Bradley T J 1973 Residual ethylene oxide in gas-sterilized, medical-grade silicones. Journal of Pharmaceutical Sciences 62: 1634–1637

Yager J W, Hines C J, Spear R C 1983 Exposure to ethylene oxide at work increases sister chromatid exchanges in human peripheral lymphocytes. Science 219: 1221–1223

Yodaikin R E 1981 The uncertain consequences of formaldehyde toxicity. Journal of the American Medical Association 246: 1677–1678

FURTHER READING

American Society for Hospital Central Service Personnel 1982 Ethylene oxide for use in hospitals. A manual for health care personnel

8

Sterilization by ionizing radiation

Radiation sterilization means treatment by gamma rays, X-rays or accelerated electrons, all of which are ionizing radiations. It excludes ultraviolet light, which is a low energy, non-ionizing radiation with very poor penetrating power.

Ionizing radiations kill all types of microorganisms and usually have enough energy for useful penetration into solids and liquids. They do not heat or wet materials significantly and are widely used for industrial sterilization of heat-sensitive medical and laboratory equipment. Space requirements, safety precautions and cost preclude the installation of large automated sterilization facilities in hospitals and laboratories. However, several small-scale batch-type facilities are now in use. Application of the process to pharmaceuticals, biological products and foods may be limited by the inactivation of some drugs and nutrients and also by development of off-flavours in foods. However, radiation pasteurization of foods, at least up to an average dose of 1 Mrad (10 kGy), to extend storage life has been shown to pose no toxicological, carcinogenic or teratogenic hazards. Low-dose irradiation is also useful for reducing the level of microbial contamination of the raw materials used in the manufacture of pharmaceuticals and cosmetics.

A brief review of the properties, mechanisms of biological action and effects of ionizing radiations on microorganisms and materials will precede a description of facilities for radiation sterilization and the main applications of the process.

UNITS AND TERMS

Energy

electron volt (eV): the energy gained by an
electron moving through a potential difference
of 1 volt. An electron volt corresponds to
1.602×10^{-19} joules (J) and is applicable to
electromagnetic and particulate radiation. One
mega electron volt (MeV) = 10^6 eV

Power (Output)

joule per second (J/s or Js^{-1}) or watt (W): expresses
the power, or output, of a radiation source

Quantity

becquerel (Bq): the quantity of radioactive isotope
that undergoes one disintegration per second.
The becquerel is the SI unit, replacing the curie
(Ci); 1 Bq = 2.7×10^{-11} Ci
1 MCi = 3.7×10^{16} Bq

Absorbed dose

gray (Gy): unit of dose defined as 1 joule of energy
absorbed per kilogram of material irradiated.
The gray is the SI unit, replacing the rad (100
ergs/g); 1 Gy = 100 rad
25 kGy = 2.5 Mrad

TYPES OF RADIANT ENERGY

Radiation may be described as energy in motion. It
may be non-particulate (electromagnetic) or particulate (accelerated electrons).

Electromagnetic radiation

Electromagnetic radiations travel at the speed of
light (3×10^8 m/s). The wavelengths and corresponding energy quantum levels of each photon in
the bands of the electromagnetic spectrum are
listed in Table 8.1. The energy level of gamma
photons is sufficient to ionize or excite atoms, but
is far below the level that could induce radioactivity in the treated material by disrupting the atomic
nucleus. Ultraviolet radiation in the range 240–

280 nm is biocidal but practical application is
limited by its lack of penetrating power to disinfection of air, clear water and clean surfaces which
are in the direct path of the radiation. Visible light
may damage bacterial nucleic acids but generally
has little effect on microorganisms, especially
those which are protected by carotenoid pigments
(Krinsky, 1976). Infrared radiation is sometimes
used as a rapid method of heat transfer in dry heat
sterilization processes but its action is limited to
heating the exposed surfaces of solid objects. Microwave energy generates heat in moist food but
has no role in sterilization.

Cobalt–60 (^{60}Co) is used as the source of gamma radiation in sterilization facilities. It is prepared
by placing the stable ^{59}Co in a nuclear reactor,
where it absorbs neutrons to yield radioactive
^{60}Co. The resulting specific activity is 10^{11}–10^{13}
Bq/g (3–400 Ci/g), depending on the time of irradiation. At each successive disintegration, gamma
radiation is emitted at two separate energy levels
of 1.333 and 1.173 MeV. The half-life of the isotope is 5.272 years, so that the quantity of radioactivity decreases by approximately 12.3 per cent
per annum. Both emissions are suitable for sterilization because they are absorbed by all materials. Penetration depends on the density of the
absorbing material; the absorbed dose falls to about one half after penetrating 12 cm of unit density
material. ^{60}Co emits 15 kJ/s (15 kW) per MCi.

Caesium–137 (^{137}Cs), emitting gamma rays at
0.662 MeV, can also be used for sterilization and
may find increasing application in future if the
need to dispose of it (as a fission product of ura-
nium–235) justifies the cost of separation (Eymery,
1974).

X-rays are similar to gamma radiation but are
produced artificially by bombardment of a heavy
metal target with an electron or cathode ray beam.
The fraction of electron beam energy that is converted to electromagnetic radiation increases
steeply with voltage; facilities have been designed
to provide the very high doses required for sterilization of medical products or food.

Particulate radiation

Electric current is a flow of electrons. When these
are accelerated to very high speeds they gain ener-

Table 8.1 Wavelengths, frequencies and energies of electromagnetic radiations[1]

Type of electromagnetic radiation	Wavelength	Frequency	Energy	
	nm	Hz	eV	J
Gamma	<0.1	$>3\times10^{18}$	$>10^4$	$>2\times10^{-15}$
X-ray	$10^{-4}-1$	$3\times10^{21}-3\times10^{17}$	10^3-10^7	$2\times10^{-16}-2\times10^{-12}$
Ultraviolet				
Extreme	1–20	$3\times10^{17}-1\times10^{16}$	$60-10^3$	$10^{-17}-2\times10^{-16}$
Far	20–200	$1\times10^{16}-1\times10^{15}$	6–60	$10^{-18}-10^{-17}$
Near	200–380	$1\times10^{15}-8\times10^{14}$	3–6	$5\times10^{-19}-10^{-18}$
Visible	380–750	$8\times10^{14}-4\times10^{14}$	1.5–3	$2\times10^{-19}-5\times10^{-19}$
Infrared	$750-10^6$	$4\times10^{14}-3\times10^{11}$	$10^{-3}-1.5$	$2\times10^{-22}-2\times10^{-19}$
Microwave	$10^6-3\times10^8$ (1mm–300mm)	$3\times10^{11}-1\times10^9$	$4\times10^{-6}-10^{-3}$	$7\times10^{-25}-2\times10^{-19}$

[1]Values provided by McKellar B H J, Physics Department, University of Melbourne

gy and penetrating power. The energy at which they are produced is restricted, in practice, to levels that do not exceed 10 MeV as higher energies may induce radioactivity in the treated material. The depth of penetration is 0.33 cm/MeV in unit density material, which is much lower than that for gamma radiation.

MECHANISM OF BIOCIDAL ACTION

The DNA target

All living cells are affected by ionizing radiation in a similar way. The main biological target is deoxyribonucleic acid (DNA), which controls the genetic constitution and reproductive process of the cell. DNA is the most vital cell constituent and it presents a relatively large volume in the microbial cell for absorption of radiation and a large surface for reaction with radiation products. The involvement of DNA as the principal target of lethal action is supported by the following observations (Haynes, 1966; Latarjet, 1972):

1. Frequency of mutations among radiation survivors is above the normal level
2. Replication of DNA, transcription of messenger RNA and synthesis of proteins, which are all controlled by DNA, are more sensitive to irradiation than are other metabolic processes such as respiration (Pollard & Davis, 1970)
3. Artificial incorporation of 5-bromouracil in DNA increases its sensitivity to irradiation but 5-fluorouracil, which is incorporated only in RNA, does not produce this effect (Kaplan et al, 1962; Myers et al, 1977)
4. Oxygen sensitizes bacteria and cell-free DNA to irradiation in a similar way
5. Proteins, such as bacterial toxins (Skulberg, 1965) and enzymes, are relatively insensitive to sterilizing doses of radiation
6. Bacteria that have an efficient mechanism for the repair of DNA damage are highly resistant to irradiation.

The action of radiation on living cells may be considered in three stages, each of extremely short duration:

1. Ionization
2. Radical formation
3. Biochemical changes.

Ionization ($10^{-16}-10^{-17}$ second)

As a gamma photon passes through a material, it interacts with some of the orbital electrons in atoms or molecules. These events are infrequent and randomly distributed along the path. The absorbed energy produces positively charged ions when the electron is ejected from an atom, or it may produce unstable excited atoms and molecules. Many of the electrons are ejected at high velocities and produce a great number of additional ions, electrons or excited states. Accelerated electrons from a machine act in the same way as the high-velocity electrons that are produced within the cell; thus the microscopic geometry of events following the passage of gamma or X-ray photons and beams of electrons is the same. Each electron produces denser ionization towards the end·of its track through the cell. The linear energy transfer (LET) value is a measure of the absorbed energy per unit length of track and hence of the number of ions and excited species. The atomic nucleus is unaffected by energy levels that are employed for sterilization.

Radical formation (10^{-12}–10^{-14} second)

The ejected electrons finally reach thermal energies of 0.025 eV and may become solvated in polar materials, such as water, giving solvated electrons (e_{aq}) or they may react with molecules present in the liquid. Meanwhile, the positive ions and excited atoms or molecules undergo reactions yielding active radicals. The reactive species, such as OH•, e_{aq} and a few H• atoms, are produced in the intracellular water or the radiation reacts directly with cell constituents that are present in high concentration, producing corresponding ions, excited states and active radicals.

Biochemical changes (10^{-8} second)

The radicals, which are extremely reactive, sometimes react with each other to give the original material, doing little more than heating it up slightly. Alternatively, they may react with cell constituents. In this way DNA, for example, may be affected by the radiolysis of the water. This is known as indirect action. If oxygen is present, it may react with e_{aq} and H• producing the perhydroxyl or superoxide radical ($HO_2^•$) or with organic radicals giving peroxy species.

Very small amounts of radiant energy may have drastic biological effects, especially in unicellular organisms, but knowledge of the exact nature of the biochemical changes, or lesions, in DNA that are caused by ionizing radiation is far from complete. Two types of DNA damage have been recognized:

1. Breaks in one or both of the DNA strands
2. Lesions in the nitrogenous bases.

One active radical may cause a double-strand break if it is directly produced in the DNA molecule. Indirect action produces single-strand breaks but if the damaged sections on the two strands overlap, the effect would be the same as a double-strand break (Miller, 1970). Death of the cell may result from about three double-strand breaks in *Escherichia coli* (Ulmer et al, 1979); 1400 may be required in *Micrococcus radiodurans* (Resnick, 1966). The principal change that has been identified in the nucleic acid bases is the opening and hydration of the 5–6 C=C double bond in the pyrimidine ring structure (Shragge & Hunt, 1974). The stable products of attack on the bond by OH• radicals include uracil glycols, uracil hydrates and dihydrouracil (Shragge et al, 1974). The purines are less sensitive, but the main radical formed results in the opening of an N=C double bond at the 2–3 or the 7–8 position (Latarjet, 1972). Direct action may involve the addition of hydrogen atoms to the opened bonds.

Repair of damaged DNA

Some microorganisms have a great capacity for repair of damage to the DNA molecule (Bridges, 1976). *Micrococcus radiodurans* and *Micrococcus radiophilus* are more resistant than are bacterial spores (Anderson et al, 1956; Lewis, 1971). Some strains of *Streptococcus faecium* also show an increase above the normal level for non-sporing bacteria (Christensen, 1964). The efficiency of a repair system is often reflected by a large increase in the dose of radiation required for sterilization. The death rate is initially slow and only increases when a dose that inactivates the repair enzymes has been absorbed. Excision repair of damage caused by ionizing radiation involves four different enzymes which, in turn, incise the strand near the damaged site (endonuclease), remove or degrade the damaged section (exonuclease), resynthesize the section using the opposite intact strand as a genetic code (DNA polymerase) and, finally, rejoin the break (polynucleotide ligase). Single-strand breaks may be repaired as the open ends are held in place by the opposite strand (Latarjet, 1972; Nair & Pradhan, 1976). Double-strand breaks present greater difficulty and the repair might not be genetically correct. The complex systems which operate to repair damage to DNA that has been caused by irradiation might have evolved to correct naturally occurring errors in replication

(Lindahl, 1982). Irradiated microorganisms do not die immediately after a lethal dose has been absorbed. Bacterial motility, respiration and fermentation may continue for several hours and spores may commence germination. Death usually ensues during the first DNA replication and conditions such as low temperature, which delay this process, favour completion of the repair process. However, some gaps which remain in the DNA strands after the first replication process has been completed can be repaired by recombination (Bridges, 1976).

STABILITY OF MATERIALS TO IRRADIATION

Many of the materials that are used in the manufacture of medical devices or for their packaging are synthetic polymers. These consist of large molecules and their physical or chemical properties may be adversely affected by small chemical changes. Although most of them are much more stable to irradiation than they are to moist or dry heat, some undergo undesirable changes during or after radiation sterilization (Chapiro, 1974; Plester, 1974; Landfield, 1980). Articles that are intended for a single use only should withstand the highest dose, including local overdose, that will be used in the sterilization process.

Types of radiation-induced changes

Cross-linking between the polymer chains may occur, eventually resulting in a three-dimensional network which changes gums to a rubber-like consistency. Crystalline polymers become hard and brittle, but only at a very high dose. Degradative changes may accompany cross-linking or they may play the predominant role. Polypropylene, nylon and pressure-sensitive adhesives are subject to oxidative degradation. Polyvinyl chloride (PVC) and polyvinylidine chloride evolve hydrochloric acid and polytetrafluoroethylene (PTFE, or Teflon) evolves hydrogen fluoride. PVC discolours at 2.5 Mrad and Teflon disintegrates to a powder. Glass darkens on irradiation; this may be useful in the preparation of bottles for storing light-sensitive chemicals or pharmaceuticals. Cotton gauze can develop a yellow colour and undergoes a decrease

in strength; electron beam radiation does not reduce strength as much as does gamma radiation (Bradbury, 1974).

Factors influencing stability

1. *Physical or chemical structure of the material*: stability is favoured by the presence of a benzene ring in the polymer, especially if it is not part of the chain structure.
2. *Additives*: the presence in the formulation of substances with aromatic ring structures, as in phenolics, improves stability.
3. *Atmosphere during irradiation*: oxygen may enhance radiation-induced degradation. Oxidative deterioration of polypropylene may be reduced by the inclusion of an antioxidant in the formulation but stabilization of Teflon has so far been unsuccessful. PVC may be stabilized by the addition of complexes containing zinc, but the problem of the instability of this material has not yet been completely overcome.
4. *Dose rate*: materials such as polypropylene that are subject to oxidative degradation may withstand exposure to a similar dose from an electron accelerator. The very high dose rate of electron beam sterilization does not allow time for diffusion of oxygen into the material to replenish the loss which occurs during irradiation.
5. *Total dose*: as the effects of irradiation are cumulative, materials that are likely to undergo multiple treatments should be tested to dose levels up to or above 100 Mrad.
6. *Post-irradiation storage*: the development of adverse changes following irradiation is attributed to long-lived radicals that persist in materials such as polyethylene, cellulose and Teflon, where they are immobilized in the rigid structure. In rubber-like polymers the radicals are mobile and short-lived.

Levels of stability

Stability is usually rated on the response of the material to a single irradiation in the dose range 2.5–5 Mrad. Teflon is unsuitable for radiation sterilization but fluorinated ethylene copolymers are more resistant. Polyisobutylene is also unsuitable because it is converted to a sticky or oily consistency.

Polyvinyl chloride (PVC) and polypropylene are borderline in their stability to a process using 2.5 Mrad. Efforts are being made to stabilize them and these appear to have had some success with polyproplene. Tygon, a PVC copolymer, is stable to 2.5–3 Mrad. The other materials that are most commonly used – polyethylene (low- and high-density) and polystyrene – present no problems; polystyrene is one of the most stable synthetic materials. Phenolics, epoxy resins and adhesives (e.g. Araldite), polyester resins and mineral oils are also stable to high doses. Silicone rubber is more stable than are other types of rubber; however, silicone oil is stable only at a single-dose level.

SUSCEPTIBILITY OF MICROORGANISMS

Types and species

Microorganisms are much more resistant to ionizing radiation than are higher forms of life. In unicellular organisms the level of resistance is closely related to the volume of the DNA target. The general order of increasing resistance is shown in Table 8.2.

The wide range of doses that may be required for equivalent levels of inactivation reflects variation between genera, species and strains but may also be attributed to variation in the conditions in which irradiation is carried out. Bacterial spores are usually no more than 10 times as resistant as are vegetative bacteria. This is a small difference by comparison with their relative resistances to heat. The DNA in the spore core appears to be protected in vivo because, when extracted from the spore, it is as susceptible to irradiation as is that obtained from vegetative bacteria (Tanooka & Sakakibara, 1968). The mechanism of protection may be similar to that which confers resistance to heat on the constituents of the spore core.

Viruses may be classed as moderately or highly resistant, depending on the DNA volume; this is of more importance than the size of the particles. D values range from 0.39–0.53 Mrad (Sullivan et al, 1971). The resistance of the relatively large pox viruses corresponds to that of bacterial spores but the very small viruses that cause poliomyelitis in humans and foot-and-mouth disease in domestic animals are highly resistant. Bacterial viruses are extremely resistant. The 'slow' viruses such as those associated with the Creutzfeld-Jakob syndrome in man and scrapie in sheep are also highly resistant.

Some exceptions to the general order of resistance among vegetative bacteria, spores and viruses may be seen in Table 8.2. Cultures of Gram-positive cocci which were isolated from dust included strains of S. faecium with resistance

Table 8.2 Sensitivity of microorganisms to ionizing radiation

Group	Organisms	Sterilizing dose[1] Mrad
Sensitive	Vegetative bacteria (excluding some micrococci and streptococci)	0.05–1
Moderately resistant	Moulds and yeasts	0.4–3
	Streptococcus faecium (suspended in buffer)	1–3
Resistant	Bacterial spores	1–5
	Bacillus pumilus	1–3
	Clostridium botulinum (some strains)	3
	Some viruses	1–3
	Streptococcus faecium (dried from serum broth)	1–4.5
	Animal viruses (except foot-and-mouth disease virus)	3–4
Highly resistant	*Moraxella* (some strains)	¯5
	Micrococcus radiodurans	5.5–7
	Bacillus spores (contrived mutants)	3.5¯8
	Foot-and-mouth disease virus	¯5
	Bacterial viruses	wide range (one dose inadequate)

[1]Based on inactivation factor of 10^8 (8D)

in the range that is characteristic of bacterial spores (Christensen, 1964). The resistance of *M. radiodurans* (Anderson et al, 1956) and *M. radiophilus* (Lewis, 1971) is equivalent to· that of the very small viruses. The micrococci are associated with food sources but the streptococcus is an opportunistic pathogen. These bacteria appear to owe their resistance to the operation of very efficient repair mechanisms and the death rate curves are frequently characterized by a broad shoulder which extends until the absorbed dose is sufficient to inactivate the repair enzymes. Gram-negative bacilli in the genus *Moraxella* may also be highly resistant to irradiation (Welch & Maxcy, 1975). Some bacterial spores (e.g. *Bacillus sphaericus*, strain C_1A) appear to have increased in resistance by mutation. This might have occurred after repeated exposure to substerilizing doses of radiation; however, this procedure could also result in decreased resistance (Ley et al, 1970).

FACTORS INFLUENCING SENSITIVITY

Much of the variation in reported D values for organisms of the same or closely related species may be attributable to the influence of the environment before, during or immediately after irradiation. Analysis of the contribution of separate factors, such as oxygen, moisture or temperature, is difficult because the actions are often interdependent.

Oxygen

The resistance of microorganisms is usually increased 2–5 times if anoxic conditions are maintained during and after irradiation. The spores of *Bacillus pumilus,* for example, give a D value of 0.175 Mrad when irradiated in air and 0.306 Mrad in the absence of oxygen (Burt & Ley, 1963a). However, a small amount of oxygen is sufficient to ensure maximum sensitivity (Roberts & Hitchins, 1969). Potassium permanganate, which is a strong oxidizing agent, can substitute for molecular oxygen; it sensitizes spores to irradiation in anaerobic conditions but does not increase their sensitivity when oxygen is available (Tallentire & Jones, 1973).

Moisture

The influence of moisture on microbial susceptibility is complex because it is interrelated with that of oxygen.

Temperature

Thermoradiation

Radiation sterilization is normally carried out at ambient temperature, although some heat is generated when radiant energy is absorbed by the material treated or extraneous materials, including air, in the environment. Increases of the order of 10°C have been shown to reduce D values by as much as 50 per cent (Pallas & Hamdy, 1976).

The combined effects of radiation and moist or dry heat are potentially useful in the food industry. Kempe (1955) showed that prior irradiation sensitized spores of *Clostridium botulinum* to moist heat; there was no sensitization to irradiation if the order of treatment was reversed. Synergism is observed under certain conditions when heat and irradiation are applied simultaneously (Fisher & Pflug, 1977; Gombas & Gomez, 1978). A synergistic action is one in which the combined effect is greater than the sum of the separate effects. Fisher & Pflug (1977) demonstrated that each agent in the combination must be able to kill spores by itself and that synergism occurs in conditions when they are equally effective as separate sterilizing agents. Synergism has also been demonstrated in certain combinations of dry heat and irradiation (Sivinski et al, 1973). However, Emborg (1974) has expressed doubt about the applicability of combined radiation and heat treatment to the sterilization of medical devices.

Subzero temperature

The effect of irradiation on microorganisms in frozen substrates is important in relation to food. When spores of *Clostridium botulinum* (strain 33A) were irradiated in phosphate buffer and in pork pea broth, there was a sharp increase in resistance when freezing occurred. This was attributed to the reduction of indirect action as the active radicals produced in water were immobilized. A further reduction occurred gradually as the temperature was reduced to −196°C by means of liquid nitrogen (Grecz et al, 1967).

Organic substrates

Protection against radiation damage is conferred by dried serum broth (Christensen & Sehested, 1964), grease films (Burt & Ley, 1963a), sucrose and other complex substrates (Dyer et al, 1966). The protective effect is reflected by tailing death rate curves.

Chemical agents

Glycerol, thiourea, dimethyl sulphoxide and cysteine protect bacteria against radiation damage, possibly by scavenging free radicals. However other chemicals, including iodoacetic acid and potassium iodide, act as sensitizers (Lewis & Kumta, 1975); the effect may be due to an increase in the number of single-strand breaks through reaction of the iodine compound with radiolytic products of water (Mullenger et al, 1967) or other cell components (Shenoy et al, 1968).

The influence of some chemical agents occurs after irradiation, when the treated microorganisms are cultured to detect survivors. The susceptibility of bacterial spores to sodium chloride in the recovery medium increases in proportion to the radiation dose (Roberts et al, 1965).

STERILIZING DOSE

A radiation sterilization process is defined by a single parameter, the minimum absorbed dose. This is the amount of energy absorbed at sites in the load where the lowest dose is received. The time of exposure required to deliver the dose depends on the power, or output, of the radiation source and also on the average density of the material treated. Times range from fractions of a second in electron beam sterilization of small packs to several hours or even days for gamma radiation. Materials of different density, such as scalpel blades and cotton dressings, should not be treated by electron beam irradiation at the same time. Products with different densities can be sterilized simultaneously by gamma radiation if the total weight of material in each container is the same and the irradiation time is based on the high density material.

The dose is maintained at the specified level by adjustment of the conveyor speed as the output of a ^{60}Co source deteriorates. Although economics dictate that a gamma radiation plant should operate 95 per cent of the time, temporary shutdowns are necessary for maintenance, repair or admittance of visitors for educational purposes. The interruptions do not affect the dose to be delivered unless the period is unduly long and the nature of the material permits multiplication of microorganisms that are still viable (Borick & Fogarty, 1967; Burt & Ley, 1963b).

The sterilizing dose must be calculated for the particular goods because it is influenced by the number and resistance of the organisms initially present. The most resistant contaminants are usually bacterial spores but resistant Gram-positive cocci (Christensen, 1964) and yeasts (Ley et al, 1972) have been isolated from medical devices prior to sterilization. Another investigation, using fractional doses, did not indicate the presence of any organisms with a comparable level of resistance among the contaminants on goods which had been stored in adverse conditions (White, 1973). However, several highly resistant organisms (spore-formers, Gram-positive rods and cocci) have been isolated from presterilized sutures in Sweden, syringe needles and their production environment in Poland, and cellulosic material in Australia. Knowledge of the most resistant bacteria in the microbial population to be sterilized is important because they may determine the dose required, even if they constitute considerably less than 1 per cent of the total number.

If the D value for *B. pumilus* spores in anoxic conditions is taken as 0.3 Mrad a minimum dose of 2.5 Mrad (8D) would be sufficient, provided the contamination level does not exceed 100 organisms per item and the microorganisms are no more resistant than spores of *B. pumilus*. As most articles are irradiated in the presence of air, a dose based on the D value in anoxic conditions provides an additional safety margin. Many disposable products manufactured in the United States are being treated with doses from 1 to 2 Mrad, depending on the bioburden and the level of sterility assurance required for safety in use. However, doses ranging from 3.2 to 5.0 Mrad, depending on the number of contaminants initially present, have been recommended in Scandinavian countries.

It is the responsibility of the manufacturer of the product to determine the initial contamination level and ensure that it does not exceed the maximum level for which the dose has been calculated. When goods are treated at an independent sterilization facility, the operator's responsibility is limited to delivering the nominated dose. Devices such as hypodermic syringes and small catheters, which are moulded at a high temperature, usually carry fewer than 100 organisms per item if they have been assembled and packaged hygienically (Cook & Berry, 1968). Catgut sutures may contain up to 10^3 organisms, which are likely to include bacterial spores. Intravenous sets may be more heavily contaminated because of their size and complexity.

INSTALLATIONS FOR RADIATION STERILIZATION

Radiation sterilization is virtually limited to industrial applications because the installations are large, the safety precautions are elaborate and the cost is high. Gamma radiation (^{60}Co) plants are usually more costly than are electron accelerators. The design and construction of ^{60}Co installations and electron accelerators will be described briefly. A comparison of the relevant characteristics is made in Table 8.3.

^{60}Co installation

The installation is located within a larger building (Eymery, 1973). It consists of:

1. Irradiation chamber and annexes
2. ^{60}Co, as source of gamma radiation
3. Mechanical load conveyors
4. Process controls and safety systems.

The general layout of an installation designed for sterilization of medical devices is shown in Figure 8.1.

Chamber and annexes

The walls are constructed of reinforced concrete, up to two metres thick. The size of the irradiation chamber is determined by that of the ^{60}Co source and the load conveyors. A storage tank below floor level for the radioactive source is also constructed from concrete, and may be lined with stainless steel; it must be independent of the chamber construction for protection against earthquake damage. The tank is filled with deionized water to a depth of five metres. Dry storage in a concrete-lined pit, covered with a removable lead plug, may be used for relatively small ^{60}Co sources but is less convenient for adding new elements. The annexes to the chamber include labyrinthine corridors to prevent escape of radiation to the environment during entry and exit of load units. Both chamber and annexes are ventilated to remove ozone and oxides of nitrogen.

Table 8.3 Performance characteristics of cobalt–60 installations and electron accelerators

Characteristics	Cobalt–60 source	Electron accelerator
Energy level	1.333 and 1.173 MeV	Electrostatic 0.2–5 MeV Microwave 2–10 MeV
Penetration (unit density material)	*Ca* 30 cm (depending on source strength)	0.33 cm/MeV
Dose rate	Slow (10 Gy/s, or 10^3 rad/s)	Fast (10^6–10^{12} Gy/s, or 10^8–10^{14} rad/s)
Processing time	Long (several hours)	Short (<1 s)
Size of packs treated	Large (final cartons)	Small (single products or small cartons)
Load conveyors	Horizontal and vertical movements	Horizontal (conveyor belt)
Process controls	Conveyor speed only	Conveyor speed Scan width Beam current, energy Pulse duration and frequency
Safety measures	Source storage tank Chamber construction External indicator/control panel Ozone removal	Machine switched off Shielding to contain X-radiation Ozone removal

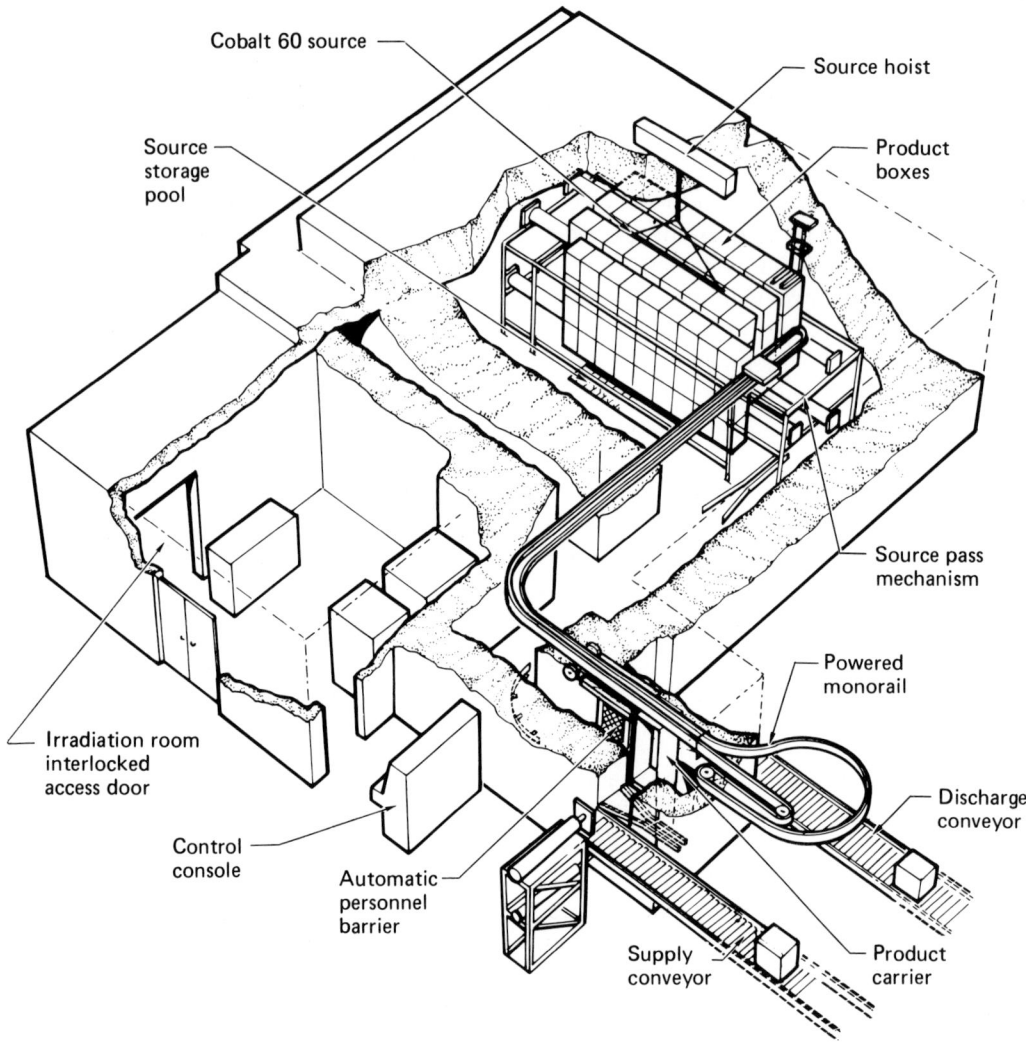

Fig. 8.1 A cobalt–60 installation for radiation sterilization (built by Atomic Energy of Canada Ltd).

^{60}Co source

The radioactive isotope is contained in metal tubes, or 'rods'. They arrive at the radiation facility in a lead transport container, which is lowered into the water-filled tank. The depth of five metres allows space for lifting the source elements from the container without emitting more than 0.1 millirad at the water surface. They are transferred by means of long-handled tools to a rectangular frame which is suspended by a mechanical hoist. The frame is not filled and rods of different ages are positioned to distribute the dose evenly to the large bulk of material. About once a year new rods are added and the necessary rearrangements are made. Spent rods are removed when all frame positions are filled. Large sources can contain 1 MCi of ^{60}Co, with a power output of 30 kilowatts or 30 kilojoules per second.

Load conveyors

The first conveyor moves standard size cartons or metal containers through a small entry port, which opens automatically at regular intervals to admit one unit, and conveys them through the approach corridors to the irradiation chamber. Here they are transferred to the irradiation conveyor, which is designed so that the load surrounds the source as completely as possible to minimize dose wastage. The cartons are moved slowly through several positions on both sides of the source until the prescribed minimum dose has been delivered. They are then transferred to another conveyor which moves them through the exit to a storage area, which is physically separated from the place where the cartons awaiting treatment are held.

Controls and safety precautions

The control panel outside the unit includes indicators of the position of the ^{60}Co source (elevated or in storage), the conveyor speed and the water level in the storage tank. The conveyor speed is adjusted periodically to compensate for source deterioration. The source elevator must be completely reliable and should return automatically to the storage position if there is any malfunction in the system. Controls are installed to ensure that the source cannot be raised to the operating position unless the chamber has been locked. Entrance of personnel to the irradiation chamber is possible only when the source is in the storage position and monitors have confirmed that the radiation has fallen to the background level. Radiation monitors should be placed at the entrance to the corridor, inside the chamber, near the air exhaust filter and the water deionizer. Monitors to verify that ozone has been effectively removed by the air-exchange system are also required.

Electron accelerators

In an electron accelerating machine low-energy electrons from the emitting surface of a hot filament are accelerated in a vacuum to high velocity and emerge through a thin window. In industrial practice, the limit is set at 10 MeV to obviate any possibility of inducing radioactivity in the irradiated material. There are two types of electron accelerators.

Electrostatic accelerators

This type operates at 0.2–5 MeV. The electrons are accelerated by travelling in an evacuated tube

through a high voltage, which may be generated by an insulating core transformer, a 'dynamitron', a Van de Graaff generator or a simple power transformer.

Microwave linear accelerators

These machines operate at 2–10 MeV. Energy is supplied to a pulse of electrons in the accelerating tube by a synchronized travelling microwave field. In pulsed systems the dose is delivered almost instantaneously (Nablo, 1974). Accessory equipment for electron accelerators includes a vacuum pump, water cooling system, operational controls and safety interlock systems.

The beam of high-energy electrons is focussed and shaped before emerging through a thin metal window. It may be rapidly scanned to and fro across the width of a horizontal conveyor belt, which carries a single layer of small packs. The operating characteristics of an electron accelerator are described by the energy (penetration), power (voltage × current), and efficiency. In pulsed systems allowance must be made for the pulse duration and pulse frequency.

Electrons penetrate effectively 0.33 cm into material of unit density but sometimes irradiation is carried out from both sides. Dual purpose machines have been designed which can readily be converted to X-ray mode to irradiate bulky packages.

Controls and safety precautions

Unlike a gamma radiation source, the electron beam can be turned off by a switch. Larger accelerators require shielding which is similar to that of a ^{60}Co installation because X-rays are produced when the electrons strike metal parts of the conveyor. Small machines may be locally shielded.

VALIDATION AND CONTROL OF RADIATION STERILIZATION

Commissioning the installation

The following procedures are involved in commissioning a gamma radiation facility:

1. Investigation of the level and distribution of activity of the radioactive source
2. Determination of the dose distribution in a load of suitable density and configuration
3. Determination of the time spent by each product unit in the various positions around the source.

The performance of conveyors and settings of timers must also be checked and recorded.

Setting the dose

The principles governing determination of the appropriate radiation dose for a particular product have been explained in an earlier section. Dose setting is based on the contamination level (bioburden) of the articles and the resistance of the microorganisms. The level of resistance may be determined by different methods (Masefield, 1982). When the average number of contaminants has been estimated, a 'worst case' distribution of resistance in the microbial population can be obtained from available tabulated data. However, detailed analysis of the bioburden may be avoided by subjection of samples of the product to incremental dosing and selection of the most resistant contaminants. D values are then determined for one or several isolates from the survivors of a dose that yielded 1 per cent of unsterile samples. The same methods apply to electron beam sterilization.

Measuring the dose

Doses may be monitored by primary or secondary dosimeters. The primary (reference) dosimeter is a chemical system that undergoes oxidation-reduction reactions in response to irradiation. A dose range of 0.1 to 4 Mrad is possible using ceric or ceric-cerous sulphate solutions as the reference dosimetry system. The radiation-induced reduction of ceric to cerous ions can be measured spectrophotometrically or electrochemically. A direct-reading dose meter is commercially available for this purpose. Calorimetry and other physical methods may also be used.

The secondary dosimeters are small strips (3 mm thick) or pellets of clear, amber or red Perspex that darken or change colour in proportion to the dose of radiation. The degree of darkening is measured in a spectrophotometer using light of a suitable wavelength. This method is reasonably accurate for doses up to 4 Mrad but each batch of Perspex must be calibrated against a reference dosimeter.

Radiochromic plastic films of nylon, polyvinyl chloride (PVC), or other material, the response of which is independent of the dose rate, may be used for electron beam or gamma sterilization. All types of secondary dosimeters must be calibrated against a reference dosimeter; however, radiation users should be aware that all reference and secondary dosimetry systems have limitations and technical problems and a completely reliable meter remains to be developed.

Process indicator discs with various dyes are commercially available. The colour changes include yellow to red, green to brown and other combinations. As these discs change colour at 1–2 Mrad, they do not verify that a dose of 2.5 Mrad has been received.

Biological indicators

If the use of biological indicators is desired, or is required by regulation, spores of a designated strain of *B. pumilus* (E601) may be used to validate or monitor processes using a dose of 2.5 Mrad. Specified strains of more resistant microorganisms (e.g. *S. faecium* $A_2 1$, a bacteriophage or spores of a mutant strain of *B. sphaericus,* $C_1 A$) are required for doses exceeding 2.5 Mrad (Christensen et al, 1969). Although biological indicators for routine control are usually considered unnecessary, the use of resistant test strains of bacteria or spores has been recommended as part of the procedure of commissioning a new radiation facility (Christensen, 1978).

Product sterility tests

The value of sterility tests on articles sterilized by irradiation is limited to situations where a gross fault in preparation, packaging or sterilization might have occurred. If contamination is detected in a sterility test, the microorganism should be identified in order to distinguish between real and accidental contamination. The packages should be inspected for integrity of the material and the sealing area before a sterility test is carried out.

Product release

Regulations governing the sterilization and release of irradiated products for distribution vary in different countries but are a continuing subject of international discussion. Reliance is placed entirely on dosimetry in the United Kingdom, Scandinavian countries and Australia, provided the production and sterilization processes have been evaluated according to the relevant code of Good Manufacturing Practice or other recommendations. Supplementary use of biological indicators is required only for validation of the process. At the other extreme, French regulations require daily use of biological indicators (Gaughran, 1982).

APPLICATIONS OF RADIATION STERILIZATION

The sterilization of medical supplies by gamma radiation from ^{60}Co or high-energy electrons commenced in parallel with the introduction of synthetic materials that do not withstand moist or dry heat sterilization. Radiation sterilization must compete with industrial ethylene oxide sterilization. The high capital costs of gamma installations and electron accelerators can be a deterrent and availability at a convenient location is also important. Some installations are operated independently, accepting goods from different manufacturers and also, on a small scale, from hospitals. Others are installed by large companies to sterilize their own products.

Advantages of radiation sterilization are:

1. The process is operated at ambient temperature
2. The materials are not wetted or significantly heated
3. Packaging materials which act as a complete bacterial barrier may be used and the articles may be packed and sealed into the outer containers
4. The process is continuous and controlled by the time of irradiation (i.e. the speed of the in-cell conveyor).

The principal disadvantage is the possibility of deleterious effects on the articles or packaging material. These may limit or preclude radiation sterilization of some electronic equipment, devices made from unstable plastics and many pharmaceuticals and foods. The low penetrability of electrons limits electron beam sterilization to small volume, low-density products.

Medical equipment

Commercially produced items of equipment for medical use are usually classed as therapeutic devices and covered by regulations similar to those that apply to pharmaceuticals. Most are intended for a single use only; if limited reuse is permissible, directions for resterilization should be specified. Polyethylene, which may be laminated with polyester, nylon, paper or metal foil is the most widely used packaging material. Tyvek, a spunbonded polyethylene, may also be used. PVC is less satisfactory and cellophane and cotton are unsuitable.

Reusable heat-sensitive equipment, which has been cleaned and packed in a hospital, may be sent to a gamma radiation facility for sterilization. This is a useful service, provided the necessary prerequisites of physical cleanliness and a low contamination level can be fulfilled, but it involves certain risks. Fine tubes, such as cardiac catheters, should not be reused because internal cleanliness cannot be verified. Knowledge of the stability of the articles and packaging material to repeated irradiation is required and the effect, if any, of irradiation on the function of electronic components. These precautions are the responsibility of the hospital authority, not of the radiation facility.

Some types of articles which may be sterilized by ionizing radiation are presented in Table 8.4. However, they represent only a small fraction of the total and no list would be complete because new heat-sensitive items may be added, while others may be altered in design or construction with the result that they can be sterilized by heat.

Pharmaceutical and biological products

Irradiation has been investigated as a method of sterilizing heat-sensitive organic materials, includ-

Table 8.4 Some articles sterilized by irradiation (Sztanyik, 1974)

Types of equipment or material	Examples	
Medical equipment	Sutures	Procedure trays
	Syringes	Urine, colostomy bags
	Needles	Inhalation therapy equipment
	Scalpels	Oxygen tents
	Lancets	Oxygen masks
	Razors	Eye droppers
	Forceps	Feeding bottles
	Infusion sets	Brushes, sponges
	Transfusion sets	Gloves
	Blood collecting sets	Dressings
	Dialysers	Bandages
	Blood oxygenators	Pads
	Endotracheal tubes	Swabs
	Cannulae	Adhesive plasters
	Catheters	Acrylic powders
	Drains	Talc
	Tracheostomy tubes	
Biological materials	Aortic valves	Enzymes
	Arterial prostheses	Vaccines
	Bone, cartilage (freeze-dried)	
Pharmaceuticals	Antibiotics (dry)	Eye drops
	Disinfectants (alcohol, QACs)	Eye ointments
	Steroids	Vitamins
Laboratory equipment	Containers	Petri dishes
	Closures	Test tubes

ing drugs, antibiotics, hormones and vaccines (Wills, 1963). Each product must be evaluated in relation to its intended use and the possible risks. Official approval of the process, based on prescribed safety tests for new pharmaceutical products, is required because chemical changes may inactivate drugs or antibiotics, destroy emulsions or produce harmful substances.

Electron beam sterilization at high dose rates, which create anoxic conditions in solutions, may be less damaging to some products than is sterilization by gamma radiation (Diding et al, 1978). Dry solids and oily preparations are generally more stable to irradiation than are aqueous solutions and suspensions. Discoloration does not necessarily indicate loss of antimicrobial or pharmacological activity. Freeze-dried penicillin and streptomycin and some other antibiotics are stable to irradiation. Cortisone and ACTH may be irradiated in solid form but suspensions and solutions are unstable. Irradiation is satisfactory for albumin, iodinated albumin and dry protease enzymes but blood plasma proteins, iodinated albumin in solution, insulin, heparin, thrombin, thyroxine and

organometal compounds are very unstable. Sodium alginate and acacia gums are stable in powdered form but lose viscosity if they are irradiated as solutions (Hartman et al, 1975). Tragacanth, which has been irradiated as a powder, gives solutions of reduced viscosity.

The vitamin B complex is stable in dry and injectable forms but the separate components are not. Vitamin C can be irradiated in dry form, in concentrated solutions and in dilute frozen solutions. Vitamin E, calciferol and ergosterol are unstable. Morphine sulphate, ergometrine maleate and procaine hydrochloride are moderately stable when dry, but atropine sulphate cannot be irradiated successfully.

Non-living graft materials, such as blood vessels, freeze-dried bone, cartilage and homograft aortic valves have given satisfactory performance after sterilization by irradiation. Some success has been achieved with vaccines and antisera.

Complex formulations of pharmaceuticals, cosmetics and toiletries, which do not have to be sterile, and some heavily contaminated raw materials, such as starch, talc and pancreatin, may be treated by a dose up to 1 Mrad to reduce the number of viable organisms to an acceptable level. Recent advances in the irradiation of drugs and antibiotics have been discussed by Diding et al (1978) and Power (1978). Among the chemical disinfectants, isopropyl alcohol and quaternary ammonium compounds, are stable to irradiation (e.g. as skin swabs) but chlorhexidine is inactivated.

Food

Interest in the use of gamma radiation for sterilization or pasteurization of food has fluctuated in the past but is now increasing as data concerning the effects of the process on nutrient quality and consumer safety become available. Three types of processes have been described (Joint FAO/IAEA/WHO Expert Committee, 1981). Low-dose treatment up to 1 kGy, or 0.1 Mrad, is adequate to inhibit sprouting, kill insects or delay ripening. Medium doses of 1–10 kGy (0.1–1 Mrad) are effective in reducing the number of microorganisms and improving the properties of food. The third type, embracing a dose range of 10–50 kGy (1–5 Mrad), is required for commercial sterilization or for the inactivation of viruses.

Studies by the Expert Committee led to the conclusions that similar reactions occur when the same food constituents (proteins, fats, carbohydrates or water) are irradiated and that the radiolytic products are predictable in nature and yield, and data obtained on one product can be applied to others of similar composition. A large amount of evidence, mainly from feeding diets that have been irradiated at doses up to 15 Mrad to half a million germfree animals, has led to the conclusion that food which has been irradiated with doses up to 10 kGy (1 Mrad) presents no danger to humans, including immunosuppressed patients. Nutritional and microbiological quality has also proved satisfactory. Irradiated food is still subject to spoilage by enzymes, but this can be prevented by mild heat treatment.

Industrial materials

Animal products such as hides, wool or hair for use in carpet manufacture, are sometimes heavily contaminated with anthrax spores and constitute a serious health risk for people who handle them. A dose of 1.5 Mrad would provide a margin of safety for *Bacillus anthracis* (Horne et al, 1959) but would not be effective against the foot-and-mouth disease virus.

REFERENCES

Anderson A W, Nordan H C, Cain R F, Parrish G, Dugg/ 1956 Studies on a radio-resistant micrococcus. I. Isol morphology, cultural characteristics, and resistance gamma radiation. Food Technology 10: 575–578

Borick P M, Fogarty M G 1967 Effects of continuous ¿ interrupted radiation on microorganisms. Applied Microbiology 15: 785–789

Bradbury W C 1974 Physical and chemical effects of ionizing radiation on cellulosic material. In: Gaughran E R L, Goudie A J (eds) Technical developments and prospects of sterilization by ionizing radiation. Multiscience, Montreal, p 387

Bridges B A 1976 Survival of bacteria following exposure to ultraviolet and ionizing radiations. In: Gray T R G, Postgate J R (eds) The survival of vegetative microbes. Cambridge University Press, p 183

Burt M M, Ley F J 1963a Studies on the dose requirement for the radiation sterilization of medical equipment. I. Influence of suspending media. Journal of Applied Bacteriology 26: 484–489

Burt M M, Ley F J 1963b Studies on the dose requirement for the radiation sterilization of medical equipment. II. A comparison between continuous and fractionated doses. Journal of Applied Bacteriology 26: 490–492

Chapiro A 1974 Physical and chemical effects of ionizing radiations on polymeric systems. In: Gaughran E R L, Goudie A J (eds) Technical developments and prospects of sterilization by ionizing radiation. Multiscience, Montreal, p 367

Christensen E A 1964 Radiation resistance of enterococci dried in air. Acta Pathologica et Microbiologica Scandinavica 61: 483–486

Christensen E A 1978 The role of microbiology in commissioning a new facility and in routine control. In: Gaughran E R L, Goudie A J (eds) Sterilization of medical products by ionizing radiation. Multiscience, Montreal, p 50

Christensen E A, Kallings L O, Fystro D 1969 Microbiological control of sterilization procedures and standards for the sterilization of medical equipment. Ugeskrift for Laeger 131: 2123 (Translation p 1–15)

Christensen E A, Sehested K 1964 Radiation resistance of *Streptococcus faecium* and spores of *Bacillus subtilis* dried in various media. Acta Pathologica et Microbiologica Scandinavica 62: 448–458

Cook A M, Berry R J 1968 Microbial contamination on disposable hypodermic syringes prior to sterilization by ionizing radiation. Applied Microbiology 16: 1156–1162

Diding N, Flink Ö, Hohansson S, Ohlson B, Redmalm G, Ohrner B 1978 Irradiation of drugs with Co–60 and electrons. In: Gaughran E R L, Goudie A J (eds) Sterilization of medical products by ionizing radiation. Multiscience, Montreal, p 216

Dyer J K, Anderson A W, Dutiyabodhi P 1966 Radiation survival of food pathogens in complex media. Applied Microbiology 14: 92–97

Emborg C 1974 Inactivation of dried bacteria and bacterial spores by means of gamma radiation at high temperatures. Applied Microbiology 27: 830–833

Eymery R 1973 Design of radiation sterilization facilities. In: Phillips G B, Miller W S (eds) Industrial sterilization. Duke University Press, Durham, ch 11, p 153

Eymery R 1974 The prospects of using cesium for radiosterilization. In: Gaughran E R L, Goudie A J (eds) Technical developments and prospects of sterilization by ionizing radiation. Multiscience, Montreal, p 173

Fisher D A, Pflug I J 1977 Effect of combined heat and radiation on microbial destruction. Applied and Environmental Microbiology 33: 1170–1176

Gaughran E R L 1982 International aspects of radiation sterilization processing. Medical Device & Diagnostic Industry 4(9): 33–35, 70, 72

Gombas D E, Gomez R F 1978 Sensitization of *Clostridium perfringens* spores to heat by gamma radiation. Applied and Environmental Microbiology 36: 403–407

Grecz N, Upadhyay J, Tang T C 1967 Effect of temperature on radiation resistance of spores of *Clostridium botulinum* 33A. Canadian Journal of Microbiology 13: 287–293

Hartman A W, Nesbitt R U Jr, Smith F M, Nuessle N O 1975 Viscosities of acacia and sodium alginate after sterilization by cobalt-60. Journal of Pharmaceutical Sciences 64: 802–805

Haynes R H 1966 The interpretation of microbial inactivation and recovery phenomena. Radiation Research Supplement 6: 1–29

Horne T, Turner G C, Willis A T 1959 Inactivation of spores of *Bacillus anthracis* by γ-radiation. Nature 183: 475–476

Joint FAO/IAEA/WHO Expert Committee 1981 Wholesomeness of irradiated food. World Health Organization Technical Report Series 659: 1–34

Kaplan H S, Smith K C, Tomlin P A 1962 Effect of halogenated pyrimidines on radiosensitivity of *E. coli*. Radiation Research 16: 98–113

Kempe L L 1955 Combined effects of heat and radiation in food sterilization. Applied Microbiology 3: 346–352

Krinsky N I 1976 Cellular damage initiated by visible light. In: Gray T R G, Postgate J R (eds) The survival of vegetative microbes. Cambridge University Press, p 209

Landfield H 1980 Radiation effects on device and packaging materials. Medical Device & Diagnostic Industry 2 (5): 45–48

Latarjet R 1972 Interaction of radiation energy with nucleic acids. Current Topics in Radiation Research Quarterly 8: 1–38

Lewis N F 1971 Studies on a radio-resistant coccus isolated from Bombay duck (*Harpodon nehereus*). Journal of General Microbiology 66: 29–35

Lewis N, Kumta U 1975 Radiosensitization of *Micrococcus radiophilus*. Radiation Research 62: 159–163

Ley F J, Kennedy T S, Kawashima K, Roberts D, Hobbs B C 1970 The use of gamma radiation for the elimination of *Salmonella* from frozen meat. Journal of Hygiene 68: 293–311

Ley F J, Winsley B, Harbord P, Keall A, Summers T 1972 Radiation sterilization: microbiological findings from subprocess dose treatment of disposable plastic syringes. Journal of Applied Bacteriology 35: 53–61

Lindahl T 1982 DNA repair enzymes. Annual Review of Biochemistry 51: 61–87

Masefield J 1982 Recent developments in radiation sterilization process controls. Medical Device & Diagnostic Industry 4 (3): 21–22

Miller D R 1970 Theoretical survival curves for radiation damage in bacteria. Journal of Theoretical Biology 26: 383–398

Mullenger L, Singh B B, Ormerod M G, Dean C J 1967 Chemical study of the radiosensitization of *Micrococcus sodonensis* by iodine compounds. Nature 216: 372–374

Myers D K, Childs J D, Jones A R 1977 Sensitization of bacteriophage T_4 to ^{60}Co-γ radiation and to low-energy X radiation by bromouracil. Radiation Research 69: 152–165

Nablo S V 1974 Developments in transformer accelerators and the technology of pulsed electron sterilization at ultra-high dose rates. In: Gaughran E R L, Goudie A J (eds) Technical developments and prospects of sterilization by ionizing radiation. Multiscience, Montreal, p 51

Nair C K K, Pradhan D S 1976 Production and rejoining of single-strand breaks in DNA of *Escherichia coli* cells after exposure to gamma-rays in the presence of iodoacetic acid under oxic and anoxic conditions. International Journal of Radiation Biology 29: 235–240

Pallas J E, Hamdy M K 1976 Effects of thermoradiation on bacteria. Applied and Environmental Microbiology 32: 250–256

Plester D W 1974 Physical and chemical effects of ionizing radiation on plastic films, laminates and packaging materials. In: Gaughran E R L, Goudie A J (eds) Technical developments and prospects of sterilization by ionizing radiation. Multiscience, Montreal, p 375

Pollard E C, Davis S A 1970 The action of ionizing radiation on transcription (and translation) in several strains of *Escherichia coli*. Radiation Research 41: 375–399

Power D M 1978 Physical-chemical changes in irradiated drugs. In: Gaughran E R L, Goudie A J (eds) Sterilization of medical products by ionizing radiation. Multiscience, Montreal, p 237

Resnick M A 1976 The repair of double-strand breaks in DNA: a model involving recombination. Journal of Theoretical Biology 59: 97–106

Roberts T A, Ditchett P J, Ingram N 1965 The effect of sodium chloride on radiation resistance and recovery of irradiated anaerobic spores. Journal of Applied Bacteriology 28: 336–348

Roberts T A, Hitchins A D 1969 Resistance of spores. In: Gould G W, Hurst A (eds) The bacterial spore. Academic Press, London, ch 16, p 611

Shenoy M A, Singh B B, Gopal-Ayengar A R 1968 Iodine incorporated in cell constituents during sensitization to radiation by iodoacetic acid. Science 160: 999

Shragge P C, Hunt J W 1974 A pulse radiolysis study of the free radical intermediates in the radiolysis of uracil. Radiation Research 60: 233–249

Shragge P C, Varghese A J, Hunt J W, Greenstock C L 1974 Radiolysis of uracil in the absence of oxygen. Radiation Research 60: 250–267

Sivinski H D, Garst D M, Reynolds M C, Trauth C A Jr, Trujillo R E, Whitfield W J 1973 The synergistic inactivation of biological systems by thermoradiation. In: Phillips G B, Miller W S (eds) Industrial sterilization. Duke University Press, Durham, p 305

Skulberg A 1965 The resistance of *Clostridium botulinum* type E toxin to radiation. Journal of Applied Bacteriology 28: 139–141

Sullivan R, Fassolitis A C, Larkin E P, Read R B Jr, Peeler J T

1971 Inactivation of thirty viruses by gamma radiation. Applied Microbiology 22: 61–65

Sztanyik L B 1974 Application of ionizing radiation to sterilization. In: Gaughran E R L, Goudie A J (eds) Technical developments and prospects of sterilization by ionizing radiation. Multiscience, Montreal, p 6

Tallentire A, Jones A B 1973 Radiosensitization of bacterial spores by potassium permanganate. International Journal of Radiation Biology 24: 345–354

Tanooka H, Sakakibara Y 1968 Radioresistant nature of the transforming activity of DNA in bacterial spores. Biochimica et Biophysica Acta 155: 130–142

Ulmer K M, Gomez R F, Sinskey A J 1979 Ionizing radiation damage to the folded chromosome of *Escherichia coli* K 12: repair of double-strand breaks in deoxyribonucleic acid. Journal of Bacteriology 138: 486–491

Welch A B, Maxcy R B 1975 Characterization of radiation-resistant vegetative bacteria in beef. Applied Microbiology 30: 242–250

White J D M 1973 Biological control of industrial gamma radiation sterilization. In: Phillips G B, Miller W S (eds) Industrial sterilization. Duke University Press, Durham, p 101

Wills P A 1963 Effects of ionising radiation on pharmaceuticals. Australian Journal of Pharmacy Supplement 44: S50–S57

FILTRATION OF LIQUIDS

Types of Filters
  Fibrous filters
  Membrane filters

The Filtration Process
  Sterilization of filters
  Pretreatment of filters or solutions
  Prefilters
  Pressure and vacuum filtration

Testing Efficiency of Filtration
  Bubble point test
  Bacteriological tests

Applications of Membrane Filtration
  Pharmaceuticals
  Biological materials
  Microbiological culture media
  Industrial applications
  Sterility tests
  Bacteriological investigations

FILTRATION OF AIR

Fibrous Depth Filters
  Mechanisms of filtration
  Factors influencing efficiency
  Design of fibrous depth filters

Granular Carbon Filters

Fibrous (Paper) Sheet Filters
  Efficiency of HEPA filters
  Disinfection of used filters

Membrane Filters

Tests for Efficiency of Air Filters
  Installations for testing
  Chemical aerosols
  Microbial aerosols

Applications of HEPA Air Filters
  Protective environments
  Mechanical ventilators
  Suction apparatus
  Compressed gases
  Laboratory effluents

9

Filtration of liquids and air

Filtration differs from other methods of sterilization as it does not involve killing microorganisms or inhibiting their growth. Living and non-living particles are removed from liquids and gases by passage through fibrous, granular or synthetic membrane filters of appropriate retention efficiency. Fibrous and granular depth filters trap small particles in tortuous channels within the filter bed. Membrane filters act as screen filters; they are traversed by channels which retain particles that are larger than the pore size. The mechanisms by which microorganisms are trapped by depth filters and screen filters are illustrated in Figure 9.1. The filtration of liquids and air will be discussed in separate sections of this chapter.

FILTRATION OF LIQUIDS

Liquids are filtered for the following purposes:

1. 'Sterile' filtration (removal of microorganisms from heat-sensitive aqueous solutions, organic solvents or oils)
2. Sterility testing of pharmaceutical products and medical devices
3. Collection of bacteria from water samples or other dilute suspensions for enumeration and identification.

TYPES OF FILTERS

Depth filters may be composed of unglazed ear-

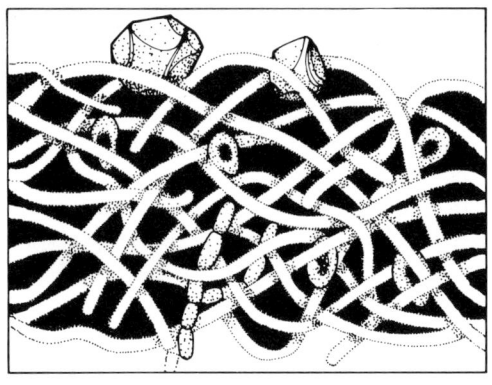

Depth filter

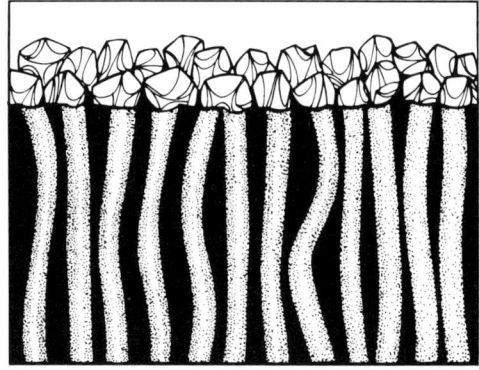

Screen filter

Fig. 9.1 Mechanisms by which microorganisms are trapped in depth and screen filters (Courtesy of Millipore Pty Ltd).

thenware or porcelain, sintered glass or compacted asbestos and cellulose fibres. Earthenware, porcelain and sintered glass filters are no longer used for microbial filtration because they are subject to cracking, clog easily and are difficult to clean for reuse. Ceramic filters are extensively used for purposes of clarification and purification but will not be discussed in the context of bacterial filtration. A brief account of fibrous depth filters, which also have limited application, will be given but the remainder of this section on liquids will be devoted to membrane filtration.

Fibrous filters

Fibrous filters are pads containing asbestos fibres mixed with cellulose filling material. Retention efficiency depends on the proportion of asbestos, to which the bacteria are selectively adsorbed. The pores are much larger than the particles removed but the channels are of uneven diameter and change direction frequently within the filter bed. The maximum pore diameter determines the size of particles retained.

The filter pads are clamped into metal holders, with perforated supporting plates, and the assembly is sterilized by steam under pressure at 121°C. The clamps are tightened after sterilization, when the filter and sterile receiver are assembled for use. Filtration may be carried out under vacuum, with an open funnel, or under positive pressure with a closed funnel. Uniform pressure is important and the pressure differential should not exceed 35–70 kPa because compression of the mat would decrease the flow rate. The liquid which remains in the filter must not be driven or sucked through because the pad will channel or crack, providing access to the filtrate for microbial contaminants. The filters are discarded after a single use.

Asbestos filters may still be used in laboratories for sterilization of heat-sensitive bacteriological culture media or concentrated solutions of heat-sensitive ingredients, such as serum or sugars, before they are added aseptically to an autoclaved solution of the heat-stable components. Large multiplate filters, which have been used in the past to produce sterile water in hospitals, are unsuitable for this purpose because the outlet invariably becomes heavily contaminated during use.

Asbestos filters have a high dirt-holding capacity but their use has declined for the following reasons:

1. Resistance to flow is high because the total pore volume is low (20–30 per cent)
2. A significant volume of the solution is lost by retention in the filter pad
3. Components of the solution (e.g. proteins, enzymes and antibiotics) may be adsorbed, reducing the concentration in the filtrate
4. Alkalinity in the filtrate may necessitate rejection of the first portion that passes through the filter
5. Fibres are shed into the filtrate
6. Penetration of microorganisms depends on the time required for filtration and some eventually pass through

7. Asbestos is a recognized health hazard.

Membrane filters

Types of membranes

Synthetic membrane filters are prepared from mixed cellulose esters (acetate and nitrate) for general use. Polytetrafluoroethylene (Teflon) and polyvinylidene fluoride are used to make more resistant, hydrophobic filters which are required for strongly acid or alkaline solutions or nonaqueous liquids, such as organic solvents and oils. Membranes with a hydrophobic edge are used for sterility tests on solutions containing antimicrobial agents. Filters with a large surface area, which are sealed into cartridges, may be made from polycarbonate or a more flexible acrylic-polyvinyl chloride (PVC) copolymer which can be pleated. The membranes are 125–150 μm in thickness and are traversed by channels of uniform diameter, without major deviations or lateral connections. The circular discs are 13–293 mm in diameter.

Membrane filters have a low dirt-handling capacity compared with fibrous depth filters and are easily clogged by particles that are just larger than the pore diameter; however, they have several advantages over the fibrous filters:

1. All particles larger than the pore diameter are retained and bacteria cannot pass through
2. A large pore volume (80 per cent of the filter) ensures an adequate flow rate
3. The volume of liquid retained in the membrane is small and can be expelled without breaking sterility
4. The quality of the filtrate is not altered by adsorption of solutes or contamination with foreign material.

Grades of membrane filters

The filters are graded according to the pore size, which is related to their intended use. Prefilters with a pore diameter of 0.8 or 1.2 μm are used to prolong the life of the high-efficiency filters. Two grades of bacterial filters are manufactured; a pore diameter of 0.45 μm is satisfactory for recovering bacteria from liquids but a diameter of 0.22 μm or 0.2 μm (depending on the brand) is required for

producing bacteria-free filtrates. Pore sizes from 0.01–0.1 μm are required for complete retention of viruses and mycoplasmas, although the latter might be successfully retained by serial passage through two bacterial grade filters.

Membrane filters are subject to blockage by particles which are just above the pore diameter in size, and some virus particles that are held in the channels may reduce the flow rate. Large particles do not affect the flow rate significantly but form a porous mat which retains many smaller particles, including viruses, as it builds up.

Membrane filter holders

Membrane filters are delicate and must be supported on a porous or perforated disc. Many types of filter holders are available from the firms that manufacture the membranes. The design and efficiency of the holder and provision for collection of the sterile filtrates are as critical to successful filtration as the quality of the membrane itself. Some types of apparatus for use with membranes ranging from 13–293 mm diameter are illustrated in Figure 9.2. The approximate scale of each diagram may be judged from the indicated size of the membrane.

Diagram A in Figure 9.2 represents a filter holder with an open funnel; this model is commonly used for filtration of volumes up to 300 ml. Filtration is operated by suction.

Diagram B shows an assembly with a closed funnel. It may be made from plastic, glass or metal and is designed for sterility testing, when the membrane must be protected from extraneous contamination. The lid is fitted with closed or filtered entry ports for introduction of the liquid, admission of air as the volume of liquid in the reservoir decreases and admission of steam for sterilization. Presterilized filters in small disposable polypropylene chambers have become available for sterility tests. The pooled sample is divided between two or three of these units, as required, by a peristaltic pump. After addition of the appropriate culture media, the units are incubated intact.

Diagram C represents a miniature line filter (Swinny or Swinnex type). It has a Luer-lock fitting on the inlet for connection to a syringe, which holds the liquid and supplies it to the filter under positive

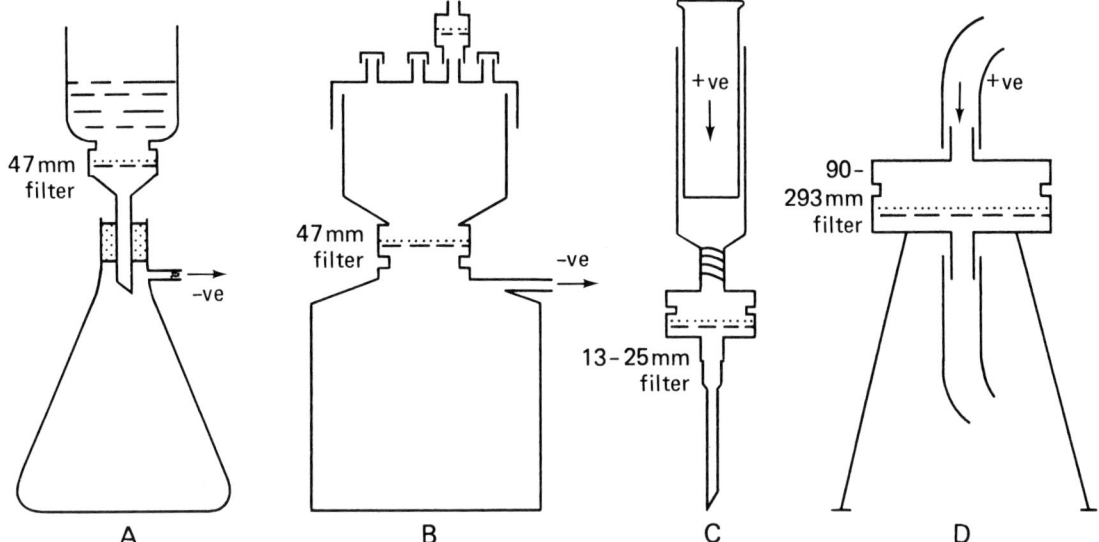

Fig. 9.2 Some types of apparatus for membrane filtration.

pressure exerted by the plunger. This type of apparatus is designed for small scale filtration of pharmaceuticals, such as intravenous additives, radioactive pharmaceuticals and eye drops in a hospital pharmacy or for similar purposes in a laboratory. Filtration should be carried out in a controlled environment.

Diagram D is a line filter, capable of filtering up to 500 litres if it is fitted with a 293 mm diameter membrane. The inlet of the circular holder is connected to the reservoir of liquid and the exit leads to the receiver. Line filters are used to sterilize relatively large volumes of bacteriological or tissue culture media. They may be operated under positive or negative pressure. Compact polycarbonate units, containing a stack of membrane filters, are now available to handle volumes up to 50 litres; this corresponds to the volume that can be handled by a conventional line filter with a 142 mm membrane. They can be autoclaved (once only) at 121°C for up to 60 minutes. Persons who are involved in performing filtration should keep in touch with developments in this rapidly advancing field.

THE FILTRATION PROCESS

Sterilization of filters

Membranes which consist of cellulose esters, Tef-

lon or polyvinylidene fluoride are sterilized by steam at 121°C for a holding time of 30 minutes. They can be placed in the holders before sterilization if the funnels are fitted with vented caps to prevent deformation of the membrane by pressure changes during the sterilization cycle. A small amount of distilled water should be added to closed systems to provide steam internally for sterilization. Line filters and cartridge filters can be sterilized in situ by inline steaming at 121°C. Filters that cannot be autoclaved and are not sold in sterile condition should be sterilized in accordance with the manufacturer's instructions.

Pretreatment of filters or solutions

Membrane filters may contain small amounts of detergent, such as Triton X100, to make them stable to autoclaving. They should be washed before filtration of tissue culture media as the growth-promoting quality of the medium may be affected by the detergent (Cahn, 1967). Some solutions for filtration may require pretreatment (e.g. centrifugation) to avoid clogging of the filter by fine particles, colloids or gels.

Prefilters

The working life of fine filters may be greatly extended by the use of a prefilter. The prefilter may be a depth filter made from fibreglass; asbestos filters are unsuitable because the fibres are toxic to tissue cultures. Alternatively, a membrane filter of 0.8 or 1.2 μm pore diameter can be used. The performance characteristics of the prefilter should be related to those of the final filter. If the latter is a membrane of 0.45 μm pore diameter the prefilter should, ideally, be capable of retaining particles above 5 μm in diameter as this is the size that is most likely to block the bacterial filter. A prefilter that is too coarse will not protect the membrane against the particles which are most likely to clog it whereas, if it is too fine, the prefilter will clog prematurely. In order to ensure an adequate flow rate the area of the prefilter should be greater than that of the final filter.

Pressure and vacuum filtration

Liquids do not run freely through bacterial filters. Positive pressure must be applied to the reservoir or the receiver must be connected to a vacuum pump. Positive pressure filtration requires more elaborate apparatus but has the following advantages over suction:

1. Higher flow rates are possible because pressure differentials greater than one atmosphere can be applied
2. Contamination of the filtrate by air leaks or backflow of water is prevented
3. Protein-containing solutions do not froth in the receiver and volatile solvents do not evaporate
4. The filter assembly can be tested for leaks by a bubble point test before and after use
5. The filtrate can be collected directly in the final containers if the outlet is enclosed in a protective shield or filtration is carried out under clean room conditions.

When filtration is operated by suction, the exit from the receiver should be protected from airborne contamination by a plug of fibrous filter material and a trap should be installed on the vacuum line to prevent backflow of water or oil from the pump. After a sterile filtration has been completed, the membrane is discarded and reusable holders should be cleaned according to the manufacturer's directions.

TESTING EFFICIENCY OF FILTRATION

The efficiency of membrane filters is not affected by thickness, velocity or the pressure differential at which filtration is carried out. Performance may be defined in terms of flow rate (volume filtered in a given time) or throughput (volume filtered before the filter clogs). The flow rate is related to the pore diameter and the total pore volume. It varies directly with the pressure differential (provided clogging does not occur) and the effective filtration area, but decreases as the viscosity of the liquid increases. Viscosity can sometimes be reduced by raising the temperature, as is recommended for filtration of ointments dissolved in isopropyl myristate (United States Pharmacopeia, 1980).

Bubble point test

The bubble point, or bubble pressure, is the pressure required to cause the first bubble of air to break through a filter that is saturated with water. The bubble point test may be performed on a membrane filter assembly before use, without breaking sterility, and repeated after filtration. This is especially important when radioactive isotopes with a short half-life are sterilized by filtration because they are used before their sterility can be tested. The bubble point method is also used to test the quality of the membranes.

To perform a bubble point test, the liquid is placed in a pressure vessel; some is transferred to the filter holder and is driven through the filter under slight positive pressure until the lower end of the delivery tube is immersed. The pressure is then increased gradually until air bubbles appear in the receiver. Membranes of 0.45 μm and 0.22 μm pore diameter have bubble pressures of 220 kPa and 380 kPa respectively. Values are higher for oils and lower for alcoholic solutions.

Bacteriological tests

Bacteriological tests are carried out by passing a suspension containing a known number of cells through the filter. *Serratia marcescens* ATCC 14756 and *Pseudomonas diminuta* ATCC 19146 (0.3 × 1.0 μm) have been recommended (Bowman et al, 1967); the latter provides the most rigorous challenge to a membrane of sterilizing grade. *Pseudomonas aeruginosa* and spores of *Bacillus subtilis* var. *niger* have also been used. Filtration should be carried out slowly and the entire filtrate should be cultured because the passage of a single cell renders the liquid unsterile. Bacteriological tests do not give an immediate result but are useful for assessing the reliability or reproducibility of particular types of membrane filters or filter holders. The efficiency of a filtration process that has been completed may be tested by passing a bacterial culture through the filter and incubating the filtrate to detect growth.

APPLICATIONS OF MEMBRANE FILTRATION

Membrane filters are more versatile than are depth filters. In addition to the primary purpose of sterile filtration, they can be used in sterility testing and bacteriological studies because the microorganisms are retained on the surface where they may be examined or cultured in situ.

Pharmaceuticals

Heat-sensitive injections and ophthalmic solutions, which comprise more than 10 per cent of the preparations listed in the different Pharmacopoeias, are sterilized commercially by filtration. A bactericide is usually included in the filtered solutions to kill or inhibit the growth of occasional contaminants that might enter during transfer to the final containers, unless the preparation is intended for intravenous administration in volumes greater than 15 ml or for intrathecal injection. If filtration of small volumes of eye drops or additives for intravenous infusions is carried out in hospital pharmacies, the use of a laminar flow cabinet is essential. Products that have been sterilized by filtration are usually subject to more stringent sterility tests than are those sterilized by autoclaving in the final containers.

The sterilization of large volume parenterals by filtration is applied mainly to solutions for total parenteral nutrition. However, intravenous solutions that are sterilized by heat require preliminary filtration through 1.2 μm and 0.45 μm membranes to remove bacteria, which are pyrogenic even

when they are killed, and a variety of other extraneous particles that commonly occur in these products. The particles arise from rubber closures, containers, ingredients of the formulation or precipitation reactions between components (Garvan & Gunner, 1963, 1964; Davis et al, 1970). If the particles are introduced into the blood stream in large numbers, they cause granulomatous lesions in the lungs, brain and other tissues. Subsequent to filtration and sterilization, particles may be introduced into the intravenous solution by additives or by the administration set. In order to overcome this problem, the use of final filters at the outlet of the set or close to the cannulation site has been suggested (Rapp et al, 1975; Wilmore & Dudrick, 1969). A 0.22 μm membrane is required because *P. aeruginosa* may pass through the 0.45 μm grade (Holmes et al, 1980). Inline filtration has also been recommended for peritoneal dialysis fluids (Sharpstone & Goldby, 1967).

Biological materials

Serum for addition to culture media for propagation of bacteria and viruses can be sterilized only by filtration, and this applies also to antisera and many other blood products. Serum and other materials that have a high content of colloidal material may require serial filtration in which the liquid is passed through a depth type prefilter or a membrane of 1.2 μm pore size and then through a 0.2 or 0.22 μm membrane. The membranes may be mounted as a stack in the same holder, held apart by spacers of porous material. Virus vaccines are passed through 0.45 μm filters to remove bacterial contaminants and tissue culture debris (Cliver, 1968).

Microbiological culture media

Most bacteriological culture media are heat-stable to varying degrees but some heat-sensitive ingredients, such as sugars and serum, are sterilized separately and added aseptically to the sterilized solution of heat-stable components. Tissue culture media, which are used for propagation of viruses, are sterilized by filtration; foetal calf serum may be prefiltered and added to the medium before the final filtration.

Industrial applications

Filtration plays a prominent part in the commercial production of antibiotics for parenteral or oral administration. After purification, the concentrated solution is filtered and then distributed aseptically into the final containers, in which it may be freeze-dried. Some heat-sensitive industrial fermentation media may be sterilized in large quantities by filtration. Membrane filters of 0.45–1.2 μm are used to remove yeast cells in the clarification of beer and wines.

Sterility tests

The important role of membrane filtration in sterility tests on commercially produced pharmaceutical products and medical devices has been discussed in Chapter 2. Membranes of 0.45 μm pore size and 47 mm diameter, with a hydrophobic edge, are used for tests on antibiotics and also on injections that contain a chemical preservative. Residues left on the filter after the liquid has passed through are removed or inactivated by washing with an appropriate diluent and the membrane is cultured for detection of bacteria or fungi. Oil-based pharmaceuticals, such as ointments, are dissolved in isopropyl myristate and the membrane is washed with a diluent containing a surface active agent to remove oil residues before the membrane is cultured. Membrane filtration has also made it practicable to perform sterility tests on relatively large samples of intravenous infusions.

Bacteriological investigations

This special application of membrane filters is not relevant to sterilization except that it is used to determine numbers and types of microbial contaminants that have been rinsed from solid objects. The main use of the filters is in the analysis of bacterial populations in water samples. An interesting development in membrane design followed reports that faecal coliform counts varied with the type or brand of membrane used (Presswood & Brown, 1973; Schaeffer et al, 1974). Examination of various membranes showed that they varied with respect to the size of the pore openings; larger openings enabled the bacteria to be immersed in liquid medium during filtration and subsequent incubation of the membrane, eliminating the adverse effect of drying on their viability. The correlation between recovery of faecal coliforms and the number of large openings on the filter surface has been confirmed by electron microscopy (Standridge, 1976), and membranes are now manufactured with enlarged openings (e.g. 2.4 μm) leading to narrower channels of 0.7 μm diameter.

FILTRATION OF AIR

The human respiratory tract acts as a filter which effectively prevents bacteria-carrying particles greater than 5 μm in diameter from reaching the alveoli of the lung. This is achieved by the tortuous course of the air stream through the bronchi and bronchioles, where the particles are trapped on the moist mucous lining. However, smaller droplet nuclei (1–2 μm) which arise when droplets of respiratory tract secretions dry in air, can penetrate this natural filtration mechanism. The surgeon's mask is also an air filter, intended to prevent outward or inward passage of droplets carrying potentially harmful bacteria or viruses. The high-efficiency particulate air filters (HEPA filters) that are now used to provide ultraclean air for medical and industrial purposes are in a different category because they have a retention efficiency of at least 99.97 per cent for airborne particles 0.3 μm or more in diameter.

Ultraclean air is required in hospital areas where patients undergo surgery or are being nursed in protective isolation, and in industrial premises where sterile pharmaceuticals or medical devices are produced. The supply of sterile air to cultures of bacteria or fungi that are used for production of antibiotics, enzymes or organic acids is a particularly exacting task, as is the aseptic assembly of presterilized components for life-detection space capsules. The following types of filters are used for the various purposes:

1. Fibrous depth filters
2. Granular depth filters
3. Fibrous (paper) sheet filters
4. Membrane filters.

FIBROUS DEPTH FILTERS

Plugs of non-absorbent cotton wool are used in microbiological laboratories to exclude microbial contaminants from culture media in test tubes or flasks. They are adequate for this purpose if they remain clean and dry but cotton wool is relatively inefficient as a filter because it has little mechanical strength and tends to channel during steam sterilization or to break down during use. Finely spun glass fibres, resin-treated natural wool or mineral slag wool are used to make depth filters for industrial fermentation processes. The glass fibres are made by heating borosilicate glass in a high-velocity air stream; they are circular in cross section and of uniform diameter in the range 0.06–6 μm. About 70 per cent of the fibres in mineral slag wool are also less than 6 μm in diameter but a small proportion of much coarser fibres adds strength to the filter.

The fibrous material is packed into tubes or larger containers, where it is held under pressure from both ends. Cartridge depth filters may be preformed slabs containing mixed fibres which are bonded together by resin. All types of filters must be packed and assembled so that air cannot pass between the medium and container wall. Large and small depth filters are usually sterilized by steam and an exposure time of 2 hours is recommended.

Mechanisms of filtration

The interspaces in fibrous filters are larger than the particles that the filter retains but contact between the particles and the fibres results in adsorption or mechanical trapping as the air flows through uneven channels, which change direction continually along their path through the filter bed. Fibrous filters are generally more efficient in removing bacteria from gases than from liquids because the microorganisms can leave the air stream more easily. The mechanisms of arrest that operate in a particular filter depend on the size, mass, electrostatic charge and velocity of the particles. The following mechanisms are recognized in fibrous depth filters:

1. Interception (direct impact)
2. Inertial impaction
3. Diffusion and gravitational settling (sedimentation)
4. Electrostatic precipitation.

These mechanisms are illustrated in Figure 9.3.

Interception

Light particles have little momentum and tend to follow the course of the air stream around the fibres but direct interception may occur. The chance of colliding with a fibre increases with particle size, and is also favoured by fine fibres. This mechanism of capture may occur at low or high velocities, but the magnitude of its contribution to filtration is uncertain.

Inertial impaction

Heavy particles tend to continue in a straight path, colliding with a fibre instead of following the air

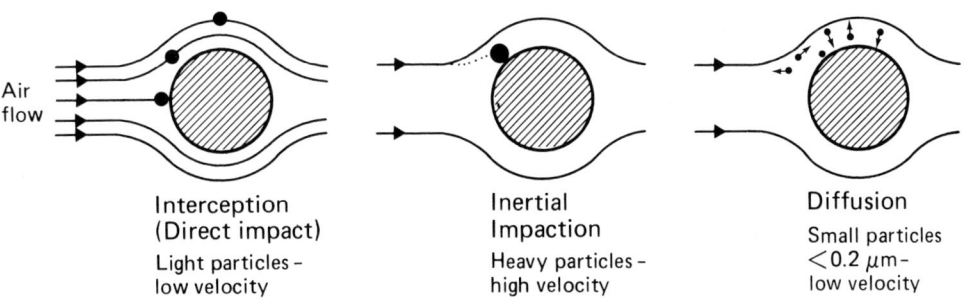

Fig. 9.3 Mechanisms by which airborne particles may be trapped in fibrous depth filters.
Note Shaded areas represent fibres in cross section.

stream around it. This mechanism of impingement is favoured by high velocity and a matrix of fine fibres which causes abrupt changes in the gaseous flow path. The chance of impaction also increases with the density and size of the particles. Inertial impaction is the principal mechanism of arrest in high-velocity filters; it does not operate at velocities below 30 cm/s.

Diffusion

Particles less than 0.3 μm in diameter, such as bacteriophage, are too small for direct interception and too light to be collected by inertial impaction. However, if the velocity is very low, they may diffuse out of the air stream by random Brownian movement. This increases the length of their path through the filter and promotes contact with the fibres, to which they adhere. Diffusion is the principal mechanism of retention in low-velocity filters (less than 30 cm/s). Very small particles (less than 0.3 μm) can be removed only by low-velocity filters. Thermal convection and gravitational settling may also participate under these conditions. Electrostatic precipitation may also be involved.

Electrostatic precipitation

Particles may be retained by the attraction of opposite charges on the filter material and the microbial cells. Electrostatic precipitation is important in resin-treated wool filters, where the charge on the resin coating is opposite to that on the wool. The impregnation of wool with resin increases filtration efficiency from 50 per cent to 99.99 per cent. Electrostatic attraction is independent of air velocity and particle size.

Factors influencing efficiency

Fibrous filters are never 100 per cent efficient because they do not act as mechanical sieves. The level of efficiency is expressed as per cent retention or per cent penetration of the airborne particles. Efficiency is governed by the following factors:

1. Air velocity
2. Filter thickness

3. Fibre diameter and packing density
4. Number and size of particles.

Air velocity

Linear velocity per second is equal to the volume of air per second divided by the area of the filter. If velocity is increased from a very low level, the efficiency of retention for particles of a given size decreases at first to a minimum, which is reached at about 30 cm (1 ft) per second. Beyond this point, efficiency increases with velocity, as shown in Figure 9.4 (curve A). The changing effect of velocity is associated with a difference in the mechanism of retention (Humphrey & Gaden, 1955; Humphrey, 1960). At low velocity, efficiency depends mainly on diffusion, but this mechanism becomes less effective as the velocity increases. Above 30 cm/s, inertial impaction starts to operate, especially for particles exceeding 1 μm in diameter. This mechanism increases in efficiency with the velocity, until a point is reached at which channelling occurs through displacement of fibres or the trapped microorganism are released by vibration. Submicron particles, such as bacteriophage and viruses, can be removed only by the mechanisms that operate in low-velocity filters, as shown in Figure 9.4 (curve B).

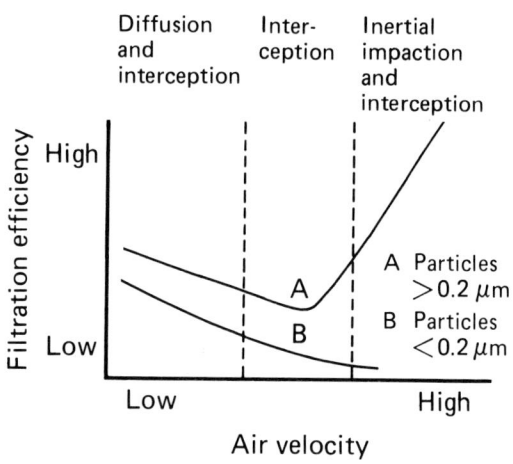

Fig. 9.4 Influence of air velocity on filtration efficiency and mechanisms of interception of microorganisms by fibrous depth filters.

Filter thickness

The proportion of particles retained at different depths in a fibrous filter bed approximates to a logarithmic relationship (Humphrey & Gaden, 1955), so that most are trapped in the proximal layers and the number decreases sharply as the depth of the filter is traversed. A penetration constant (k) and the reciprocal X_{90} value (the depth required for 90 per cent retention) may be derived from the following formula:

$$\log \frac{N}{N_0} = -kX,$$

where N_0 is the number of particles entering the filter, N is the number that penetrate to a given depth, and X is the depth at which the count was determined. Glass fibre and slag wool filters operating below 15 cm/s usually achieve 99.99 per cent retention at a depth of 76 mm. When two depth filters are connected in series, the combined efficiency for particles of a given size is the product of their separate efficiencies.

Fibre diameter and packing density

Fine fibres which are densely packed provide minimum pore size with maximum surface for adsorption of particles. Ideally, the fibre diameter should be less than that of the smallest particles to be filtered, but in practice a range of 1–6 μm is satisfactory in glass fibre and slag wool filters. If the packing is too dense, the resistance to air flow is excessive and the fibrous structure may be damaged; if it is too loose, channelling may occur. A suitable packing density is 190–400 kg/m^3. Bonding resins may be used to maintain porosity and to prevent shifting of the filter material during sterilization. The efficiency of a filter is lost if it becomes wet.

Number and size of particles

The bacterial content of filtered air is directly related to the number of microorganisms initially present. Thus the chance of producing sterile air is greatly increased if the air intake is sited high above ground level and prefilters are used.

Single bacteria (cocci and bacilli) range from 0.3 μm to about 1 μm in diameter. Bacterial viruses and the large animal viruses are 100–250 nm, but most viruses are 20–100 nm. However, as airborne microorganisms are usually associated with dried residues of non-living material, the particles are larger than the actual size of the microorganisms they contain. Particle size influences filtration efficiency through its effect on the mechanism of retention. The most difficult size to remove is 0.3 μm; larger and smaller particles are both removed with greater efficiency.

Design of fibrous depth filters

The depth of a filter depends on the degree of reduction of the microbial contaminants that is required. This may be calculated from an estimate of the number of bacteria-carrying particles in the incoming air, the volume of air that will pass the filter in a given time, and the maximum acceptable chance of a viable microorganism penetrating the filter. For example, if the initial contamination level of the air is 175 viable particles/m^3 and 14 m^3 of air per minute will pass the filter during a 3 day cycle, the total number entering the filter is 10^7. If the maximum acceptable chance of penetration is 10^{-3}, a reduction factor of 10^{10} is required. Other design parameters, such as optimum diameter, air velocity and pressure drop involve complex calculations because these factors are interrelated.

Low-velocity filters

These operate at 5–12 cm/s. They have a low pressure drop and are large in cross section to give adequate flow rates. They are moderately efficient and relatively insensitive to changes in velocity that occur during operation; a decrease in velocity increases their efficiency. This is the only type of filter that is capable of removing particles less than 0.3 μm in diameter.

High-velocity filters

These operate above 0.6 m/s. They are more compact than are low-velocity filters and are cheaper to instal but they are more costly to operate because they have much greater resistance to air flow and a large pressure drop is required to achieve adequate flow rates. If the air velocity decreases below 0.6 m/s during operation, the efficiency may fall below the level for which the filter has been designed.

GRANULAR CARBON FILTERS

Filters packed with granular carbon of particle size 1–2 μm and mesh range 10–60 are frequently used to provide sterile air for industrial fermentations (Cherry et al, 1963). They are large, low-velocity filters with a pressure drop of 6.9–34.5 kPa (1–5 lb.f/in^2). The factors governing their efficiency have not been fully investigated but, as with fibrous filters, it depends on the depth of the filter bed and the initial contamination level of the air. As carbon filters work best under dry conditions, the air should be delivered at a temperature above the dew point to prevent condensation. The carbon may spontaneously ignite if air is passed through the filter while it is still hot after steam sterilization.

FIBROUS (PAPER) SHEET FILTERS

High-efficiency (HEPA) filters with a low resistance to air flow and a large surface area are required to provide air with an extremely low bacterial count to industrial premises where sterile pharmaceuticals are manufactured, operating rooms and protective isolation facilities in hospitals, and aseptic work areas in microbiological laboratories. Ultraclean environments ('clean rooms') were developed initially for aseptic assembly of presterilized spacecraft components. The highest clean room standard is designated Class 100; the number of airborne particles of 0.5 μm or more should not exceed 3.5/l or 100/ft^3. Particles over 5 μm diameter should not be detected. The role of air filtration in meeting the standard is limited to removal of bacteria-carrying particles from fresh or recirculated air that is introduced into the room. A conventional or a unidirectional ('laminar') flow system must be established to remove microorganisms that arise from equipment or persons, or work activity within the room, away from the sensitive

area and ultimately to the exhaust system.

The HEPA filters that are used for these purposes are large paper sheets, made from glass or cellulose fibres and ranging from less than 1 μm to 5 μm in diameter. They may be used separately or in combination. Esparto grass from South America is a source of long cellulose fibres. Continuous glass fibre may be formed into sheets of graduated density, with relatively loose packing at the inlet surface to prevent clogging and denser packing towards the outlet side to provide mechanical strength and filtration efficiency. The very large fibrous sheets that are required to give adequate velocities and flow rates are pleated around suitable supporting material and are sealed at all edges in a frame to form a compact filter unit. The integrity of the filter depends on absence of pinholes in the paper and perfect edge sealing. Single units are installed in air ducts or, in 'laminar' flow systems, they form a bank of parallel units occupying the whole area of a ceiling or wall.

Efficiency of HEPA filters

HEPA filters have efficiencies ranging from 99.97 to 99.997 per cent retention for particles averaging 0.3 μm in size. Larger and smaller particles may be retained with 100 times greater efficiency. Filtration efficiency may be reduced below the rated level by increased air velocity, neutralization of electrostatic charges on the particles, or relative humidities over 95 per cent (Harstad & Filler, 1969).

HEPA filters have a working life up to 3–4 years if they are used in conjunction with prefilters with a lower pressure drop. The prefilters remove large particles and some of the smaller ones. The prefilter should be changed several times before the final filter is replaced (Fig. 9.5). Indications for replacement of the HEPA filter are:

1. An inadequate flow rate, which is not remedied by changing the prefilter
2. A pressure drop that exceeds the capacity of the blower fans
3. A leak that cannot be sealed.

Disinfection of used filters

HEPA filters installed in the exhaust systems of

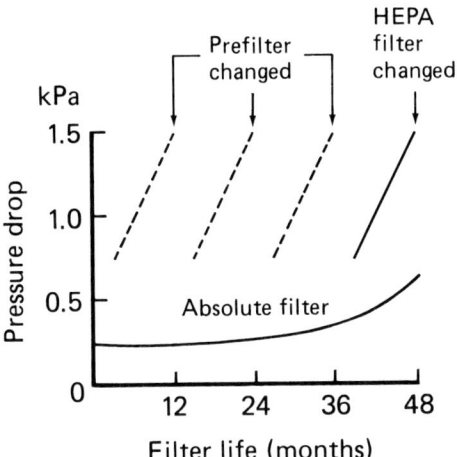

Fig. 9.5 The role of prefilters in extending the working life of a high-efficiency (HEPA) filter.

rooms or safety cabinets where pathogenic microorganisms have been dispersed should be disinfected in situ, or removed by a person wearing protective clothing and then incinerated or autoclaved. Disinfection in situ may be accomplished by heating elements in the exhaust duct if the filter is fireproof. However, this method is applicable only to safety cabinets and very small rooms. Disinfection by formaldehyde vapour is recommended. Formalin (37–40 per cent w/v formaldehyde) should be vaporized in the duct for 30 minutes at a temperature of at least 24°C, and adequate humidity must be provided by introduction of steam or water spray.

MEMBRANE FILTERS

The properties of membrane filters have been described in the section of this chapter that deals with their role in the filtration of liquids. They may be used for air filtration at pressures exceeding the bubble pressure but the high pressure drop which is required restricts their use mainly to some of the small scale applications. As electrostatic forces are generated in air filtration, a membrane of 0.8 μm pore diameter can retain particles with a diameter of 0.5 μm. An inline filter with a 90 mm diameter membrane has been used for sterilization of air supplied to a tissue culture system (Vosseller et al,

1971). The filter was sterilized by admitting steam at 110°C for at least 2 and up to 20 hours to both sides of the membrane and air-drying it thoroughly afterwards.

TESTS FOR EFFICIENCY OF AIR FILTERS

Filters are tested by determining the per cent penetration of high-density aerosols with a known particle size distribution. Standard tests are based on chemical dusts with a high proportion of 0.3 μm particles, as this size is most difficult to filter. Bacteriological tests are unnecessary if a filter passes the more rigorous chemical tests, but may be used to compare different types of filters for efficiency in removing bacteria or viruses, or for a check on reproducibility of performance in a particular type or brand of filter.

Installations for testing

The various test methods are similar in principle, regardless of the type of filter or aerosol used. For tests with chemical dusts, the filter is installed in a duct which should be of adequate size and length upstream and downstream of the filter to allow the aerosol to be dried and mixed uniformly and to permit the withdrawal of samples for analysis. In bacteriological tests, the filter to be tested may be installed in a line filter holder; the bacterial aerosol is passed into a mixing chamber before it enters the line to the test filter.

Chemical aerosols

Chemical dusts consisting of sodium chloride or dioctyl phthalate are commonly used. A fluorometric method, in which aerosolized rhodamine B was used as the fluorescent dye, has also been described (Sullivan et al, 1967). In the sodium chloride flame test, dried particles of 0.01–1.5 μm diameter are generated from a 2 per cent solution of sodium chloride. The sodium content of the filtered and unfiltered air is measured by the intensity of colour produced in a hydrogen flame photometer. The mean particle size in dioctyl phthalate (DOP) smoke is 0.3 μm. The amounts in upstream and downstream samples are measured photoelectrically and the lower limit of detection is 0.001 per cent penetration. The chemical tests provide an immediate result. The DOP smoke test is also used to detect pinholes or imperfect seals in the filter face of laminar flow installations.

Microbial aerosols

Aerosols containing bacteria or bacterial viruses (bacteriophage) are considered to be more sensitive than chemical tests for critical evaluation or comparison of filters with an efficiency rating near 100 per cent. *B. subtilis* var. *niger* spores (approximately 1 μm in diameter) may be generated as predominantly single- or two-celled particles by a DeVilbis nebulizer. *P. aeruginosa* or *S. marcescens* may also be used but these vegetative bacteria tend to die in the air stream. Aerosols of bacteriophage T$_1$ (Harstad & Filler, 1969) and an actinophage (Roelants et al, 1968) have been used to determine the efficiency of virus retention. In a less orthodox method, susceptible chickens were used as an indicator of the in-use effectiveness of filters in removing Marek's disease virus, an avian pathogen, from the effluent air of an enclosure containing infected birds (Burmester & Witter, 1972).

APPLICATIONS OF HEPA AIR FILTERS

High-efficiency air filters made from cellulose or glass fibres have a wide range of applications in hospitals, microbiological laboratories and industrial processes, as shown in Table 9.1.

Protective environments

Operating theatres are always supplied with filtered air but the benefit of replacing conventional plenum ventilation with a laminar flow system is difficult to evaluate because it must be assessed by the incidence of infections, rather than by its effect on the number of airborne contaminants. When a laminar flow enclosure is installed in an operating theatre, it is usually for orthopaedic surgery, which incurs a high risk of infection because the operation field is usually large and the time is prolonged. Laminar flow units in which the filters

Table 9.1 Applications of high-efficiency air filters

Locations	Applications
Hospitals	Ventilation of operating theatres and protective isolation facilities
	Decontamination of inspired or expired air in mechanical ventilators and suction apparatus
	Filtration of compressed gases (e.g. O_2) administered to patients
	Filtration of air admitted to steam or gas sterilizers
Microbiological laboratories	Ventilation of safety cabinets and 'sterile' rooms
	Decontamination of exhaust air from cabinets or rooms where aerosols of pathogenic microorganisms have been generated
	Decontamination of effluent air from aerated bacterial or fungal cultures
Industrial premises	Ventilation of rooms or enclosures for aseptic filling of liquids sterilized by filtration
	Ventilation of rooms for sterility testing
	Ventilation of rooms for assembly of micro-electronic equipment

are located in a panel behind the head of the bed or in an overhead canopy are used for individual leukaemia patients.

Mechanical ventilators

Mechanical ventilators are used in anaesthesiology and, over longer periods, by patients requiring intensive care. Installation of bacterial filters in the inspiratory and expiratory limbs of the breathing circuits of mechanical ventilators and anaesthetic apparatus is intended to protect the patient from infection, to decrease the need for frequent disinfection of the complex apparatus or to prevent the discharge of pathogenic bacteria, such as *P. aeruginosa*, from the patient's respiratory tract into the ward environment.

The filters must be small, cheap, disposable or autoclavable and of low air resistance. They should not absorb anaesthetic gases, and residual ethylene oxide must be removed if it has been used to sterilize the circuit (Bryan-Brown, 1972). Glass fibre filters can fulfil these requirements. The inspiratory side of the breathing circuit poses no problems if the filter precedes the humidifier. However, effective filtration of exhaled gases is difficult because moisture increases the resistance of the filter and may block it completely. A wet filter can support growth of Gram-negative bacteria which may be pathogenic to debilitated patients. Backflow of condensate from tubes beyond the filter may also be responsible for contamination of the circuit and wetting of the filter (Martin & Ulrich, 1969). Methods that have been recommended to maintain the filter in a dry condition include the use of siliconized (hydrophobic) filter material (Lumley et al, 1976) and the provision of an electrically heated mantle to maintain the filter at 56–76°C during use (Pyle et al, 1969; Holdcroft et al, 1974). Disposable fibreglass filters have been described by Dyer et al (1970) and Shiotani et al (1971).

The advantages of incorporating filters in mechanical ventilators used by patients in intensive care do not appear to be questioned. However, recent surveys by Garibaldi et al (1981) and Feeley et al (1981) have indicated no significant differences in the incidence of postoperative pneumonia in patients on whom anaesthetic circuits with and without filters were used.

Suction apparatus

Filtration is necessary to prevent dissemination of bacteria, directly to the room air or through the vacuum system, from bottles that trap mucus and purulent secretions from the respiratory tracts of tracheostomy patients and premature infants. The liquid in the trap should contain an antifoam agent. Disinfectants are not recommended because they tend to promote frothing. A line filter, made from two layers of fibreglass paper sealed in an aluminium container has been described (Marshall, 1964). Constant performance over a period of four months has been reported, but the filter is useless if it becomes wet.

For high-vacuum suction apparatus that is used in surgical emergencies, a filter of not less than 50 per cent efficiency, prepared by packing 8 g of non-absorbent (bleached) cotton wool in a cylinder of 7.5 cm length and 5.5 cm diameter, is acceptable (British Standards Institution, 1967).

Compressed gases

Compressed gases are drawn from cylinders at high pressure, and low-resistance filters are therefore unnecessary. The Linde filter, designed for use with clinical oxygen, consists of a tubular brass case, 10.5 cm long and 2.8 cm diameter, divided into five compartments by mesh copper screens which are supported by perforated Teflon discs (Mortensen & Hill, 1964). The compartments are packed with Pyrex glass wool to a density of $0.3 \ g/cm^3$ and the ends are closed with caps adapted to fit standard oxygen connectors.

Laboratory effluents

Filters fitted to the exhaust ducts of safety cabinets which are used for containment of harmful microorganisms must be designed to cope with the maximum air flow rate and the expected contamination level. The filtration of effluents from aerated cultures of pathogenic microorganisms is complicated by their high moisture content. An ingeniously designed filter overcomes this problem by trapping the microorganisms in a heat-resistant mineral fibre filter pad, which is maintained at 200°C by a thermostatically controlled heating element in an adjacent compartment (Cameron & Favelle, 1967).

REFERENCES

Bowman F W, Calhoun M P, White M 1967 Microbiological methods for quality control of membrane filters. Journal of Pharmaceutical Sciences 56: 222–225

British Standards Institution 1967 Specification for Surgical Suction Apparatus Part 1. Electrically operated surgical suction apparatus of high vacuum and high air displacement type. British Standard 4199: Part 1: 1967

Bryan-Brown C W 1972 Bacterial filters. International Anesthesiology Clinics 10: 147–156

Burmester B R, Witter R L 1972 Efficiency of commercial air filters against Marek's disease virus. Applied Microbiology 23: 505–508

Cahn R D 1967 Detergents in membrane filters. Science 155: 195–196

Cameron J, Favelle H K 1967 An effluent-air filter. Journal of Applied Bacteriology 30: 261–263

Cherry G B, Kemp S D, Parker A 1963 The sterilization of air. Progress in Industrial Microbiology 4: 35–60

Cliver D O 1968 Virus interactions with membrane filters. Biotechnology and Bioengineering 10: 877–889

Davis N M, Turco S, Sively E 1970 A study of particulate matter in I.V. infusion fluids. American Journal of Hospital Pharmacy 27: 820–826

Dyer E D, Maxwell J G, Peterson D E, Mitchell C R 1970 Disposable fiberglass filter to counter bacterial contamination of intermittent positive pressure breathing equipment. Anesthesia and Analgesia 40: 140–147

Feeley T W, Hamilton W K, Xavier B, Moyers J, Eger E I 1981 Sterile anesthesia breathing circuits do not prevent postoperative pulmonary infection. Anesthesiology 54: 369–372

Garibaldi R A, Britt M R, Webster C, Pace N L 1981 Failure of bacterial filters to reduce the incidence of pneumonia after inhalation anesthesia. Anesthesiology 54: 364–368

Garvan J M, Gunner B W 1963 Intravenous fluids: 'A solution containing such particles must not be used'. Medical Journal of Australia 2: 140–145

Garvan J M, Gunner B W 1964 The harmful effects of particles in intravenous fluids. Medical Journal of Australia 2: 1–6

Harstad J B, Filler M E 1969 Evaluation of air filters with submicron viral aerosols and bacterial aerosols. American Industrial Hygiene Association Journal 30: 280–290

Holdcroft A, Lumley J, Gaya H, Adams D, Darlow H M 1974 Respiratory filters in clinical practice. Lancet ii: 25–26

Holmes C J, Kundsin R B, Ausman R K, Walter C W 1980 Potential hazards associated with microbial contamination of in-line filters during intravenous therapy. Journal of Clinical Microbiology 12: 725–731

Humphrey A E 1960 Air sterilization. Advances in Applied Microbiology 2: 301–311

Humphrey A E, Gaden E L Jr 1955 Air sterilization by fibrous media. Industrial and Engineering Chemistry 47: 924–930

Lumley J, Holdcroft A, Gaya H, Darlow H M, Adams D J 1976 Expiratory bacterial filters. Lancet ii: 22–23

Marshall M 1964 Bacterial filter for suction apparatus. Lancet ii: 21

Martin J T, Ulrich J A 1969 A bacterial filter for an anesthetic circuit. Anesthesia and Analgesia 48: 944–946

Mortensen J D, Hill G 1964 Clinical and bacteriologic evaluation of a new filter designed specifically for bacteriologic decontamination of oxygen used clinically. Diseases of the Chest 45: 508–514

Presswood W G, Brown L R 1973 Comparison of Gelman and Millipore membrane filters for enumerating fecal coliform bacteria. Applied Microbiology 26: 332–336

Pyle P, Darlow M, Firman J E 1969 A heated ultra-high-efficiency filter for mechanical ventilators. Lancet i: 136–137

Rapp R, Bivins B, Schroeder H, DeLuca P P 1975 Evaluation of a prototype air-venting inline intravenous filter set. American Journal of Hospital Pharmacy 32: 1253–1259

Roelants P, Boon B, Lhoest W 1968 Evaluation of a commercial air filter for removal of viruses from the air. Applied Microbiology 16: 1465–1467

Schaeffer D J, Long M C, Janardan K G 1974 Statistical analysis of the recovery of coliform organisms on Gelman and Millipore membrane filters. Applied Microbiology 28: 605–607

Sharpstone P, Goldby F S 1967 Peritoneal dialysis with in-line sterilization of dialysate by filtration. British Medical Journal 4: 728

Shiotani G M, Nicholes P, Ballinger C M, Shaw L 1971 Prevention of contamination of the circle system and ventilators with a new disposable filter. Anesthesia and Analgesia 50: 844–854

Standridge J H 1976 Comparison of surface pore morphology of two brands of membrane filters. Applied and Environmental Microbiology 31: 316–319

Sullivan J F, Songer J R, Mathis R G 1967 Fluorometric method for determining the efficiency of spun-glass air filtration media. Applied Microbiology 15: 191–196

United States Pharmacopeia 1980 20th rev. Mack Publishing Company, Easton, p 882

Vosseller G V, Chian E S K, Mirzahi A, Moore G E 1971 In situ steam sterilization of membrane filters. Biotechnology and Bioengineering 13: 591–596

Wilmore D W, Dudrick S J 1969 An in-line filter for intravenous solutions. Archives of Surgery 99: 462–463

10

Chemical disinfectants

This chapter contains brief descriptions of the properties and main applications of chemical antimicrobial agents that are commonly used as solutions in water or alcohol for disinfection of equipment, surfaces and intact skin or mucous membranes. General discussion of mechanisms of biocidal action, microbial susceptibility, factors influencing efficiency in use and potential toxicity will be found in Chapter II, together with the evaluation of disinfectants and the consequences of incorrect use.

ALCOHOLS

General properties

Ethyl alcohol ($CH_3.CH_2OH$) and isopropyl alcohol ($CH_3.CHOH.CH_3$) are colourless liquids, boiling at 78.5°C and 82.3°C respectively. They evaporate at room temperature, leaving no residue. The low surface tension of alcohol-water mixtures confers wetting ability and they penetrate well into crevices of the human skin or inanimate objects. These alcohols are miscible with water. They are flammable at the concentrations which are recommended for disinfection.

Microbial susceptibility

| Gram-positive bacteria | highly susceptible |
| Gram-negative bacteria | highly susceptible |

Acid-fast bacteria	susceptible
Bacterial spores	resistant
Lipophilic viruses	susceptible
Hydrophilic viruses	resistant

Formulation

Water must be added to alcohols to obtain the maximum rate of biocidal action, which depends on protein denaturation. Recommended concentrations of alcohol range from 60–90 per cent but the method of preparing the solutions (by weight or volume) is rarely stated. Price (1939) recommended 70 per cent ethyl alcohol by weight for skin disinfection. In 1945, Archer recommended 80 per cent by volume which is approximately 70 per cent by weight. The same recommendation is made in this book as it ensures that the concentration of alcohol will be neither too high nor too low for effective bactericidal action. The precise optimum concentration for disinfection varies over a wide range depending on the moisture content of the bacteria. Isopropyl alcohol is generally assumed to be equally effective at slightly lower concentrations (e.g 60–70 per cent v/v). The additional carbon atom would confer increased activity, as is usual in the series of water-miscible alcohols, but the difference is reduced by the fact that isopropyl alcohol is a secondary alcohol, whereas ethyl alcohol is a primary alcohol.

Factors influencing efficiency

Alcohols coagulate or precipitate proteins in serum, pus, sputum and other biological materials. This action may protect microorganisms from effective contact with the alcohol. The concentration of alcohol diminishes as it evaporates and the action may be bacteriostatic at concentrations below 50 per cent. There is no residual action after the alcohol has completely evaporated.

Adverse effects

Alcohols are irritant and toxic to tissue cells and are generally unsuitable for application to mucous membranes. Skin conditioners, such as glycerol or resins, must be added to alcohol-based skin disinfectants if they are applied frequently to the hands because dryness, roughness or cracking of the skin may result from the removal of lipids.

Rubber swells and plastics may be hardened by frequent or prolonged contact with alcohol; contact times should be limited to 10 minutes. The lens cement of optical equipment, such as endoscopic instruments, is weakened by disinfection with alcoholic solutions.

Applications

Alcohols, which are non-selective bactericides, are used in situations where continuing action is not required and the lack of solid residues is an advantage. They are more frequently used as solvents for non-volatile disinfectants, such as chlorhexidine or iodine compounds.

Skin disinfection

Ethyl alcohol (80 per cent v/v) or isopropyl alcohol (60–70 per cent v/v) is suitable for skin disinfection before routine injections. A contact time of at least 15 seconds should be allowed.

Surface disinfection

Ethyl alcohol (80 per cent v/v) may be used to disinfect cleaned clinical thermometers and is the agent of choice if contamination with *Mycobacterium tuberculosis* or other pathogenic acid-fast bacteria is likely. It may also be used to disinfect the surface of glass ampoules containing local anaesthetics, cleaned surfaces of hospital trolleys, dental bracket tables and the interior of laboratory safety cabinets. Precautions are required to prevent accidental ignition.

ALDEHYDES

General properties

Formaldehye (H.CHO) and glutaraldehyde (CHO.CH$_2$.CH$_2$.CH$_2$.CHO) are available as aqueous solutions which have a characteristic pungent odour. Formaldehyde polymerizes to form a white deposit (paraformaldehyde) in the concentrated stock solution (formalin) and on articles after prolonged immersion in diluted solutions. Polymerization of glutaraldehyde occurs more slowly but is accelerated when the acid stock solution is rendered alkaline to activate it for use as a disinfectant (Stonehill et al, 1963). Gorman et al (1980) have reviewed the present status of glutaraldehyde.

Microbial susceptibility

Gram-positive bacteria	highly susceptible
Gram-negative bacteria	highly susceptible
Acid-fast bacteria	moderately susceptible
Bacterial spores	susceptible (slow killing, species variation)
Lipophilic viruses	susceptible
Hydrophilic viruses	moderately susceptible
Fungi	fungistatic or fungicidal

Formulation

Formalin is an aqueous solution containing 37–40 per cent w/v formaldehyde. It may be diluted with water or alcohol to the concentration required for use. If alcohol is used, its final concentration should be 70–80 per cent v/v.

Glutaraldehyde is sold as a 2 per cent w/v aqueous solution, to be used undiluted as a broad spectrum disinfectant or sterilant for heat-sensitive instruments. The acid stock solution (pH 4) is accompanied by a liquid or powdered activator which must be added to adjust it to pH 7.5–8.5 before use. The whole of the contents (usually 2–5 litres) must be activated when the container is opened for use. A working life of 14–28 days (depending on the brand) is usually specified, but care must be taken to avoid the introduction of organic material or water by uncleaned or excessively wet instruments. If only part of the activated solution is required for a single use, the used portion should be discarded.

Factors influencing efficiency

Formaldehyde is active at acid or alkaline pH but glutaraldehyde must be alkalinized for biocidal action at room temperature. Alkaline solutions slowly decrease in activity as polymerization occurs. The difference between the activity of acid and alkaline solutions diminishes if an acid solution is heated but disinfection is normally carried out at ambient temperature.

Glutaraldehyde reacts with proteins in nutrient broth, with the production of a reddish colouration and a loss of activity at low concentrations. However, most reports indicate that deposits of proteinaceous material on the articles to be disinfected do not present a significant barrier to penetration.

Adverse effects

Formaldehyde vapour and, to a lesser degree, glutaraldehyde vapour are extremely irritant to the eyes and the mucous membranes of the respiratory tract. Cases of contact dermatitis have occasionally been reported in nurses who removed instruments from glutaraldehyde solutions with their hands (Sanderson & Cronin, 1968).

An unusual case of formaldehyde toxicity involved haemolysis in a patient undergoing haemodialysis. The source of formaldehyde was traced to the filters in a newly installed water filtration system (Orringer & Mattern, 1976). Its significance lies in the fact that formaldehyde is widely used as a disinfectant for haemodialysis equipment.

In common with other alkylating agents, aldehydes are potentially carcinogenic and precautions against unnecessary inhalation of the vapours should be taken. Formaldehyde has caused squamous cell carcinomas in rats (Yodaikin, 1981) but extensive surveys of persons who were occupationally exposed to uncontrolled levels of formaldehyde vapour for many years in industry have produced no evidence of a relationship with human cancer (Editorial Lancet, 1983). However, concentrated formaldehyde must not be mixed with chlorine disinfectants or any other source of free chlorine because a potent carcinogen, bis-(chloromethyl) ether, is produced (Drew et al,

1975). Some simple precautions that should be taken in pathology and microbiology laboratories have been outlined by Clark (1983).

Aldehyde disinfectants do not damage stainless steel instruments or loosen the lens cement of endoscopes, but the articles should be rinsed thoroughly before use. Prolonged immersion may result in deposition of polymer that is difficult to remove.

Applications

The use of aldehydes as disinfectants is limited to situations in which action against bacterial spores, viruses, acid-fast bacilli or fungi is required. They provide an alternative to strong chlorine disinfectants when these are likely to damage instruments or other equipment. The sporicidal action of glutaraldehyde is superior to that of formaldehyde but it may be less effective against acid-fast bacteria (Rubbo et al, 1967; Bergan & Lystad, 1971). A wide range of viruses is susceptible, including both lipophilic and non-enveloped types (Klein & Deforest, 1963; Saitanu & Lund, 1975). Fungi may be inhibited or killed.

Disinfection of heat-sensitive instruments

Heat-sensitive endoscopic instruments, such as cystoscopes and laparoscopes, should be sterilized by a gaseous process but the necessary time is not available when an instrument is required for repeated use on the same day. If a method of pasteurization by hot water or subatmospheric steam is not available, the disassembled and thoroughly cleaned instrument should be immersed in alkaline glutaraldehyde for 20–30 minutes. A vertical jar should be used to ensure that air is not trapped in the tubes. The instruments must be rinsed three times with sterile distilled water before use.

Sterilization of heat-sensitive instruments

When time is available for sterilization and a gaseous process is not available, immersion in alkaline glutaraldehyde for 10 hours is recommended.

Decontamination of soiled instruments

All blood-stained instruments are potentially contaminated with hepatitis B virus. They can usually be cleaned safely by trained staff wearing protective clothing but glutaraldehyde is a suitable disinfectant if heat treatment is not practicable.

Disinfection in microbiological laboratories

Solutions or sprays containing formaldehyde or glutaraldehyde may be used to disinfect safety cabinets after work involving hazardous microorganisms. Formaldehyde vapour, generated within the cabinet, is recommended for disinfection before replacement of exhaust filters. The aldehydes are also effective in decontaminating incubators, cold rooms or benches which have become contaminated with fungi or bacterial spores. Solutions are more effective than vapours; in either case, safety precautions are required.

CHLORHEXIDINE

General properties

Chlorhexidine is a cationic biguanide, with the following formula:

$$Cl-\bigcirc-NH.C.NH.C.NH.(CH_2)_6.NH.C.NH.C.NH-\bigcirc-Cl$$

The potential of chlorhexidine as a bactericide was discovered during a survey to find new anti-malarial agents related to proguanil (Davies et al, 1954). It is a basic substance, forming salts with inorganic and organic acids. The hydrochloride and acetate are white powders; the hydrochloride is virtually insoluble in water and the acetate has a solubility limit of 1.9 per cent w/v, but both are soluble in alcohol. The gluconate is produced as a 20 per cent w/v aqueous concentrate which may be diluted with water or alcohol. Aqueous solutions of chlorhexidine salts are moderately surface active. They are colourless and odourless but have a bitter, unpleasant taste.

Microbial susceptibility

Gram-positive bacteria	highly susceptible
Gram-negative bacteria	moderately susceptible
Acid-fast bacteria	resistant
Bacterial spores	resistant
Lipophilic viruses	may be susceptible
Hydrophilic viruses	resistant

Formulation

Aqueous and alcoholic solutions of chlorhexidine, ranging in strength from 0.02–1 per cent w/v, can be prepared from a stock solution containing 20 per cent w/v chlorhexidine gluconate. Distilled water should be used because anions in tap water, such as chloride and sulphate, can precipitate the bactericide. A coloured 5 per cent w/v stock solution contains a surface active agent to counteract precipitation by hard water, but this has limited application. The problem of precipitation may also be encountered when colouring agents are added by the user to identify the concentration or to distinguish between aqueous and alcoholic solutions. When it is necessary to adjust the tonicity of a chlorhexidine solution for application to injured tissue, sodium acetate must be used instead of sodium chloride.

Ethyl alcohol, or a mixture of ethyl and isopropyl alcohols to a total concentration in the range 60–90 per cent, is used to prepare solutions for skin disinfection. Several chlorhexidine formula-tions are available commercially. Alcoholic solutions usually contain 0.5 per cent chlorhexidine, with or without glycerol or resins as skin conditioners. A bactericidal skin cleanser contains 4 per cent chlorhexidine, providing 1 per cent in available form (Lowbury & Lilly, 1973). Obstetric lubricant creams contain 1 per cent of the active agent. Mouth rinses or gels for use in the control of dental plaque are complex formulations containing ingredients to mask the unpleasant taste.

Aqueous solutions containing a low concentration of chlorhexidine, or a 1:10 mixture of chlorhexidine and cetrimide (e.g. Savlon), are sterilized commercially, in appropriate volumes for the intended use, to overcome the problem of survival and growth of Gram-negative bacteria which may be introduced by contaminated distilled water or dirty containers when dilutions are prepared in the hospital. This precaution applies particularly to the 0.02–0.05 per cent w/v aqueous solutions which are used for urinary catheterization and bladder irrigation. The solutions are stable to autoclaving at 115–121°C at pH 5–6 but chlorhexidine is extensively inactivated if heated in poor quality glass bottles that release alkali. Chlorhexidine is inactivated by gamma radiation but can be sterilized by filtration if the first 10 ml of filtrate is discarded to allow for adsorption by the membrane.

Factors influencing efficiency

Chlorhexidine is active in the pH range 5.5–8; the optimum is usually on the alkaline side because this promotes the availability of anionic groups on the bacterial surface to react with the cationic chlorhexidine. The free base precipitates above pH 8. Precipitation by inorganic anions has already been mentioned. Soaps and other anionic detergents react with chlorhexidine and inactivate it. Nonionic detergents may also be incompatible; polysorbate 80 (Tween 80) is used as an inactivator in bactericidal tests.

Adverse effects

Chlorhexidine is remarkably free from toxicity and its potential for skin irritation and sensitization is very low (Rosenberg et al, 1976). Acute oral toxicity is low because chlorhexidine is poorly absorbed from the alimentary tract. Animal tests for chronic toxicity resulted in decreased consumption of the unpalatable drinking water, but the effects of long-term consumption are not serious, and are usually reversible. No adverse effects on reproduction and no brain changes of the type associated with hexachlorophene have been detected. Tests for dermal absorption in neonatal monkeys and human volunteers have revealed no detectable amounts in the blood or urine and, in the monkeys, no adverse changes in the brain tissue (Gongwer et al, 1980). A few cases of haematuria following bladder irrigation with 0.02 per cent w/v aqueous chlorhexidine have been reported but this also occurred with other irrigating solutions. The complication can be avoided if the volume of each instillation is limited to 25 ml (Pearman, 1971). Chlorhexidine does not delay healing when applied to wounds or abrasions. However, it should never be used in surgery on the middle ear or the brain because it may cause sensorineural deafness, as do many other antiseptics (Bicknell, 1971). Risks of similar magnitude are also associated with brain surgery.

A small amount of *p*-chloroaniline is produced during heat sterilization of aqueous chlorhexidine but the quantity in a dilute solution is unlikely to present a hazard (Goodall et al, 1968).

The possibility of changes in the resident skin flora, resulting in an increase of Gram-negative bacteria or yeasts, has been investigated. Frequent body bathing with chlorhexidine may increase the number of Gram-negative bacteria in the axillae or groin, but pathogens were not found (Aly & Maibach, 1976).

In summary, chlorhexidine may be regarded as a non-toxic, non-irritant and rarely sensitizing substance in its recommended uses as a skin and mucous membrane disinfectant and wound antiseptic (Gardner & Gray, 1983).

Applications

Chlorhexidine is used mainly as a disinfectant of skin and mucous membranes. When applied to the skin, it combines the immediate action of iodine compounds with the residual and cumulative action of hexachlorophene.

Disinfection before surgery or venepuncture

A chlorhexidine skin cleanser may be used, locally or for washing the whole body (Davies et al, 1977) in advance preparation for surgery. At the time of surgery, alcoholic chlorhexidine (0.5 per cent w/v in 80 per cent v/v ethyl alcohol) should be applied to the operation site for 2 minutes prior to incision.

Disinfection of hands

A distinction is made between surgical hand disinfection, where the resident bacteria must be reduced to a very low level, and disinfection of the hands of staff in patient care areas where the danger of transmitting infection is usually limited to transient contamination with pathogenic microorganisms.

Two types of chlorhexidine preparations may be used before surgery. The regular use of a chlorhexidine skin cleanser (e.g. Hibiscrub, Hibiclens) is most convenient; a reduction in the resident bacteria by more than 80 per cent occurs after the first application and more than 99 per cent reduction can be maintained by regular use (Lowbury & Lilly, 1973). Alternatively, 5–10 ml of alcoholic chlorhexidine (0.5 per cent w/v in aqueous alcohol) containing skin conditioners may be applied to the hands and forearms for 2 minues after they have been washed with ordinary soap, rinsed and dried. However, Lowbury et al (1974) reported that application of a solution containing 0.5 per cent w/v chlorhexidine in 95 per cent alcohol to the dry hands was more effective and more convenient than washing with the chlorhexidine skin cleanser, giving 97.9 per cent reduction of the resident flora after a single application and 99.7 per cent reduction after repeated use.

Hand washing by staff working in hospital wards and nurseries, diagnostic departments and other patient care areas needs only to remove transient contaminants that may have been acquired from attending to the previous patient. Although thorough washing can sometimes achieve this without the use of antibacterial agents, a disinfectant should be used as pathogenic microorganisms, such as *Pseudomonas aeruginosa,* may be involved (Lowbury et al, 1964a). Use of a chlorhexidine skin cleanser is most convenient when the hands must be washed but, if the hands are dry and have not been soiled, an alcoholic solution with skin conditioners can be used without washing (Lowbury et al, 1974).

In microbiological laboratories, clinics and dental surgeries routine handwashing with a liquid soap that is hygienically dispensed is usually satisfactory. In the event of accidental contamination in the laboratory or after treatment of a dental patient who is suspected of harbouring pathogenic microorganisms, immediate application of an alcoholic chlorhexidine solution containing skin conditioners is recommended. Care should be taken not to contaminate the dispenser or the wash basin fittings prior to disinfection.

Antiseptic skin care

After the discovery of the harmful effects of bathing premature infants or those with skin abnormalities with emulsions or dusting powders containing hexachlorophene, alternative bactericides were investigated (Hnatko, 1977). A chlorhexidine skin cleanser, at a dilution of 1:10, has been used on more than 3000 infants without any adverse reactions and a powder containing 1 per cent chlorhexidine hydrochloride was also satisfactory (Gardner & Gray, 1983).

Disinfection of mucous membranes

Chlorhexidine is widely used for the prevention of infection in urinary catheterization and bladder irrigation. An aqueous solution containing 0.02–0.05 per cent w/v chlorhexidine is used and it should be sterile for instillation into the bladder. Chlorhexidine skin cleanser or a cetrimide and chlorhexidine solution may be more effective in obstetrics and gynaecology, where mucous secretions and fatty exudates may protect the bacteria.

The oral mucous membranes may be disinfected before surgery by aqueous chlorhexidine (0.2–0.5 per cent w/v), alcoholic chlorhexidine being used to disinfect the neighbouring skin. Special formulations containing 0.2 per cent w/v chlorhexidine and substances which mask the unpleasant taste are in use for the control of dental plaque (Ainamo, 1977).

Disinfection of contaminated wounds

The objective is to remove microbial contaminants and foreign material. An aqueous solution containing chlorhexidine and cetrimide, which is an effective detergent, is suitable. A cream containing chlorhexidine and silver sulphadiazine is among the preparations that are used to prevent contamination of burn wounds; burned patients may also be bathed in a dilute solution of a cetrimide-chlorhexidine solution.

Surface disinfection

Surface disinfection has a minor role in the applications of chlorhexidine. The reduction of activity by organic matter limits its use to cleaned objects or surfaces. Aqueous or alcoholic solutions may be used for wiping or spraying trolley tops or bracket tables. Aqueous chlorhexidine (0.1 per cent w/v) has been used for disinfection of cystoscopes but it does not kill tubercle bacilli and might not be effective against *P. aeruginosa*. A cetrimide-chlorhexidine solution may be used for cleaning and disinfecting the breathing tubes of mechanical ventilators if a method of pasteurization is not available.

CHLORINE COMPOUNDS

General properties

The biocidal activity of elemental chlorine (Cl_2) and a variety of organic and inorganic chlorine-releasing compounds is mediated by hypochlorous acid (HOCl), which is formed in aqueous solutions at pH 5–8. Hypochlorite ions (OCl^-), which predominate in strongly alkaline solutions, are virtually devoid of activity. Chlorine dioxide (ClO_2), which does not depend on production of HOCl for its biocidal action, is included in a later section of this chapter.

Chlorine compounds are oxidizing agents and the end products of their reaction with microorganisms and associated organic material are inactive chlorides (e.g. sodium chloride). The following types of chlorine compounds are most commonly used as disinfectants:

Sodium hypochlorite, NaOCl
Calcium hypochlorite (chloride of lime), $Ca(OCl)_2$
Lithium hypochlorite, LiOCl
Chlorinated trisodium phosphate (sodium hypochlorite in water of crystallization of the strongly alkaline phosphate)
Chlorinated isocyanurates, e.g. sodium dichloroisocyanurate (NaDCC, or SDIC):

Microbial susceptibility

Gram-positive bacteria	highly susceptible
Gram-negative bacteria	highly susceptible
Acid-fast bacteria	moderately susceptible
Bacterial spores	susceptible (optimum pH 7.6)
Lipophilic viruses	susceptible
Hydrophilic viruses	susceptible (high concentration)
Amoebic cysts, algae	susceptible
Fungi	moderately susceptible

Formulation

Sodium hypochlorite is available only as aqueous solutions, which are usually prepared by adding chlorine to caustic soda:

$$Cl_2 + 2NaOH \rightarrow NaOCl + NaCl + H_2O$$

Commercial sodium hypochlorite usually contains 12–14 per cent available chlorine when manufactured. When preparing dilutions, allowance should be made for deterioration of the stock solution: a 14 per cent solution may be reduced to 10 per cent or less in about 4 weeks. An electrolytically prepared solution containing 1 per cent available chlorine, used mainly for disinfection of infants' feeding bottles, is more stable.

The strongly alkaline solution is diluted with water to concentrations, ranging from 200 parts per million (p.p.m.) to 5000 p.p.m. (0.5 per cent), as required for its various uses. However, sporicidal action is greatly accelerated by buffering the solution to pH 7.6 (Death & Coates, 1979). Calcium and lithium hypochlorites are white solids.

Chlorinated trisodium phosphate and the various chlorinated isocyanurates are marketed as powders; the organic compounds usually contain compatible detergents. They vary in water solubility and it is important to ensure that the solid is completely dissolved before the solution is used. It may be difficult or impossible to prepare concentrated solutions (above 1000 p.p.m.) of chlorine disinfectants from the powdered forms.

Concentrations of chlorine-based disinfectants refer to available chlorine, which is a measure of oxidizing power. Available chorine is equivalent to the amount of elemental chlorine (Cl_2) that is required to produce a molecule of hypochlorite (NaOCl). It is therefore double the amount that is present in the hypochlorite molecule because one of the chlorine atoms is included in the inactive sodium chloride. The available chlorine content of a powder is expressed as per cent w/w and that of a concentrated solution as per cent w/v or parts per million (p.p.m.) depending on the strength. One per cent corresponds to 10 000 p.p.m. When a powdered disinfectant contains mixed active and inactive solids, the manufacturer's directions regarding the weight of powder to be dissolved in a stated volume of water must be followed.

Available chlorine content is determined in the laboratory by titration. A solution of sodium arsenite with starch indicator is used. The titration in millilitres of 0.141N sodium arsenite corresponds to the available chlorine content as grams per litre (Ayliffe et al, 1984).

Factors influencing efficiency

Concentration and pH

The effects of concentration and pH are interrelated and the latter may be more important; for example, 100 p.p.m. at pH 7.6 kills spores of *Bacillus subtilis* as rapidly as does 1000 p.p.m. at pH 9. The strong alkalinity of sodium hypochlorite solutions favours stability during storage but the pH must be in the range 6–8 for effective biocidal action. The solution decomposes at pH 4, evolving chlorine. The dilution factor (e.g. from 10 per cent available chlorine to 1000 p.p.m.) may be sufficient to achieve the optimum range of pH but buffering to pH 7.6 is required for rapid and reliable sporicidal action of dilute solutions.

The influence of temperature has practical significance because hypochlorite solutions may be used for hot cleaning and sanitization in the food and dairying industries. An increase of 10°C halves the time required for sporicidal action.

Organic material

Chlorine disinfectants react readily with all types of organic matter, including blood, faeces and tissues. Nitrogenous components are converted to organic chloramines (N-chloro compounds), which retain some activity; however, these are eventually destroyed by oxidative reactions if sufficient chlorine is available. The concentration of available chlorine that is used for disinfection should be high enough to provide an effective residual of the active agent after the chlorine demand of the organic material associated with the microorganisms has been satisfied.

Hard water

The calcium and magnesium ions in hard water do not inactivate chlorine disinfectants but ferrous or manganous cations, and nitrite or sulphide anions reduce active hypochlorous acid to inactive chloride. Small amounts of potassium bromide may potentiate the action of hypochlorite (Shere et al, 1962). However, this effect is less obvious at the high concentrations of available chlorine that are used for disinfection in hospitals.

Adverse effects

Strong hypochloride solutions have a penetrating and irritant odour due to release of gaseous chlorine. They bleach and damage the texture of fabrics and corrode many metals; silver and aluminium are most susceptible but stainless steel instruments and utensils are damaged by the high concentrations that are required for general disinfection in hospitals. Food cans withstand 10 p.p.m. available chlorine in the cooling water (Malpas, 1971).

Chlorine disinfectants are approved for use in the catering, food and dairying industries because the relatively weak solutions (200–300 p.p.m.) that are used as sanitizers produce no toxic residues. Chlorine in swimming pools may cause eye irritation. Chlorinated trisodium phosphate, which is strongly alkaline, is unsuitable for the cleaning of dairy equipment when this is done manually because it is too irritant to the skin.

Applications

Chlorine disinfectants have a wide range of uses, from the treatment of water supplies to inactivation of hepatitis B virus in blood.

Disinfection of water

Chlorine is used for the disinfection of public water supplies, swimming pools and water used for cooling canned foods or washing fresh foods such as fish or poultry (Table 10.1). Sewage may also be treated with chlorine but reliance must be placed on the production of chloramines as the high chlorine demand of the organic materials cannot, in practice, be satisfied. Residual free chlorine in water supplies and swimming pools should be about 0.6 p.p.m. and should fall to 0.3 p.p.m. by the time the water reaches the consumer. Levels of 5–10 p.p.m. are required for ice-water mixtures used in the food industry. Tablets of halazone or other N-chloro compounds may be used for disinfection of suspect drinking water by individual consumers.

Sanitization

Chlorine disinfectants are widely used in the dairying, food production and catering industries because they do not leave toxic residues. The recommended concentration for use on precleaned equipment and work surfaces is 200–300 p.p.m. If

Table 10.1 Water disinfection with chlorine (Malpas, 1971; Trueman, 1971)

Application	Available chlorine concentration (p.p.m.)
Public water supplies	0.5 (holding time 1–2 h)
New water mains	20 (2 h)
Swimming pools	0.6, dropping to not less than 0.3, continuous treatment
Industrial process water	
Can cooling	4–5 (free chlorine must be present)
Poultry processing	10–20 (200 for 10 min for ice-water)
Abbatoirs	10 (free residual)
Sea water	40
(fish and trawlers)	
Washing salads, fruit, raw meat, fish	100 (soak 10–15 min and rinse well)
Fish and shellfish from polluted water	200–6000
Potable water for aircraft	10 (30 min, then dechlorinate)
Drinking water (small scale or individual)	20–30 (15 min)
Algal control	0.2–2.0
Slime control (paper industry, power station cooling water)	Example: 3–5, for 15–20 min every 3 h
Soft drinks industry	Virtual sterility required; super chlorination and dechlorination

detergent-sanitizers are used on uncleaned equipment or surfaces a higher concentration may be required to allow for inactivation by organic matter. Infant feeding bottles may be disinfected by the use of a 1: 80 dilution of a purified 1 per cent w/v stock solution (i.e. 125 p.p.m.) after they have been thoroughly cleaned.

General disinfection

Sodium hypochlorite, at an available chlorine concentration of at least 5000 p.p.m. (Sehulster et al, 1981), is recommended for decontaminating blood that has been splashed or spilled on equipment or floors. If the articles (e.g. instruments) or material cannot withstand the high concentration, alkaline glutaraldehyde must be used for inactivating the hepatitis B virus. Solutions containing 1000 p.p.m. available chlorine are suitable for general disinfection of environment and equipment in hos-

pitals. A buffered solution (pH 7.6), containing only 100 p.p.m. available chlorine, has proved effective in disinfecting fibreoptic endoscopes (Coates & Death, 1982). A concentration of 1000 p.p.m. may be used in laboratory discard jars in bacteriological laboratories but 5000 p.p.m. is required in virus laboratories. A lower concentration may provide temporary safety if the contaminated equipment is autoclaved in the container before it is emptied.

HEXACHLOROPHENE

General properties

Hexachlorophene is a bisphenol, in which two chlorinated phenol molecules are linked by a methylene bridging group:

The white solid has low solubility in water but is more soluble at alkaline pH. It forms emulsions with soap and detergents.

Microbial susceptibility

Gram-positive bacteria	susceptible (killed slowly)
Other microorganisms	resistant

Formulation

Hexachlorophene is used as a 3 per cent w/w skin cleansing emulsion, formulated with non-alkaline detergents (e.g. pHisoHex). It is also incorporated in dusting powder and bar soaps.

Factors influencing efficiency

Hexachlorophene maintains its activity against

pathogenic staphylococci in the presence of soap and alkaline or neutral detergents. The initial action on the skin bacteria is slow but adsorption of hexachlorophene to the skin provides the sustained and cumulative action that is required for surgical hand disinfection.

Adverse effects

Accidental ingestion of a hexachlorophene emulsion has caused death in adults and children on several occasions (Wear et al, 1962; Lustig, 1963). The use of hexachlorophene as a skin disinfectant or antiseptic can cause an oedematous condition of the brain, which may result in convulsions and even death. The threshold blood level for brain changes in rats is about 1.2 μg/ml (Kimbrough, 1973). High blood levels and clinical symptoms have occurred in humans only when hexachlorophene preparations were applied to small premature infants, diseased skin, mucous membranes or injured tissues, such as burn wounds. It has not resulted in excessive blood levels or clinical symptoms when used on normal infants (Plueckhahn, 1973) or the hands of doctors and nurses (Butcher et al, 1973). An isolated episode, involving many fatalities among the infants affected, resulted from an error in the formulation of a hexachlorophene dusting powder (Martin-Bouyer et al, 1982).

Applications

Preparation for surgery

Hexachlorophene detergent emulsions are used for cleansing the skin of patients in preparation for elective surgery. However, a more rapidly acting bactericide, such as chlorhexidine or an iodophor, must be used for disinfecting the operation site immediately before surgery.

Disinfection of hands

The use of a hexachlorophene emulsion by surgeons and nurses is effective in killing *Staphylococcus aureus* within 1 hour. The resident skin bacteria are reduced by 90 per cent or more after several days if the preparation is used regularly (Lowbury et al, 1963). The immediate result of a single application is no more effective than that obtained with plain soap and water.

Antiseptic skin care

The application of hexachlorophene emulsions or creams to the skin of newborn infants to prevent staphylococcal infections in hospital nurseries has been effective in curtailing the spread of staphylococcal infections in many hospitals. Suspension of the practice in American hospitals while its safety was being evaluated showed that the incidence of infections increased in many hospitals while its use was discontinued (Kaslow et al, 1973).

IODOPHORS

General properties

Iodophors are organic complexes containing iodine trapped within the micelles of a surface active agent. The amount of free iodine in a concentrated solution is low but it is released from the micelles as the solution is diluted. Further dilution, after all of the iodine has been liberated, results in decreasing activity. The organic carrier may be polyvinylpyrrolidone (PVP), another nonionic surface active compound or a cationic detergent. Povidone-iodine (PVP-I) is a brown, water-soluble powder containing approximately 10 per cent w/w iodine. Iodophors are also soluble in ethyl and isopropyl alcohols. Iodine-based disinfectants are stable in acid solutions but decompose, releasing iodine vapour, if heated above 40°C.

Microbial susceptibility

Gram-positive bacteria	highly susceptible
Gram-negative bacteria	highly susceptible
Acid-fast bacteria	susceptible
Bacterial spores	susceptible
Protozoan cysts	susceptible
Lipophilic viruses	susceptible
Hydrophilic viruses	susceptible
Fungi (yeasts)	susceptible

Formulation

Povidone-iodine may be used as an aqueous or alcoholic solution. A povidone-iodine antiseptic solution contains 1 per cent w/v available iodine and a surgical scrub, incorporating added detergents, contains 0.75 per cent. Low-foaming products, strongly acidified with phosphoric acid, are used in the dairy industry.

Factors influencing efficiency

The optimum pH is in the neutral and acid range. The influence of temperature on activity is irrelevant because decomposition occurs above 40°C, with evolution of iodine vapour. Soft or hard water may be used to prepare solutions for use as surface disinfectants or sanitizers. Iodine reacts more slowly than chlorine with organic matter because it is a weaker oxidizing agent; this property may outweigh its slower biocidal action.

Adverse effects

In their principal use as skin disinfectants, iodophors have several advantages over the solutions of free iodine which they have replaced. The incidence and severity of hypersensitivity reactions is greatly reduced and stains on clothing or dressings can be removed by washing. However, caution should be exercised in their application to sensitive tissues. Wlodkowski et al (1975) reported that povidone-iodine can cause changes of genetic significance in DNA and Ahrenholz et al (1979) found that human neutrophil function was depressed as a result of application to the peritoneal cavity.

Applications

Disinfection of operation sites

Povidone-iodine surgical scrub may be used for advance preparation of operation sites, followed by disinfection with an aqueous or alcoholic iodophor before incision. The use of an iodophor to disinfect the skin before collection of blood, cerebrospinal fluid or bone marrow is recommended. The broad spectrum action of iodine makes it particularly suitable for the maintenance of intravenous infusion sites, especially in long-term procedures such as parenteral nutrition where fungaemia caused by *Candida albicans* is a common complication.

Povidone-iodine, applied as a wet compress for at least 15–30 minutes, reduces but does not eliminate the risk of infection by *Clostridium perfringens* during surgery on the lower bowel or thighs (Lowbury et al, 1964b; Drewett et al, 1972). Instillation of a povidone-iodine powder or spray into the peritoneal cavity, or application to the sutured wound after abdominal surgery, is a subject of controversy. Gilmore and Sanderson (1975) reported a decrease in the incidence of postoperative infections, with no sign of bacterial resistance or other harmful effects. Morgan (1979) and others have also reported a significant decrease in the infection rate. However, several investigators (Pollock & Evans, 1975; Galland et al, 1977; De Jong et al, 1982) found the incidence of wound infection to be no different from that when a saline irrigation was used as a control.

Disinfection of hands

A povidone-iodine skin cleanser was found by Lowbury and Lilly (1973) to be slightly inferior to a chlorhexidine skin cleanser in its immediate and cumulative action on the resident flora. The iodophor achieved 68 per cent and 97.7 per cent reductions respectively, compared with 86.7 per cent and 99.2 per cent for chlorhexidine. However, the iodine preparation would be more effective against viruses.

General disinfection

Iodophors may be used to disinfect clinical thermometers used by tuberculosis patients; the thermometers should be rinsed after 10 minutes immersion and stored dry. Iodophors may be used as an alternative to chlorine compounds for disinfection of clean ward equipment or room surfaces in hospitals.

Sanitization

Iodophors are suitable for disinfection of clean equipment, utensils and work surfaces in the food production, catering and dairying industries, although chlorine disinfectants are more widely used. The recommended concentrations of available iodine are 50–150 p.p.m. The presence of iodine can be detected by colour to the lower limit of its bactericidal activity. A strongly acid iodophor is used to prevent or remove milkstone from milking machines and other dairy equipment. Iodophors may also be used for disinfection of cows' udders as part of a mastitis control programme.

STRONG OXIDIZING AGENTS

Chlorine dioxide, peracetic acid and hydrogen peroxide form a diverse group of chemical compounds which are used mainly for their sporicidal activity. They are highly reactive and the solutions may be unstable. Each has a broad spectrum of biocidal action, which includes bacterial spores.

Chlorine dioxide

Chlorine dioxide (ClO_2) is a stronger oxidizing agent than other chlorine disinfectants. It also differs from them as it does not give rise to hypochlorous acid and does not combine with ammonia or organic nitrogen compounds to produce amines. Chlorine dioxide is prepared by mixing dilute solutions of chlorine and sodium chlorite. Strong solutions are not prepared because explosion might occur. The dilute solutions, containing 4–5 per cent w/v of the active agent, may be stabilized by addition of boron compounds.

The bactericidal activity of chlorine dioxide is similar to that of other chlorine disinfectants and the sporicidal action is independent of pH over the range 6–10. Applications are limited to water treatment, where it is useful for removing tastes and odours by breaking down phenolic compounds. It is used to control slime in paper pulp processing.

Peracetic acid

Pure peracetic acid ($CH_3CO.OOH$) is a colourless liquid, miscible with water and organic solvents. It has a pungent odour and is highly explosive. A 40

per cent w/w solution of peracetic acid is prepared commercially from acetic acid and hydrogen peroxide, using sulphuric acid as catalyst. It contains 39 per cent acetic acid, 5 per cent hydrogen peroxide, 1 per cent sulphur dioxide and 15 per cent water. A detergent (sodium alkylaryl sulphonate, 0.1 per cent) may be added. The solution can be stabilized for transportation but it should be stored in containers with vented caps to prevent pressure building up as oxygen is released. A 2 per cent v/v solution may be used as an aerosol.

Peracetic acid is more active than is hydrogen peroxide against bacteria and their spores (Baldry, 1983). Some activity is retained at subzero temperatures. The surfaces to be treated should be clean, and a relative humidity around 80 per cent is required when it is used as a vapour (Portner & Hoffman, 1968). The breakdown products are water, acetic acid and oxygen.

The solution is irritant and corrosive; the vapour is also irritant but is easily removed from a ventilated area. Dense fogging may damage surfaces by accumulation of liquid. The 2 per cent v/v solution damages iron and steel; rubber is affected but still usable. Stainless steel, glass and plastics are resistant. The agent is a weak carcinogen, and produces tumours in mice.

Peracetic acid is used mainly in germfree animal technology to disinfect or sterilize animal isolators and entry locks. It is also suitable for laboratory safety cabinets and air filters, which must be flushed with air after treatment.

Hydrogen peroxide

Hydrogen peroxide (H_2O_2) exists only in solution. It is a slow oxidizing agent. Dilute solutions are unstable, especially in the presence of tissue which contains the enzyme catalase. Concentrated solutions containing 90 per cent w/v H_2O_2, which are prepared electrochemically using inert containers and piping, are stable. These may be diluted to 3–6 per cent w/v for disinfection and the container may be opened daily without loss of the peroxide. A 6 per cent solution withstands heating. There are no toxic decomposition products.

There is some activity against most types of microorganisms but enteric viruses and bacterial spores require a high concentration for lethal action. An initial lag in the rate of sporicidal action may be shortened by an increase in the concentration or temperature. Fungi are relatively resistant.

Uses that have been proposed for hydrogen peroxide include spray disinfection of mechanical ventilators (Ayliffe et al, 1984), acrylic resin implants, plastic eating utensils and soft contact lenses. The absence of toxicity is attractive to the food industry and hydrogen peroxide is used to disinfect cartons which are aseptically filled with 'sterilized' milk (Swartling & Lindgren, 1968).

PHENOLS

General properties

Phenol ('carbolic acid') is the parent compound of the substituted phenols which are used to formulate phenolic disinfectants. The substituents may be alkyl groups (methyl, ethyl), halogen atoms (Cl, Br, F) or aromatic ring structures (phenyl, benzyl). All of the compounds retain the alcohol (OH) group of the parent phenol, which is no longer used as a disinfectant because of its irritant nature and lower activity. The formulae of some substituted phenols that are commonly used to formulate the disinfectants are shown below.

Alkylphenols are obtained by collecting coal tar distillate in three fractions with increasing boiling points. Cresols predominate in the first, xylenols in the second, and high-boiling tar acids in the third fraction. Bactericidal activity generally increases and skin irritancy decreases as the boiling point rises. The crude phenols are usually dark brown. Halogenated phenols, which may also contain alkyl or aromatic substituents, are prepared synthetically and are white solids which are insoluble in water. They are generally more active than phenols containing alkyl groups only.

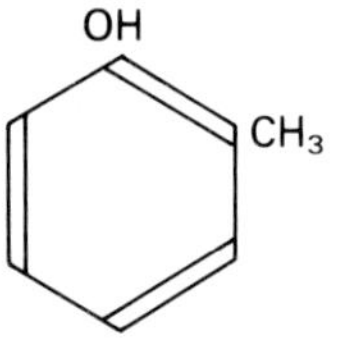

o-cresol 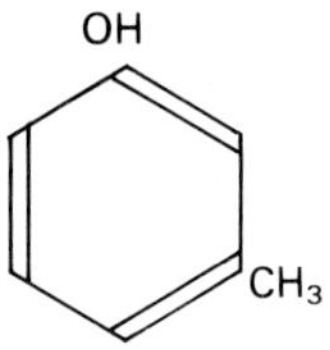　　*m*-cresol 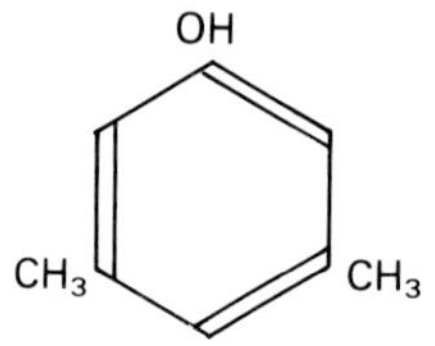　　*m*-xylenol

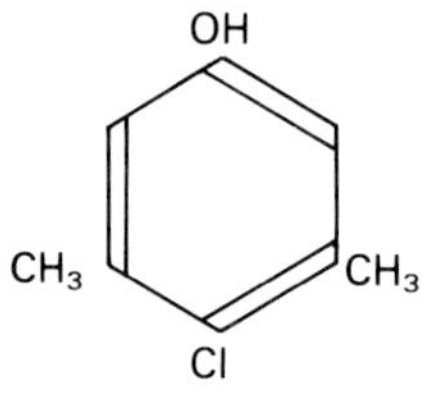

p-chlor-*m*-xylenol 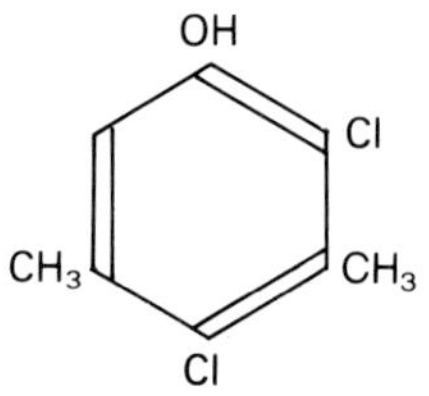　　*di*-chlor-*m*-xylenol

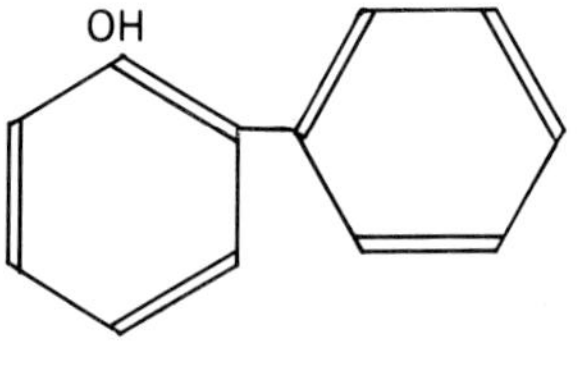

o-phenylphenol

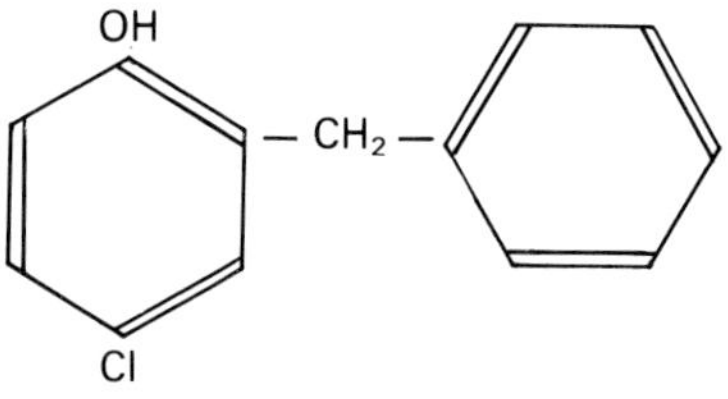

o-benzyl-*p*-chlorphenol

Microbial susceptibility

Gram-positive bacteria	highly susceptible
Gram-negative bacteria	highly susceptible
Acid-fast bacteria	may be susceptible
Bacterial spores	resistant
Lipophilic viruses	susceptible
Hydrophilic viruses	resistant

Formulation

Most formulations contain mixed phenols, the types and proportions being selected to yield products with a desired spectrum of activity. The coal tar phenols act non-selectively against Gram-positive and Gram-negative bacteria but the chloroxylenols are deficient in activity against Gram-negative organisms, especially *Pseudomonas, Proteus* and *Klebsiella*. Activity in this area has been greatly improved by the inclusion of aromatic phenols, such as *o*-phenylphenol and *o*-benzyl-*p*-chlorphenol. The formulae are usually trade secrets and only the total phenol content is specified. Some products now on the market are more active against the Gram-negative bacilli than they are against Gram-positive cocci.

Phenolic disinfectants are formulated with surface active agents or emulsifiers because the active ingredients are insoluble in water. 'Clear soluble fluids' contain natural soaps or synthetic anionic detergents. The relative concentrations of phenols and surfactant are critical because the phenols must escape from their location within molecular aggregates (micelles) of the carrier to the aqueous phase, where they exert their bactericidal action. Clear soluble fluids can be made from crude or refined coal tar phenols, chloroxylenols or complex mixtures of synthetic phenols.

'Black fluids' and 'white fluids' are crude coal tar disinfectants. The former are clear liquids in concentrated form but the latter are emulsions. The black fluids produce emulsions on dilution. Hydrocarbons are used to stabilize the emulsions but they are liable to break down as the solutions age. Use-dilutions of phenolic disinfectants are prepared on a volumetric basis as the exact composition is usually not known.

Factors influencing efficiency

Phenols have relatively high concentration coefficients and a small reduction in the concentration causes a large increase in the killing time. They are most active at neutral or slightly acid pH because the unionized molecule is the active form. The activity of chloroxylenols against Gram-negative bacilli is low but it may be increased by formulation with ethylenediamine tetraacetic acid (Russell & Furr, 1977).

Organic matter has little effect on the activity of coal tar disinfectants. The synthetic phenols are affected to some extent but their activity is less affected than is that of chlorine compounds, chlorhexidine and quaternary ammonium compounds. Oils and fats reduce activity by extracting the phenols from the aqueous solution.

Natural soaps and anionic detergents are compatible with phenols, subject to being formulated in the correct proportions. Nonionic detergents, such as polysorbate 80 (Tween 80) reduce activity and cationic detergents (quaternary ammonium compounds) are incompatible. Hard water is unsuitable for preparing dilutions; formulae that contain soap are affected more than are those that contain synthetic detergents.

Adverse effects

All phenolic disinfectants are poisonous if swallowed (Joubert et al, 1978). Crude coal tar disinfectants, such as lysol, cause chemical burns if the concentrated solution comes in contact with the skin. Synthetic formulations are less irritant but chlorinated phenols have caused allergic photocontact dermatitis. The odour of coal tar disinfectants is objectionable and is no longer associated in the mind of the user with efficiency. However, its place has been taken by the perfume of added pine oils, which do not contribute significantly to the bactericidal activity. Phenols may stain wool, cotton and synthetic fabrics and cause damage to copper, nickel and zinc.

Applications

The phenols are general purpose disinfectants for use on inanimate objects and surfaces where bactericidal action in the presence of organic soils is required. They are also effective against lipophilic viruses. Some formulations kill *M. tuberculosis* but they are less effective against acid-fast bacteria than are alcohols, aldehydes and halogen-based disinfectants. Accuracy in dilution is important because a small decrease in concentration results in a large increase in the time required for disinfection.

Hospital uses

Clear soluble phenolics are suitable for disinfection of used instruments if this is necessary and heat treatment is not available. They may be used for disinfecting floors, walls, furniture and fittings in high risk areas such as operating theatres, delivery rooms, nurseries, intensive care wards and dialysis or renal transplant units. They are also appropriate for dealing with spillage of biological material other than blood. If sinks, slop-hoppers or wash basins are suspected of being a source of bacteria causing hospital-acquired infection, a strong phenolic may be poured into the waste pipe and left overnight.

Laboratory uses

Phenolic disinfectants are appropriate for routine disinfection in laboratory animal units and of benches that have been contaminated with non-sporing bacteria. They may be used, as an alternative to chlorine compounds, in discard jars in bacteriology, but not in virology, laboratories (Maurer, 1978).

General hygiene

Relatively cheap coal tar disinfectants may be used in unoccupied premises or outdoor situations.

QUATERNARY AMMONIUM COMPOUNDS (QACs)

General properties

The quaternary ammonium compounds are cationic (positively charged) surface active disin-

fectants. Both characteristics contribute to their bactericidal activity by promoting uptake of the molecules by the microorganisms. The complex cations form salts with chloride or bromide; the anions play no part in the antimicrobial action. The active cations may be regarded as derivatives of an ammonium ion (NH_4^+), in which the four hydrogen atoms have been replaced by organic groups. At least one of these groups is a long hydrocarbon chain derived from fatty acids in vegetable oils. The water-repellant chain causes the molecules to concentrate as an oriented layer at the surface of the solution and at all interfaces with colloidal protein, suspended particles and solid surfaces. The charged nitrogen-containing group has a high affinity for water and prevents the QAC from separating out of the aqueous solution. There are many types of quaternary ammonium compounds; the formulae of cetrimide and benzalkonium chloride are shown.

The QACs are non-crystalline solids, soluble in water and alcohols. The solutions are slightly alkaline, colourless and, with the exception of pyridine-based compounds, odourless. They are stable to heat and radiation sterilization.

Microbial susceptibility

Gram-positive bacteria	highly susceptible
Gram-negative bacteria	moderately susceptible
Acid-fast bacteria	resistant
Bacterial spores	resistant
Lipophilic viruses	susceptible
Hydrophilic viruses	resistant

Formulation

QAC disinfectants are sold as concentrated solutions (10–50 per cent w/v) containing a single active agent (e.g. benzalkonium chloride) or they may also contain a biguanide, such as chlorhexidine. These are used to prepare dilute solutions in water or 80 per cent v/v ethyl alcohol. Detergent-santizers are formulated with compatible nonionic detergents. Many of these can be regarded only as expensive cleaning agents, but some meet the

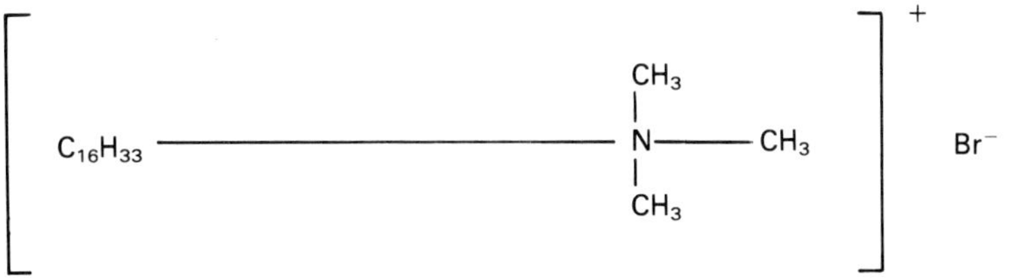

$$[C_{16}H_{33} \underline{\hspace{4cm}} \overset{\displaystyle CH_3}{\underset{\displaystyle CH_3}{N}} \underline{\hspace{1cm}} CH_3]^+ \quad Br^-$$

Cetrimide

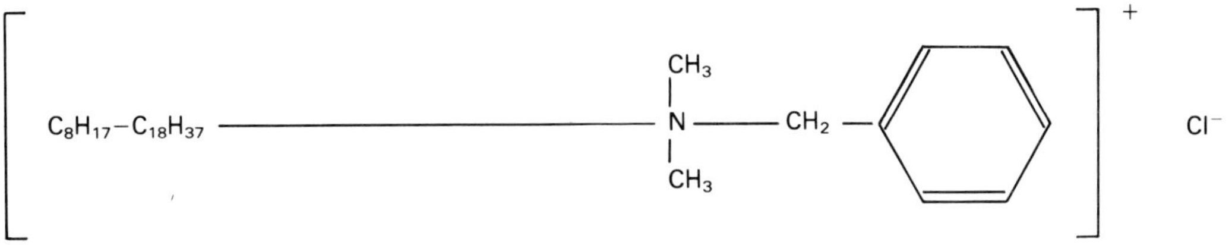

$$[C_8H_{17}-C_{18}H_{37} \underline{\hspace{4cm}} \overset{\displaystyle CH_3}{\underset{\displaystyle CH_3}{N}} \underline{\hspace{1cm}} CH_2 \underline{\hspace{0.5cm}} \bigcirc]^+ \quad Cl^-$$

Benzalkonium chloride

standard of hospital grade disinfectants. Each product must be evaluated by microbiological tests, regardless of the QAC content.

Factors influencing efficiency

Types of microorganisms

The quaternary ammonium compounds have a narrower antibacterial spectrum than the synthetic phenols and chlorhexidine. They are very active against Gram-positive cocci but are unreliable for killing Gram-negative bacteria. If the latter gain access to the solutions during preparation, storage or use, they may multiply in dilute solutions, producing a large population within a few days. *P. aeruginosa, Pseudomonas cepacia* and species of *Achromobacter* or *Serratia* are the most frequent contaminants.

Concentration and pH

The concentration coefficients of QACs are low, so that halving the concentration approximately doubles the time for a specified level of inactivation. The optimum pH is on the alkaline side (9–10); values below 7 are unfavourable.

Organic and synthetic materials

The proteins in blood, serum and milk inactivate

QACs by adsorption; the colloidal protein in serum has an adsorbing surface of about 1 m^2/ml. A three- to fourfold increase in the concentration of a QAC is required for activity in the presence of colloidal or particulate organic matter. Cotton gauze adsorbs QACs (Kundsin & Walter, 1957). Cellulosic and synthetic materials used in containers or cleaning utensils, such as sponges and mops, also inactivate QACs by adsorption (Maurer, 1978). Anionic soaps and synthetic detergents inactivate by chemical reaction between the molecules which carry opposite electric charges. Many nonionic detergents (e.g. polysorbate 80) also inactivate QACs; calcium, magnesium, ferric and possibly aluminium ions reduce activity.

Adverse effects

The quaternary ammonium compounds are popular disinfectants and sanitizers because of their freedom from toxicity and other undesirable effects. The chronic oral toxicity of dilute solutions is low, but human death may be caused by swallowing a concentrated solution. Skin irritation and sensitization are reported occasionally.

Cement, synthetic rubbers and aluminium may be damaged by quaternary ammonium disinfectants, especially if an antirust compound has been added to the solution.

Applications

Surface disinfection

The quaternary ammonium compounds are suitable for disinfection of clean surfaces and are widely used as detergent-sanitizers. Lack of toxicity enables them to be used as sanitizers in the dairying, food production and catering industries as an alternative to chlorine compounds but the latter generally retain their established position.

QACs are not recommended for routine cleaning in hospitals but a high level of activity against pathogenic staphylococci may be useful if these bacteria are found to be colonizing or infecting patients.

Skin disinfection

The QACs are unreliable skin disinfectants because microorganisms may be trapped between the surface of the skin and the inactive side of the molecular film. A product containing cetrimide and chlorhexidine is an effective wound cleanser.

REFERENCES

Ahrenholz D H, Marxen L, Simmons R L 1979 Depression of human neutrophil function by povidone iodine: a mechanism for the effect of betadine in *E. coli* peritonitis. Federation Proceedings 38: 1427

Ainamo J 1977 Control of plaque by chemical agents. Journal of Clinical Periodontology 4(5): 23–35

Aly R, Maibach H I 1976 Effect of antimicrobial soap containing chlorhexidine on the microbial flora of skin. Applied and Environmental Microbiology 31: 931–935

Archer G T L 1945 Bactericidal effect of mixtures of ethyl alcohol and water. British Medical Journal 2: 148–151

Ayliffe G A J, Coates D, Hoffman P N 1984 Chemical disinfection in hospitals. Public Health Laboratory Service, London

Baldry M G C 1983 The bactericidal, fungicidal and sporicidal properties of hydrogen peroxide and peracetic acid. Journal of Applied Bacteriology 54: 417–423

Bergan T, Lystad A 1971 Antitubercular action of disinfectants. Journal of Applied Bacteriology 34: 751–756

Bicknell P G 1971 Sensorineural deafness following myringoplasty operations. Journal of Laryngology and Otology 85: 957–961

Butcher H R, Ballinger W F, Gravens D L, Dewar N E, Ledlie E F, Barthel W F 1973 Hexachlorophene concentrations in the blood of operating room personnel. Archives of Surgery 107: 70–74

Clark R P 1983 Formaldehyde in pathology departments. Journal of Clinical Pathology 36: 839–846

Coates D, Death J E 1982 Use of buffered hypochlorite solution for disinfecting fibrescopes. Journal of Clinical Pathology 35: 296–303

Davies G E, Francis J, Martin A R, Rose F L, Swain G 1954 1:6-di-4'-chlorophenyldiguanidohexane ('Hibitane'). Laboratory investigation of a new antibacterial agent of high potency. British Journal of Pharmacology and Chemotherapy 9: 192–196

Davies J, Babb J R, Ayliffe G A J, Ellis S H 1977 The effect on the skin flora of bathing with antiseptic solutions. Journal of Antimicrobial Chemotherapy 3: 473–481

Death J E, Coates D 1979 Effect of pH on sporicidal and microbicidal activity of buffered mixtures of alcohol and sodium hypochlorite. Journal of Clinical Pathology 32: 148–153

De Jong T E, Wierhout R J, Vroonhoven T J van 1982 Povidone-iodine irrigation of the subcutaneous tissue to prevent surgical wound infections. Surgery, Gynecology & Obstetrics 155: 221–224

Drew R T, Laskin S, Kuschner M, Nelson N 1975 Inhalation carcinogenicity of alpha halo ethers. 1. The acute inhalation toxicity of chloromethyl methyl ether and bis (chloromethyl) ether. Archives of Environmental Health 30: 61–69

Drewett S E, Payne D J H, Tuke W, Verdon P E 1972 Skin distribution of *Clostridium welchii*: use of iodophor as sporicidal agent. Lancet i: 1172–1173

Editorial 1983 Formaldehyde and cancer. Lancet ii: 26

Galland R B, Saunders J H, Mosley J G, Darrell J H 1977 Prevention of wound infection in abdominal operations by peroperative antibiotics or povidone-iodine. Lancet ii: 1043–1045

Gardner J F, Gray K G 1983 Chlorhexidine. In: Block S S (ed) Disinfection, sterilization, and preservation, 3rd edn. Lea & Febiger, Philadelphia, ch 12, p 251

Gilmore O J A, Sanderson P J 1975 Prophylactic interparietal povidone-iodine in abdominal surgery. British Journal of Surgery 62: 792–799

Gongwer L E et al 1980 The effects of daily bathing of neonatal rhesus monkeys with an antimicrobial skin cleanser containing chlorhexidine gluconate. Toxicology and Applied Pharmacology 52: 255–261

Goodall R R, Goldman J, Woods J 1968 Stability of chlorhexidine solutions. Pharmaceutical Journal 200: 33–34

Gorman S P, Scott E M, Russell A D 1980 A review Antimicrobial activity, uses and mechanism of action of glutaraldehyde. Journal of Applied Bacteriology 48: 161–190

Hnatko S I 1977 Alternatives to hexachlorophene bathing of newborn infants. Canadian Medical Association Journal 117: 223–226

Joubert P, Hundt H, Du Toit P 1978 Severe Dettol (chloroxylenol and terpineol) poisoning. British Medical Journal 1: 890

Kaslow R A et al 1973 Staphylococcal disease related to hospital nursery bathing practices — a nationwide epidemiologic investigation. Pediatrics 51: 418–425

Kimbrough R D 1973 Review of recent evidence of toxic effects of hexachlorophene. Pediatrics 51: 391–394

Klein M, Deforest A 1963 The inactivation of viruses by germicides. Chemical Specialities Manufacturers Association Proceedings 49: 116–118

Kundsin R B, Walter C W 1957 Investigations on adsorption of benzalkonium chloride U.S.P. by skin, gloves, and sponges. Archives of Surgery 75: 1036–1042

Lowbury E J L, Lilly H A 1973 Use of 4% chlorhexidine detergent solution (Hibiscrub) and other methods of skin disinfection. British Medical Journal 1: 510–515

Lowbury E J L, Lilly H A, Ayliffe G A J 1974 Preoperative disinfection of surgeons' hands: use of alcoholic solutions and effects of gloves on skin flora. British Medical Journal 4: 369–372

Lowbury E J L, Lilly H A, Bull J P 1963 Disinfection of hands: removal of resident bacteria. British Medical Journal 1: 1251–1256

Lowbury E J L, Lilly H A, Bull J P 1964a Disinfection of hands: removal of transient organisms. British Medical Journal 2: 230–233

Lowbury E J L, Lilly H A, Bull J P 1964b Methods for disinfection of hands and operation sites. British Medical Journal 2: 531–536

Lustig F W 1963 A fatal case of hexachlorophane ('pHisoHex') poisoning. Medical Journal of Australia 1: 737

Malpas J F 1971 The use of chlorine for water disinfection in industry. Chemistry and Industry p 111–115

Martin-Bouyer G, Lebreton R, Toga M, Stolley P D, Lockhart J 1982 Outbreak of accidental hexachlorophene poisoning in France. Lancet i: 91–95

Maurer I M 1978 Hospital hygiene, 2nd edn. Edward Arnold, London

Morgan W J 1979 The effect of povidone-iodine (Betadine) aerosol spray on superficial wounds. British Journal of Clinical Practice 33: 109–110

Orringer E P, Mattern W D 1976 Formaldehyde-induced hemolysis during chronic hemodialysis. New England Journal of Medicine 294: 1416–1420

Pearman J W 1971 Prevention of urinary tract infection following spinal cord injury. Paraplegia 9: 95–104

Plueckhahn V D 1973 Infant antiseptic skin care and hexachlorophene. Medical Journal of Australia 1: 93–100

Pollock A V, Evans M 1975 Povidone-iodine for the control of surgical wound infection: a controlled clinical trial against topical cephaloridine. British Journal of Surgery 62: 292–294

Portner D M, Hoffman R K 1968 Sporicidal effect of peracetic acid vapour. Applied Microbiology 16: 1782–1785

Price P B 1939 Ethyl alcohol as a germicide. Archives of Surgery 38: 528–542

Rosenberg A, Alatary S D, Peterson A F 1976 Safety and efficacy of the antiseptic chlorhexidine gluconate. Surgery, Gynecology & Obstetrics 143: 789–792

Rubbo S D, Gardner J F, Webb R L 1967 Biocidal activities of glutaraldehyde and related compounds. Journal of Applied Bacteriology 30: 78–87

Russell A D, Furr J R 1977 The antibacterial activity of a new chloroxylenol preparation containing ethylenediamine tetraacetic acid. Journal of Applied Bacteriology 43: 253–260

Saitanu K, Lund E 1975 Inactivation of enterovirus by glutaraldehyde. Applied Microbiology 29: 571–574

Sanderson K V, Cronin E 1968 Glutaraldehyde and contact dermatitis. British Medical Journal 3: 802

Sehulster L M, Hollinger F B, Dreesman G R, Melnick J L 1981 Immunological and biophysical alteration of hepatitis B virus antigens by sodium hypochlorite disinfection. Applied and Environmental Microbiology 42: 762–767

Shere L, Kelley M J, Richardson J H 1962 Effect of bromide-hypochlorite bactericides on microorganisms. Applied Microbiology 10: 538–541

Stonehill A A, Krop S, Borick P M 1963 Buffered glutaraldehyde. A new chemical sterilizing solution. American Journal of Hospital Pharmacy 20: 458–465

Swartling P, Lindgren B 1968 The sterilizing effect against *Bacillus subtilis* spores of hydrogen peroxide at different temperatures and concentrations. Journal of Dairy Research 35: 423–428

Trueman J R 1971 The halogens. In: Hugo W B (ed) Inhibition and destruction of the bacterial cell. Academic Press, London, ch 3E, p137

Wear J B Jr, Shanahan R, Ratliff R K 1962 Toxicity of ingested hexachlorophene. Journal of the American Medical Association 181: 587–589

Wlodkowski T J, Speck W T, Rosenkranz H S 1975 Genetic effects of povidone-iodine. Journal of Pharmaceutical Sciences 64: 1235–1237

Yodaikin R E 1981 The uncertain consequences of formaldehyde toxicity. Journal of the American Medical Association 246: 1677–1678

11
Principles of chemical disinfection

Aqueous solutions of antimicrobial agents were associated with two landmarks in the prevention of hospital-acquired infection during the nineteenth century. In 1847, Semmelweiss showed that the incidence of puerperal sepsis in a maternity hospital in Vienna could be greatly reduced if the doctors rinsed their hands in chloride of lime between performing post mortem examinations and attending to their living patients. His recommendation did not receive full cooperation from the doctors and hospital authorities but Lister's method of antiseptic surgery, reported in the British Medical Journal in 1867, fared better. He achieved a dramatic reduction in post-operative infection, which previously killed up to 50 per cent of surgical patients, by disinfecting instruments with 5 per cent phenol and spraying a 2.5 per cent solution on the wound and adjacent skin.

Chemical disinfection of instruments was replaced by sterilization when the emphasis shifted from antiseptic to aseptic surgery but chemicals are still required for disinfection of operation sites and the skin of surgeons and nurses. They are used to make contaminated equipment safe to clean and to prepare some types of equipment for reuse. They are sometimes required to disinfect areas of the hospital environment which have been contaminated with material containing pathogenic microorganisms. They may also be used as an adjunct to cleaning in rooms where patients who are abnormally susceptible to infection are nursed. The selection of appropriate chemical disinfectants for specified purposes and the provision of instructions for their preparation and use should be assisted by a clearly defined hospital policy.

Simple guidelines formulated by Kelsey & Maurer (1967) recommend that chemical disinfectants should not be used if:

1. Sterilization is required
2. Disinfection by hot water or steam is applicable
3. Cleaning alone is adequate.

This chapter discusses the limitations of disinfectants and precautions which must be taken to prevent the solutions from becoming a potential or actual source of hospital-acquired infection through the survival and multiplication of bacteria which are relatively resistant to their action. Methods that may be used to evaluate bactericidal action and confirm their in-use effectiveness are explained.

MECHANISMS OF BACTERICIDAL ACTION

Chemicals that are used for disinfection of inanimate objects or intact body surfaces are selected for rapid bactericidal action against susceptible microorganisms and may be termed general protoplasmic poisons. It is difficult to identify any particular component or structure as the primary target of a rapidly lethal action. However, initial damage to the cell membrane resulting in the loss of important cell constituents, such as purines, pyrimidines, ribose, amino acids and potassium, has been demonstrated in studies on chlorhexidine and quaternary ammonium compounds, phenols and alcohols. These are commonly termed 'membrane active' disinfectants. Glutaraldehyde on the other hand, appears to seal the cell membrane against leakage of intracellular components.

Membrane active disinfectants

The cell membrane regulates the uptake of essential nutrients, including amino acids, and prevents the escape from the cell of vital protein and nucleic acid precursors. It is also the site of action of respiratory enzymes and coenzymes and of systems involved in the synthesis of cell wall components including peptidoglycan.

Investigations by Hugo and Longworth on the effects of chlorhexidine on Gram-positive and Gram-negative bacteria, and their conclusions regarding the mechanisms of bacteriostatic and bactericidal action, have been summarized by Longworth (1971).

Chlorhexidine is strongly adsorbed to the surface of *Staphylococcus aureus* and *Escherichia coli*, reducing the negative charge on the cells. The subsequent changes in cell structure or metabolism depend on the concentration of chlorhexidine in the solution. Leakage of cytoplasmic constituents occurs at bacteriostatic concentrations and the rate increases with the amount of chlorhexidine adsorbed by the cells until the minimum bactericidal concentration is reached. Leakage then ceases abruptly as chlorhexidine penetrates to the interior of the cells and precipitation occurs within the cytoplasm. Studies with the electron microscope have shown clearly that the bacteria are transformed into 'ghost' cells at low concentrations and changes indicative of coagulation occur when the concentration reaches 0.05 per cent w/v.

Support for the conclusion that the cell membrane is the primary site of action of chlorhexidine has been provided by studies on protoplasts and spheroplasts, produced from Gram-positive and Gram-negative bacteria respectively. These are fragile cells which have been deprived partially or completely of their rigid cell wall component. They can survive only in a suspending fluid containing a high concentration of sucrose to balance the osmotic pressure within the cytoplasm; they lyse on dilution with water. Treatment with a low concentration of chlorhexidine causes them to lyse while they are still in the protective solution. A bactericidal concentration precipitates proteins in the cell membrane and lysis does not occur even when the suspending fluid is diluted.

The mechanism of action of quaternary ammonium disinfectants closely resembles that of chlorhexidine in the pattern of leakage at bacteriostatic, and precipitation of cell contents at bactericidal, concentrations (Davies et al, 1968). Inhibition of respiration, probably through action on the cytochrome system, by cetyltrimethylammonium bromide and also by hexachlorophene has been reported (Wiseman, 1971; Frederick et al,

1974). The failure of hexachlorophene to cause cytoplasmic precipitation, even at a high concentration, accounts for its lack of rapid bactericidal action.

Gram-positive bacteria are more sensitive to membrane active disinfectants than are the Gram-negative species because of differences in cell wall composition. Gram-negative bacteria are relatively resistant because they contain complex lipoproteins and lipopolysaccharides which impede access of antibacterial agents to the underlying membrane. If these cell wall components are disaggregated by treatment with ethylenediamine tetraacetic acid (EDTA) or by removal of magnesium ions, the susceptibility of the Gram-negative bacteria is greatly increased.

Aldehydes

Glutaraldehyde and formaldehyde are alkylating agents which probably owe their ability to kill spores to reaction with nucleic acids as well as with proteins. If protoplasts and spheroplasts are treated with glutaraldehyde, they fail to lyse on dilution of the suspending medium. This indicates hardening of the cell membrane (Munton & Russell, 1970; 1973) or cell wall (McGucken & Woodside, 1973). Leakage of cell constituents has not been observed. The mechanism of action of glutaraldehyde has been reviewed by Gorman et al (1980).

Halogens

The halogens are oxidizing agents, chlorine being stronger than iodine. Evidence for the role of oxidation in the bactericidal action of halogen-based disinfectants is provided by the conversion of about 90 per cent of the iodine which has been taken up by the cells to inactive iodide (Brandrick & Newton, 1967). However, participation of direct halogenation of cell constituents is suggested by the fact that hydrogen peroxide and potassium permanganate are stronger oxidizing agents but less efficient bactericides than are the halogen-based disinfectants.

SUSCEPTIBILITY OF MICROORGANISMS

Vegetative bacteria

Gram-positive and Gram-negative bacteria are readily killed by all types of hospital grade disinfectants, although some of the Gram-negative bacteria are capable of survival and growth in phenolic, quaternary ammonium and biguanide disinfectants if the solutions are too dilute or have been inactivated by mixture or contact with incompatible materials. Species of *Klebsiella*, *Proteus*, *Serratia*, *Pseudomonas*, *Achromobacter* and *Flavobacterium* have been isolated from contaminated disinfectants and outbreaks of infections caused by them. These bacteria owe their ability to grow in diluted disinfectants or in water containing traces of organic and inorganic impurities to very simple nutritional requirements and the ability to multiply at ambient temperatures (Favero et al, 1971).

The natural resistance of Gram-negative bacteria to disinfectants which damage the cell membrane is associated with relative inaccessibility of the membrane. Disaggregation of the outer cell wall by EDTA, which binds magnesium, enhances their susceptibility to quaternary ammonium and phenolic disinfectants (Russell & Furr, 1977). The cell wall of *Pseudomonas aeruginosa* is especially rich in magnesium.

The resistance of Gram-negative bacteria varies with the conditions in which they have grown. *Pseudomonas cepacia (syn. P. multivorans)* which has grown in water or dilute disinfectant at ambient temperature undergoes a dramatic decrease in resistance when re-exposed to the disinfectant after a single laboratory subculture in nutrient broth at 37°C (Bassett et al, 1970). The pH of the disinfectant may also determine whether bacterial multiplication occurs. The same organism, which was isolated from a solution containing a quaternary ammonium compound and chlorhexidine that had been diluted in the hospital with distilled water (pH 6), was easily killed by the same disinfectant concentration when prepared with tap water in the laboratory at pH 7.2. This is close to the optimum pH for activity of cationic disinfectants (Bassett, 1971a).

The possibilities of increased resistance in bacteria as a result of exposure to disinfectants and of a relationship to multi-antibiotic resistance have been investigated. Both are considered unlikely because disinfectants act as general protoplasmic poisons, and operation of the mutation-selection process that may lead to antibiotic resistance would not be expected. However, Gillespie et al (1967) reported that 10 out of 13 strains of *Proteus mirabilis* isolated from patients who had received numerous applications of chlorhexidine for urinary catheterization had minimum inhibitory concentrations of 125–500 μg/ml. Stickler and Thomas (1980) examined 802 isolates of Gram-negative bacteria causing urinary tract infections in patients who were subject to extensive contact with chlorhexidine for urinary catheterization. *Escherichia coli* strains were uniformly sensitive but some strains of *Proteus, Providencia* and *Pseudomonas* were above the normal m.i.c. range for cationic disinfectants and several antibiotics.

Laboratory investigations have confirmed that an increase in the resistance of certain Gram-negative bacteria to chlorhexidine can occur if they are serially subcultured in gradually increasing concentrations of the disinfectant. Prince et al (1978) obtained an increase in the resistance of strains of *Proteus, Pseudomonas* and *Serratia* to chlorhexidine. With *Proteus*, the resistance was lost after further subcultures without the disinfectant but it was stable in *Pseudomonas* and *Serratia*. A slight increase in resistance to benzalkonium chloride was also detected. A similar experiment with povidone-iodine did not produce any strains with increased resistance to this compound. Stickler (1974) observed significant increases in the minimum inhibitory concentration of chlorhexidine for two strains of *Proteus mirabilis* from 20 μg/ml to 200 μg/ml and 800 μg/ml using the same technique.

In view of these findings, the possibility of increased resistance, acquired during repeated exposure to chlorhexidine or quaternary ammonium compounds, cannot be ruled out. Martin (1969) reported that none of 205 isolates of *Proteus*, including the most resistant species *P. mirabilis*, survived exposure to 0.02 per cent w/v chlorhexidine, the lowest concentration used in practice. However, O'Flynn & Stickler (1972) reported that 39 per cent of 45 strains of *P. mirabilis* which were

isolated from patients were resistant to this concentration.

Some of the isolates of *Proteus, Providencia* and *Pseudomonas* which were relatively resistant to chlorhexidine (Stickler & Thomas, 1980), were also resistant to several antibiotics. However, Russel (1972) found that two strains of *P. aeruginosa* which were resistant to several antibiotics were as susceptible as antibiotic sensitive strains to chlorhexidine, cetrimide, glutaraldehyde, chloroxylenol and lysol. There is no evidence of genetic change resulting in resistance to aldehyde or halogen disinfectants, or of any relationship between multi-antibiotic resistance in *S. aureus* and increased resistance to a disinfectant.

Acid-fast bacteria

This group includes *Mycobacterium tuberculosis* and several other human pathogens. The organisms have a high lipid content, including waxes, which impedes penetration of aqueous solutions unless they contain a high concentration of soap or other detergent (Hegna, 1977). Some phenolic formulations are effective. Ethyl alcohol (80 per cent v/v) is the most rapidly acting tuberculocide. The activity of alkaline glutaraldehyde is slower than that of phenols, alcohol and iodine (Rubbo et al, 1967), although Collins & Montalbine (1976) gave a more favourable report. However, chemical disinfection should not be undertaken unless heat treatment, to which these organisms are extremely sensitive, is inappropriate.

Bacterial spores

In situations where sterilization by moist or dry heat is inappropriate, bacterial spores may be killed by aldehydes or halogen disinfectants although high concentrations and prolonged exposures may be required. Glutaraldehyde is more rapidly sporicidal than is formaldehyde. The spores of *Bacillus subtilis* var. *niger* (NCTC 10073) and other species may be killed very rapidly by 100 p.p.m. available chlorine if the solution is buffered to pH 7.6–8.1 (Death & Coates, 1979). There are wide differences between species of bacterial spores in their susceptibility to sporicidal chemical agents as, indeed, to heat treatment.

Viruses

These obligate intracellular parasites can survive in the environment although they do not multiply outside their specific host cells. They may be divided into lipophilic and hydrophilic groups, which differ in their susceptibility to chemical disinfectants. The lipophilic (enveloped) viruses are inactivated by most types of disinfectants. This group includes vaccinia, herpes, influenza and measles viruses and also the non-enveloped adenoviruses. The more resistant hydrophilic (non-enveloped) group includes the hepatitis viruses and many enteric pathogens, such as coxsackie, ECHO and polio viruses. The aldehydes and halogen-based disinfectants are the only effective agents against this group. Alkaline glutaraldehyde is used at 2 per cent w/v and chlorine disinfectants up to 0.5 per cent (5000 p.p.m.) available chlorine, to allow for protection by blood, faeces and tissue culture debris.

The few studies (Brown et al, 1982; Walker et al, 1983) that have been carried out to determine the susceptibility of the agent causing Creutzfeldt-Jakob disease (a virus-induced spongiform encephalopathy) have led to recommendations that heat-stable instruments should be autoclaved at 121°C for times ranging from 30–90 minutes. Heat-sensitive material can be rendered safe by treatment with sodium hypochlorite (0.5–1.0 per cent available chlorine). Tests on glutaraldehyde have not been reported.

Fungi

These eucaryotic, usually multicellular organisms present special problems in disinfection as all vegetative cells and spores must be killed to prevent regrowth. Antifungal agents are more often fungistatic than fungicidal and species susceptibility varies widely. Alkaline glutaraldehyde has antifungal activity (Gorman & Scott, 1977), and hypochlorites may control growth in some situations. The filamentous fungi that cause tinea (ringworm) in' man and animals are inaccessible to disinfectants because they are located within the keratinized skin scales shed into the environment.

Appropriate types of chemical disinfectants for use against the different groups of microorganisms are shown in Table 11.1

Table 11.1 Appropriate disinfectants for particular microorganisms

Types of microorganisms	Effective chemical disinfectants (alphabetical order)
Gram-positive bacteria (non-sporing)	Any potent bactericide
Gram-negative bacteria (particularly *Proteus, Klebsiella, Pseudomonas*)	Alcohols Halogens (chlorine, iodine) Phenolics (clear soluble type with high level of activity; not chloroxylenols)
Acid-fast bacilli (*M. tuberculosis*)	Alcohols Aldehydes Halogens Phenolics (some clear soluble formulations)
Bacterial spores	Aldehydes (prolonged exposure) Halogens (strong solutions) Peracetic acid (applications limited)
Viruses — hydrophilic and lipophilic groups	Aldehydes Halogens (strong solutions)
Viruses — lipophilic group only	Alcohols Chlorhexidine Phenolics (clear soluble type) Quaternary ammonium compounds
Fungi	Aldehydes Halogens (strong solutions)

FACTORS AFFECTING IN-USE EFFECTIVENESS

Each type of chemical disinfectant has a characteristic potential for biocidal action which is determined by its antimicrobial spectrum and mechanism of action. However, its efficiency in the conditions of use may be influenced, often adversely, by many factors. Some of these relate to the number and condition of the microorganisms and others to changes in the effective concentration of the disinfectant.

Number of microorganisms

Chemical disinfection has a low margin of safety and the rate of killing often slows in the later stages, producing tailing curves. Low initial contamination levels, which may be achieved by pre-cleaning the articles or surfaces to be disinfected, are therefore very important.

Conditions of growth

The conditions in which natural populations of microorganisms have grown is usually unknown. However, certain Gram-negative bacteria, such as the pseudomonads, are more resistant to disinfectants when they have been grown in water or some other nutritionally deficient medium at ambient temperature than when they have been cultured in a laboratory medium at 37°C (Bassett et al, 1970). Bacteria that are actively multiplying in the logarithmic phase of population growth are usually more susceptible than are physiologically old cells of the stationary phase.

Accessibility of microorganisms

Dried or clotted blood, pus, excreta, oil films or milk residues can protect microorganisms from effective contact with liquid disinfectants. Proteins are coagulated or precipitated by alcohols and hardened by aldehydes. Virus particles or their infective nucleic acid core may be protected by accompanying particulate matter or by hardening of the protein coat when they are treated with

formalin to prepare a killed vaccine (Gard, 1959). Moisture is always essential for antimicrobial action; microorganisms are not killed by dried disinfectant residues on floors (Ayliffe et al, 1966) or blankets (Rubbo et al, 1969).

Some articles harbour contaminants in pores, crevices or cracks, such as may occur in wood (Gilbert & Watson, 1971), concrete and damaged metalware, or between closely mated metal surfaces (e.g. hinged instruments). The human skin has a population of resident bacteria which multiply between the outer layers of the keratinized epithelium and cannot be reached by disinfectants.

Concentration of disinfectant

The rate of killing increases with the concentration of the antimicrobial agent. The magnitude of the effect is expressed by the concentration coefficient (n), which is calculated from the equation $k = tc^n$, where k is a death rate constant, c is the concentration and t is the time of disinfection (minutes) for a specified reduction in the viable count. For many types of disinfectants the concentration coefficient is unity, so that halving the concentration doubles the time. Phenols, however, have an unusually high coefficient (up to 6) so that a small change in concentration results in a large difference in killing time, as shown in Figure 11.1.

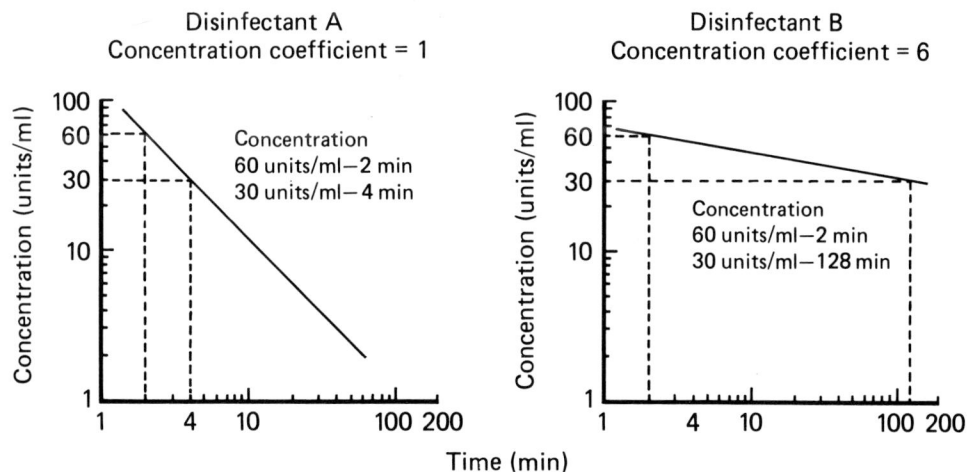

Fig. 11.1 Influence of concentration on the time required for biocidal action of a disinfectant (A) with a low concentration coefficient and (B) with a high concentration coefficient.

Temperature

Chemical disinfectants are commonly used at room temperature but some are suitable for use in conjunction with hot cleaning processes.

$$\text{Temperature coefficient} = \frac{\text{Time to kill at } x°C}{\text{Time at } (x + 10°C)}$$

The term 'to kill' implies, as usual, some specified degree of reduction in viable microorganisms. Temperature coefficients range from 2 to 14. Alkaline glutaraldehyde has a temperature coefficient of 4, so that a 10°C increase in temperature effects a fourfold reduction in the time to kill. Phenols have coefficients of 2–6. The sporicidal activity of sodium hypochlorite is increased by more than 50 per cent when the temperature is raised by 10°C. A temperature coefficient may apply within a limited temperature range only.

Hydrogen ion concentration (pH)

The effect of pH on bactericidal action may be exerted on the disinfectant, the microorganisms or both. Quaternary ammonium compounds and chlorhexidine are active as cations. The optimum pH for their action is on the alkaline side of neutrality because this increases the number of negatively charged groups on the proteins of the bacterial surface with which the antibacterial agent may combine. Phenols are also most active at alkaline pH because they act as negatively charged anions, which are suppressed by an acid pH.

Glutaraldehyde is active only at pH 7.5–8.5 at ambient temperature (20°C). The dependence on alkalinity is reduced as the temperature is raised to 70°C, when the acid solution becomes as rapidly sporicidal as the alkaline solution at room temperature (Sierra & Boucher, 1971). The reason is not clear because no difference in the proportions of the monomeric aldehyde, hydrated ring structures and polymer in the solution over a pH range 1–8 has been found (Holloway & Dean, 1975). The effect of pH is therefore attributed to a change in the condition of the microorganisms (Munton & Russell, 1970).

The halogen-based disinfectants are most active in the pH range of 6–8. The active form of chlorine disinfectants is unionized hypochlorous acid and ionic forces are not involved in the reaction of the disinfectant with microorganisms. Hypochlorite anions, which predominate in alkaline solutions, are virtually devoid of activity. The relationship between pH and per cent of Cl_2, HOCl and OCl^- is shown in Table 11.2. Iodine, in the molecular form I_2, is also active in neutral or acid solutions.

Formulation

Most disinfectants are used as aqueous solutions but some skin disinfectants contain a high concentration (60–80 per cent v/v) of ethyl or isopropyl alcohol, which contributes to the immediate biocidal action and promotes penetration of skin furrows and folds. Alcoholic solutions of formaldehyde and glutaraldehyde are not always more active than their aqueous solutions of similar strength (Willard & Alexander, 1964; Rubbo et al, 1967).

Phenolic disinfectants contain detergents to promote solubility of the active compounds. Quaternary ammonium compounds may also be formulated with detergents but only some of the nonionic types are compatible and the activity of the final formula must be confirmed by microbiological tests. Chlorhexidine is not used as a detergent-sanitizer but is formulated as a bactericidal skin cleanser (Lowbury & Lilly, 1973). An excess of the active agent is required to ensure that sufficient (1 per cent w/v) is available for biocidal action. The compatibility of detergents for combination with chlorine disinfectants and iodophors must also be verified. Unauthorized mixing of different disinfectants may result in inactivation.

The antibacterial spectrum of phenolic formulations is influenced by the types and amounts of phenols used. Some are more active against Gram-

Table 11.2 Influence of pH on availability of undissociated hypochlorous acid, the active agent in chlorine disinfection

pH	% Cl_2	% HOCl	% OCl^-
4	0.5	99.5	0
5	0	99.5	0.5
6	0	96.5	3.5
7	0	72.5	27.5
8	0	21.5	78.5
9	0	1.0	99.0
10	0	0.3	99.7

positive and others against Gram-negative bacteria.

Organic matter

Organic material, such as blood, serum, pus, faeces, and oils or fats, which may be introduced into diluted solutions by the materials being treated, inactivates all disinfectants to some extent (Gélinas & Goulet, 1983). The effect is greatest with quaternary ammonium compounds, which are adsorbed to colloidal and particulate material, and halogen disinfectants, which are converted to inactive chloride or iodide by oxidative reactions. Phenolics are less susceptible to inactivation by organic matter but those prepared from synthetic alkyl and halogenated phenols are affected more seriously than are the crude coal tar formulations containing cresols and xylenols. Aldehydes are partially inactivated by reaction with proteins. Allowance must be made for inactivation by soiling materials when determining the concentration of a disinfectant to be recommended for use on objects or surfaces that have not been cleaned.

Cellulosic and synthetic materials

Cotton materials and a wide range of synthetics may come in contact with disinfectants in the form of cotton wool, gauze dressing, cleaning cloths, sponges or mops and plastic containers for storage or use of the disinfectant. Both types of material reduce the activity of the surface active quaternary ammonium compounds and chlorhexidine by adsorption but other disinfectants are not affected significantly (Maurer, 1978).

CONTAMINATED DISINFECTANTS

This term may appear to be a contradiction. However, a large quantity of published literature concerning the survival and growth of bacteria in diluted disinfectants, including reports of associated hospital-acquired infections, has accumulated over three decades (Lowbury, 1951; Bean & Farrell, 1967; Bassett, 1971b). The types of microorganisms and disinfectants involved and the causes of contamination are now well known. The

problem is avoidable if recommended precautions, which are set out in Table 11.3, are taken.

Contamination is most often encountered in dilute solutions of quaternary ammonium compounds, chlorhexidine, synthetic phenolic disinfectants and in creams or emulsions containing hexachlorophene. However, contamination of an iodophor with *Pseudomonas aeruginosa* during production has been reported (Berkelman et al, 1984). The bacteria, which are invariably Gram-negative bacilli, include *P. aeruginosa, P. cepacia* and species of *Proteus, Klebsiella, Achromobacter, Alcaligenes, Serratia* and *Enterobacter*. The microorganisms are opportunistic pathogens, common in hospital environments, which may

Table 11.3 Growth of bacteria in disinfectants

Causes	Remedies
Inaccurate dilution	Give clear instructions for preparation
Contaminated water used for preparing dilutions (Guinness & Levey, 1976; Morris et al, 1976; Wishart & Riley, 1976)	Check bacteriological quality of distilled or deionized water
Unclean containers (Cockcroft et al, 1965; Burdon & Whitby, 1967; Thomas et al, 1972)	Avoid 'topping up'; discard unused solution, wash and sterilize or disinfect bottles or other containers before refilling with freshly prepared solution
Incompatible containers (Maurer, 1978)	Consult disinfectant manufacturer about compatibility of plastic containers
Unsuitable closures (Lowbury, 1951; Anderson & Keynes, 1958; Linton & George, 1966; Simmons & Gardner, 1969)	Do not use cork stoppers or caps with cork or plastic liners
Unfavourable pH of solution (Bassett, 1971a)	Check pH of solution (e.g. with QAC, chlorhexidine, sodium hypochlorite)
Stale solution (Maurer, 1978)	Prepare solutions daily
Inactivation by organic matter, cotton or plastics (Kundsin & Walter, 1957; Plotkin & Austrian, 1958; Malizia et al, 1960; Lee & Fialkow, 1961; Maurer, 1978)	Prevent or allow for inactivation by rayon, cotton wool or gauze swabs, cotton mops and synthetic sponges, brushes or mops
Recommended concentration very low (e.g. 0.02% chlorhexidine for bladder irrigation)	Purchase sterile solution

cause serious or fatal illness in patients who are abnormally susceptible to infection as a result of natural disorders of the immune system or medical treatment. If they are introduced into the solution during preparation or use, their non-exacting nutritional requirements enable them to multiply, producing cell populations up to 10^7/ml within 2 days at room temperature in stale water or disinfectants. A strain of *P. aeruginosa* was found to utilize benzalkonium chloride as a carbon source when the solution was buffered with ammonium acetate, which served as a nitrogen source (Adair et al, 1969). Unused solutions in stock bottles may become contaminated as well as those that have been used. Dilute solutions of some disinfectants at the concentration required (e.g. 0.02 per cent w/v chlorhexidine) are now available commercially in suitable volumes for a single use. Chlorhexidine and quaternary ammonium disinfectants are sterilized by autoclaving. Skin swabs impregnated with a QAC solution are stable to gamma radiation but chorhexidine solutions are decomposed by this process.

IN-USE TEST

The simple In-use test described by Maurer (1978) should be used regularly in hospitals to detect heavy contamination of disinfectants before they cause infection of patients. A 1 ml sample of the solution to be tested (used or taken directly from the stock bottle) is added to 9 ml of a suitable diluent. Ten drops, each of 0.02 ml volume, of the diluted sample are placed on each of two nutrient agar plates; one is incubated at 37°C for 3 days and the other at room temperature for 7 days. Five or more colonies on either plate indicate a problem that requires investigation. The method is illustrated in Figure 11.2.

Contamination usually results from faults in the preparation or use of the disinfectant. The type or brand should not be changed unless a fault cannot be found. A pass result in the In-use test demonstrates that the liquid disinfectant is unlikely to be a reservoir of infection but it does not prove that the articles that were treated by it have been disinfected. The test should be performed frequently when a new product or method of use has been

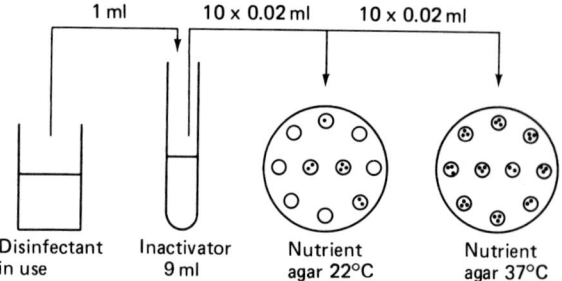

Fig. 11.2 Diagram of procedure of an In-use test for detecting bacterial multiplication in a chemical disinfectant (Maurer, 1978).

introduced into the hospital policy, but the intervals may be extended when confidence in a product and its correct use has been established.

TOXICITY OF DISINFECTANTS

Acute toxicity

Acute toxicity usually results from accidental ingestion or accidental contact of strong solutions with the skin. All disinfectants are labelled as poisons, with a warning to prevent access by children. Acute oral toxicity is customarily expressed by an LD_{50} value, which is the dose that kills half of a group of test animals. Phenolic disinfectants are acutely toxic if ingested. Hexachlorophene emulsions have caused some fatal accidents in hospital patients, who have misunderstood instructions to wash with them because the emulsion, which resembles milk of magnesia, was given to them in a drinking cup (Wear et al, 1962; Lustig, 1963). Crude coal tar phenolic disinfectants, such as lysols, cause serious burns if the concentrated liquid comes in contact with the skin. This danger is greatly reduced by the use of purified alkyl and halogenated phenols in the manufacture of clear soluble fluids for hospital use.

The incidence of skin irritation, hypersensitivity reactions and systemic toxicity, which may be associated with frequent application of antibacterial preparations to skin or mucous membranes, is usually not discovered or assessed until the disinfectant has been in use for several years. The assessment of irritancy is very subjective; a trial of two batches of bar soap, which were identical apart from a hole bored through the bars in one group, resulted in approximately half of the participants favouring one batch while the rest expressed a preference for the other batch (Blank, 1969). A sensation of dry skin may result from the removal of oils by detergents or alcohol. Real damage to the skin is manifested by reddening and soreness; it may be caused by the strongly alkaline detergents in some skin disinfectants. A successful skin disinfectant must have a low incidence of hypersensitivity reactions but it is always likely that a few individuals will be allergic to the active agent or to accompanying detergents. Patients receiving only occasional treatment before surgery or injections are unlikely to suffer adverse reactions, except with solutions containing a high concentration of elemental iodine. Iodophors are now preferred as they are less likely to sensitize and are also less irritant. Povidone-iodine has been shown to be capable of causing alteration of DNA (Wlodkowski et al, 1975). Formaldehyde, glutaraldehyde, substituted phenols and quaternary ammonium disinfectants are subjects of occasional reports of contact or photocontact dermatitis. Photocontact dermatitis may be caused by simple phenolic compounds in soaps (Adams, 1972).

Chronic toxicity

The chronic systemic toxicity of hexachlorophene, resulting from absorption into the blood from the skin, was not discovered until the agent had been widely used for 20 years to disinfect the hands of hospital staff and patients and to reduce the incidence of staphylococcal infections among infants in hospital nurseries. The potential of hexachlorophene for systemic toxicity was revealed by animal feeding tests that were done to assess its safety for use as a food preservative (Kimbrough, 1973). The animals developed paralysis in the limbs and the white matter of the brain showed spongiform encephalopathy, indicative of oedema. This condition is not unique to hexachlorophene. The mean blood level in rats with paralysis and brain changes is 1.2 μg/ml (Curley et al, 1971).

Retrospective examination of relevant hospital records and determination of blood levels in adults and infants have shown that hexachlorophene may be used safely for regular hand washing by adults (Butcher et al, 1973) and for bathing of normal, healthy infants in hospital nurseries (Plueckhahn, 1973). However, it can cause convulsions, and frequently death, in infants of low birth weight or those with abnormal or diseased skin (Kopelman, 1973; Powell et al, 1973). The death of several healthy infants was caused by a gross error in the formulation of a hexachlorophene-containing dusting powder (Martin-Bouyer et al, 1982).

Formaldehyde has recently become a focus of attention as an occupational and community health hazard. Occupations that involve exposure to formaldehyde vapour include pathology and the manufacture of ion-exchange resins, organic chemicals, brake linings and urea-formaldehyde insulating material. Occupants of private homes and other premises that contain urea-formaldehyde insulation are also exposed to significant concentrations of the vapour (Dally et al, 1981).

As an alkylating agent, formaldehyde is potentially carcinogenic and squamous cell carcinomas have been produced experimentally in rats (Yodaikin, 1981). A potent carcinogen, bis-(chloromethyl) ether, is produced if formaldehyde reacts with any source of free chlorine, including chlorine disinfectants (Drew et al, 1975). However, retrospective investigation of large numbers of persons who were occupationally exposed to formaldehyde vapour for many years, often at levels that would not be permitted now, has provided no evidence of a link between formaldehyde and human cancer. The risk of cancer from occupational exposure is therefore considered to be minimal in view of the much stricter controls that are now exercised (Editorial Lancet, 1983). Clark (1983) has provided guidelines for minimizing exposure in pathology laboratories.

EXPRESSION OF DISINFECTANT CONCENTRATIONS

The concentration of active agents in solids and solutions are expressed in different ways, which may be confusing if they are not clearly stated and understood.

1. Per cent weight/weight (w/w)

The available chlorine content of a powdered chlorine disinfectant, in a pure state or mixed with inactive substances, is expressed as grams per 100 g of the powder. The concentration of alcohol in an alcohol-water mixture may also be expressed as per cent w/w. The commonly recommended concentration of 70 per cent ethyl alcohol originally referred to w/w; 70 per cent w/w is equivalent to 77 per cent v/v and 80 per cent v/v is recommended for most uses.

2. Per cent weight/volume (w/v)

The concentration of aldehydes, chlorhexidine and QACs is expressed as per cent w/v (grams of active agent per 100 ml of solution). This method should be used for concentrated stock solutions and also for use-dilutions. If a 20 per cent w/v chlorhexidine stock solution is diluted by a factor of 1 in 200 v/v, the concentration in the diluted solution is 0.1 per cent w/v.

3. Per cent volume/volume (v/v)

Phenolic formulations and other disinfectants which contain several active ingredients are diluted by volume. The dilution factor may be expressed as per cent v/v, 1 in X or 1:X. Per cent v/v refers to ml of concentrated solution per 100 ml of diluted solution. One in X means that 1 ml of the concentrated solution is made up to a total volume of X ml. One:X means that 1 ml of the concentrated solution is added to X ml of diluent, making a total volume of X + 1 ml. The label on a diluted solution should identify the original solution and indicate which method has been used to express the dilution.

The calculations involved in the preparation of dilute solutions may be tedious or time-consuming. A helpful 'dilution without tears' formula was provided by Ware (1958): if the strong solution contains X per cent (w/v or v/v) of the active substance and a more dilute solution containing Y per cent is required, y ml of the strong solution should be measured and made up to x ml. For example, if X is 10 per cent w/v and 1 per cent

is desired, 1 ml of X would be made up to a total volume of 10 ml.

EVALUATION OF DISINFECTANTS

The complete profile of a chemical disinfectant includes information about the types and species of susceptible microorganisms, the influence of organic matter and other materials or conditions of use on its performance, and advice concerning any adverse effects on materials or personnel. These aspects have already been discussed; the types of microbiological tests that are used to investigate the rate of biocidal action and determine effective concentrations of a disinfectant for use will be outlined in this section. Chemical disinfectants cannot be evaluated on the basis of the quantity of active agent because this does not allow for changes in biocidal activity that may result from interaction with other components of the formulation or from the influence of dilution, pH, organic matter and other materials.

Microbiological tests require technical skill, combined with regular practice, and should be performed only in manufacturers' quality control laboratories, authorized independent laboratories or the laboratory of a regulatory authority. Disinfectant testing in hospitals should be limited to performance of the In-use test described earlier in this chapter.

All disinfectants intended for use on inanimate objects, intact skin or mucous membranes must be tested for biocidal action; reversible growth inhibition (biostasis) has no relevance to the evaluation of disinfectants. A biocidal test must include the following sequence of steps:

1. The test organism is exposed to a suitable concentration of the disinfectant
2. Samples are taken at specified times and added immediately to a diluent or culture medium containing the appropriate disinfectant inactivator
3. The treated samples are cultured for surviving microorganisms.

General purpose disinfectants are subjected to bactericidal tests against selected Gram-positive and Gram-negative species by methods that are officially recognized or recommended by the regulatory authority. Modified methods are required for evaluating activity against other microorganisms, such as acid-fast bacteria, spores, viruses and fungi.

Bactericidal tests

A general description of the design and performance of a bactericidal test will be followed by examples of some tests that are used in the United Kingdom or the United States of America.

Test organisms

Specified strains of *S. aureus, P. aeruginosa, Proteus vulgaris* and *E. coli* are usually recommended. A single species, or one Gram-positive and one Gram-negative species, may be selected if a preliminary bactericidal or bacteriostatic screening test is carried out to ascertain which is most resistant to the disinfectant to be tested. Other species or strains of bacteria that are causing contamination or infection in a hospital may be included.

Preparation of inoculum

The test organisms are preserved as freeze-dried (lyophilized) cultures in sealed glass ampoules. These are opened, as required, to inoculate nutrient agar slopes which are incubated for 24 hours. The slopes may be kept in the refrigerator for one month as working stock cultures. A synthetic broth (Wright & Mundy, 1960) is recommended for preparing a series of daily subcultures to be used in the tests. Any freshly prepared culture from the fifth to the fifteenth in a series may be used in a test.

The 24 hour broth culture may be used without further treatment; however, it is usually filtered, if necessary, to remove slime and centrifuged to eliminate remaining constituents of the culture medium. The washed bacteria are resuspended in hard water (342 p.p.m. hardness) to which autoclaved yeast or serum may be added to simulate dirty conditions of use. Finally, the suspension is homogenized by shaking with glass beads on a Vortex mixer and a viable count is set up immediately before performing the test.

Suspension tests and surface tests

The suspension of bacteria may be added directly to the disinfectant or dried on small carriers made from glass, stainless steel or porcelain, as appropriate to the articles or surfaces on which the disinfectant will be used. Although suspension tests may favour the disinfectant because the bacteria are uniformly exposed, they give the most reproducible results. The level of challenge can be adjusted to represent the conditions of use by varying the size of the inoculum and the type and amount of organic matter included. In a capacity test (Cantor & Shelanski, 1951), the disinfectant is challenged repeatedly by successive addition of the bacterial suspension until its capacity to kill has been exhausted.

Surface disinfection tests are more realistic than are suspension tests in simulating the conditions of use but the reagents and conditions are more difficult to standardize and the results are less reproducible. A serious disadvantage of surface disinfection tests is that they do not distinguish between bactericidal action and the removal of bacteria from the carriers during immersion in the disinfectant, diluent or inactivator.

Disinfectant inactivators

The validity of a disinfectant test depends on terminating the bactericidal action in samples which are taken for detecting or enumerating surviving bacteria. It is also necessary to prevent bacteriostatic action in the recovery medium by small amounts of the disinfectant that are carried over by the sample. If the survivors are to be assayed by plate counts, the appropriate inactivator is added to the diluent that is used to prepare the first dilution. The recovery medium contains the inactivator if the samples are added to it directly.

A nonionic detergent, such as polysorbate 80 (Tween 80) may be used, alone at a high concentration or at a lower concentration in combination with lecithin, to inactivate quaternary ammonium compounds, chlorhexidine, phenols and hexachlorophene. Egg lecithin or soya bean lecithin of 90 per cent purity should be used; it is insoluble in water but may be dispersed by mixing with the warm detergent before the solution is made up to volume. Lecithin produces cloudiness in the medium which may interfere with the detection of growth by turbidity.

Every test must include controls to demonstrate that the disinfectant has been inactivated and that the inactivator does not kill or inhibit the test organism. Sodium thiosulphate inactivates chlorine and iodine disinfectants but is inhibitory to staphylococci; the concentration in the recovery medium should not exceed 0.1 per cent w/v (Kayser & van der Ploeg, 1965; Gross et al, 1973). Green & Litsky (1974) added 0.1 per cent sodium sulphite to an agar medium and found it less toxic than thiosulphate to the bacteria. However, low concentrations of chlorine and iodine are inactivated by the proteins in nutrient broth, without the need for addition of a specific inactivator (MacKinnon, 1974).

Disinfectants containing formaldehyde or glutaraldehyde are difficult to inactivate because the excess sodium bisulphite that is required inhibits growth of bacteria and germination of spores. A combination of dimedone and morpholine has been used for formaldehyde (Nash & Hirch, 1954), and glycine (1 per cent w/v) was superior to other inactivators of glutaraldehyde which were tested by Gorman & Scott (1976). However, Cheung & Brown (1982) found that 1 per cent glycine failed to inactivate 0.5 per cent w/v alkaline glutaraldehyde and recommended that a glycine concentration of at least 2 per cent w/v should be used to inactivate 2 per cent glutaraldehyde effectively.

Preparation of disinfectant

The concentrations or dilutions of the disinfectant to be tested may be based on the manufacturer's recommendations for use but a preliminary trial is usually required to determine a suitable range for testing. The solutions should be prepared on the day of the test unless the effect of ageing is to be investigated. Distilled water or W.H.O. standard hard water (342 p.p.m.) is used for preparing the solutions; tap water is unsuitable because it contains chemicals which may precipitate some disinfectants (e.g. chlorhexidine).

Recovery of surviving bacteria

The medium used to culture bacteria that have survived exposure to the disinfectant, but have probably been damaged, must be favourable for growth and free from traces of inhibitory substances. A good quality meat broth or nutrient agar is commonly used. A non-toxic inactivator (e.g. a nonionic detergent) may be included in the recovery medium. A low incubation temperature (32°C) may increase the number of survivors recovered. The cultures should be incubated for 48 hours.

The killing of all the microorganisms added to the disinfectant cannot be proven. Bactericidal tests may be designed to follow the killing process by plate counts until the counts are no longer accurate. A reduction of 99.9999 per cent of the inoculum can be determined provided the initial bacterial count was at least 10^8 per ml of disinfectant. If this level is reached with 30 minutes, the performance is usually deemed to be satisfactory.

An alternative system uses the Most Probable Number (MPN) method of estimating the number of viable bacteria. Each sample is subdivided to inoculate several tubes of recovery medium. When some positive and some negative cultures are observed in a set, it is probable that the volume of sample that was added to each tube contained only one survivor. The per cent kill can be calculated from the number of bacteria added to the disinfectant. The MPN method is more sensitive than are plate count methods for detecting the end point but it does not measure the progress of the bactericidal action.

British Standards Institution test (BS 3286: 1960)

This suspension test was designed for the evaluation of quaternary ammonium compounds when the necessity to use chemical inactivators to distinguish bactericidal from bacteriostatic action became apparent. It is applicable to any disinfectant or microorganism (including bacterial spores) if the appropriate inactivator is used and a uniform suspension can be prepared. The inactivator recommended for QACs is a mixture of 3 per cent w/v nonionic detergent and 2 per cent lecithin, included in the diluent used for the plate counts. Alternatively, the detergent may be used alone at a concentration of 10 per cent. The bacterial suspension (*S. aureus*, *P. aeruginosa*, or *E. coli*) is added to the disinfectant and samples are taken at regular intervals, usually from 2 minutes to 30 minutes. Extended sampling times are required in sporicidal tests. The survivors are estimated by plate counts. There is no specified pass/fail criterion but death rate curves may be prepared to compare the activity of different disinfectants or concentrations.

The controls for the test are set up as follows:

1. Inactivator and disinfectant are mixed in the ratio to be used in the test
2. Inactivator alone is made up to the same volume with water
3. Water alone is measured to the same volume.

Each of the three tubes is inoculated with 1000–5000 bacteria and samples are removed immediately, after 30 minutes and after 60 minutes for colony counts. The number of colonies on all plates should be similar. The method of performing the B.S.I test is illustrated in Figure 11.3.

Kelsey-Sykes test (Kelsey & Maurer, 1974)

The Kelsey-Sykes test is a triple challenge capacity test, designed to determine concentrations of a disinfectant that will be effective in clean and dirty conditions. The disinfectant is challenged by three successive additions of a bacterial suspension; during the course of the test, which takes just over 30 minutes to perform, the concentration of the disinfectant is reduced by half and organic matter (autoclaved yeast cells) builds up to a final concentration of 0.5 per cent (dry weight). Thus it simulates conditions that are relevant to many uses in hospitals and laboratories. A single test organism may be selected from specified strains of *S. aureus*, *P. aeruginosa*, *P. vulgaris* and *E. coli* by comparing the minimum inhibitory concentration (m.i.c.) of the disinfectant for each organism. *P. aeruginosa* is usually most resistant to chlorhexidine and QACs but *S. aureus* may be more resistant to some phenolic formulations. The test procedure is illustrated in Figure 11.4.

The replicate cultures corresponding to each organism addition are incubated at 32°C for 48 hours and growth is assessed by turbidity. Sets that contain two or more negative cultures are recorded as a negative result. The disinfectant passes

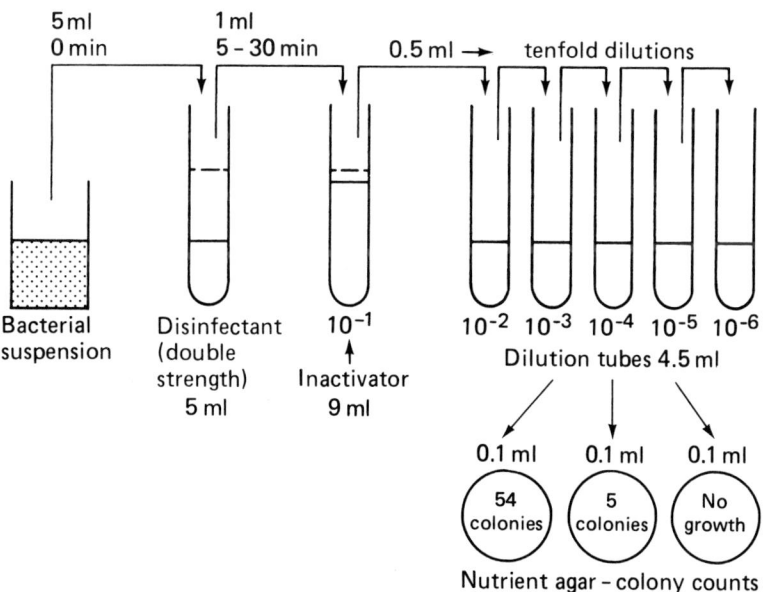

Fig. 11.3 Diagram of procedure of the British Standards Institution test (1960) for evaluation of quaternary ammonium compounds.

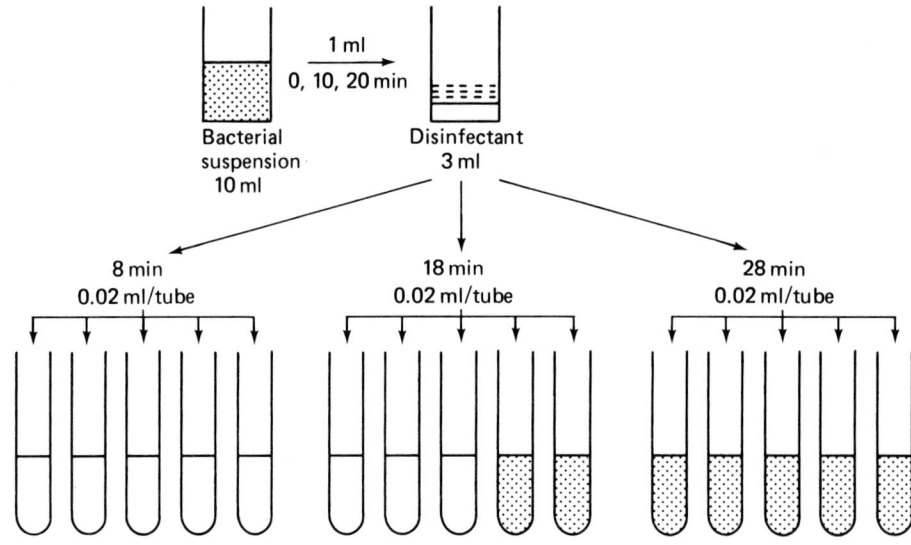

Fig. 11.4   Diagram of procedure of the Kelsey-Sykes capacity test for general disinfectants (Kelsey & Maurer, 1974).

at the dilution tested if a negative result is obtained after the first and second challenges. The third challenge is not included in the pass/fail criterion but positive cultures serve as control, showing that the recovery medium is capable of growing a small number of bacteria which have actually been exposed to the disinfectant. If there are no positive cultures after the third challenge, a lower concentration of the disinfectant should be tested.

Three concentrations of the disinfectant should be run simultaneously and separate tests are required to determine the effective concentrations for clean and dirty conditions. All the tests must be repeated on three separate days with freshly prepared bacterial suspensions and freshly diluted disinfectant, and all of the tests must be successful. Specimen results are shown in Table 11.4.

Test for Stability and Long-term Effectiveness (Maurer, 1969)

Recommended concentrations based on the Kelsey-Sykes test apply only to freshly prepared solutions. If the stock solutions are likely to be kept for more than 24 hours, the effectiveness of these concentrations must be confirmed by a supplementary test for stability of the unused solution and for the ability of freshly prepared or stale solutions to prevent multiplication of a small number of bacteria which may have survived the short-term exposure. *P. aeruginosa* is used as the test organism.

Sufficient disinfectant solution is prepared for two tests. One portion is inoculated immediately and tested for growth after holding for 7 days at room temperature. The other portion is kept at

Table 11.4   Specimen result of a Kelsey-Sykes test on a clear soluble phenolic, with *P. aeruginosa* as test organism in the presence of yeast (dirty conditions)

Concentration (% v/v)	Inoculum (count per ml)	Challenge No. 1	2	3	Result
1.0	2×10^9	+++++	+++++	+++++	Fail
1.5	2×10^9	----+	--+++	+++++	Pass
2.0	2×10^9	-----	-----	----+	Pass

room temperature for 7 days and then inoculated with a freshly prepared suspension of test organism. It is also tested for growth 7 days after inoculation. If growth is detected, a higher concentration of the disinfectant must be tested in the same way. The test for stability and long-term effectiveness is illustrated in Figure 11.5

AOAC surface disinfection tests (Crémieux & Fleurette, 1983)

Tests approved by the Association of Official Analytical Chemists form the basis for testing disinfectants in the United States. Three surface disinfection tests are included.

1. The use-dilution test is performed to confirm the efficacy of a concentration that has passed a preliminary suspension test. The test organism is dried from nutrient broth on small stainless steel cylinders. These are immersed in individual quantities of disinfectant for 5, 10 and 15 minutes. They are then transferred to individual tubes of recovery medium, a second transfer being carried out if bacteriostatic activity is suspected. The disinfectant dilution passes the test if each set of 10 carriers yields negative cultures.
2. The sporicidal test is performed on two species (*B. subtilis* and *Clostridium sporogenes*), each dried on 30 porcelain cylinders and 30 silk suture loops. Two positive cultures are permitted in a claim for disinfection but all of the 120

must be negative to justify a claim for sterilization.
3. A preliminary test for tuberculocidal activity is performed on *Mycobacterium smegmatis* dried on 10 porcelain cylinders. If all yield negative cultures after 10 minutes contact, the result is confirmed using *Mycobacterium bovis* (BCG strain).

Virucidal tests

There are several problems to be solved before virucidal tests can be standardized to a level suitable for official recognition (Chen & Koski, 1983):

1. The number of surviving virus particles that is required to initiate infection of the host cells is usually unknown
2. Residual disinfectant in the samples, or the disinfectant inactivator, may be toxic to egg embryos or tissue cultures which are used to demonstrate infectivity
3. The natural association of viruses with blood or tissue cells causes unpredictable test results.

Suspension tests are generally used because many viruses are inactivated by drying. The test virus should be stable in the cell-free state and easy to grow in high titre, so that the samples can be diluted to remove inhibitory substances before they are inoculated into tissue cultures or embryonated eggs. It should also have low pathogenicity for man and animals.

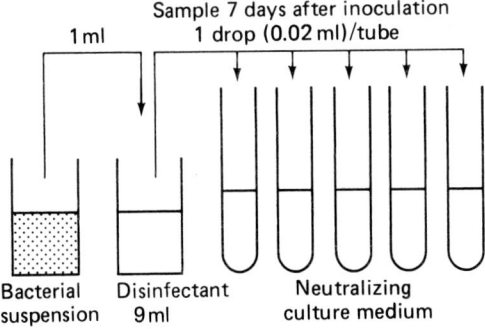

Stage 1   Disinfectant freshly diluted

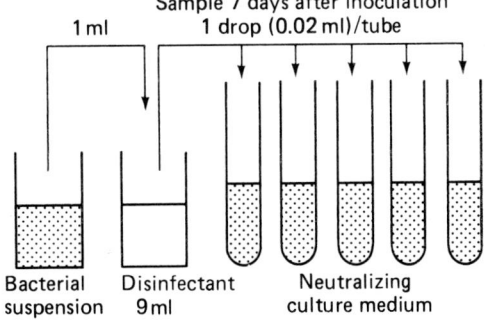

Stage 2   Disinfectant dilution stored 7 days before inoculation

Fig. 11.5   Diagram of procedure In Maurer's test for Stability and Long Term Effectiveness of chemical disinfectants (Maurer, 1969).

Fungicidal test

Filamentous fungi are difficult to test because it is not easy to prepare uniform suspensions of fragmented hyphae or spores. A suspension of microconidia of *Trichophyton mentagrophytes* is used in the AOAC fungicidal test (Czerkowicz, 1983). Strain ATCC 9533 is a suitable test organism. The growth is detached from the agar medium after 10 days incubation, homogenized in a tissue grinder, filtered to remove hyphal fragments and adjusted to contain 5×10^6 spores/ml. The suspension is added to dilutions of the fungicide and samples are cultured in dextrose broth after different exposure times. Inactivators are included in the recovery medium, or a second transfer is made to fresh medium before incubation. The highest dilution which kills in 10 minutes is the minimum requirement for a product that is intended for disinfection of inanimate surfaces.

Evaluation of skin disinfectants

The efficacy of disinfectants which are intended for application to living tissues (intact skin and mucous membranes or contaminated wounds) cannot be determined by in vitro tests. Evaluation procedures involve human volunteers, usually drawn from hospital or laboratory staff but sometimes from the community. Many different methods have been devised but standard tests, giving reproducible results, have not been achieved. The evaluation of a product depends on designing a test that is relevant to its intended use and subjecting the result to statistical interpretation. It may be helpful to perform comparative tests on one or more preparations that have demonstrated their effectiveness in use.

Preparations intended for disinfection of surgeons' hands and patients' operation sites must be tested for their ability to reduce the resident bacteria to a very low level (90–98 per cent reduction). Tests are usually carried out on the hands, samples being taken before and at different times after the test preparations have been used. A sampling method that is frequently used, with minor variations, involves rinsing or scrubbing the hands in a standard manner with a volume of liquid that contains a wetting agent (e.g. Tween 80 or Triton X–100) and appropriate disinfectant inactivators. When the samples have been treated to disperse clumps of bacteria, viable counts are performed and the per cent reduction is calculated (Lowbury et al, 1963). If residual, or sustained, action is to be tested, gloves are worn for 1–3 hours after the preparation has been used. Less precise methods of sampling include the use of cotton wool or alginate swabs; the latter dissolve and liberate the bacteria for counting.

Disinfectants intended for use by staff in hospital wards, clinics, dental surgeries or microbiological laboratories are tested for their ability to kill or remove transient contaminants that have been acquired from patients or the work environment. As the natural contaminants vary in types and may not be numerous, an easily identifiable test organism is usually applied to a marked area of skin. The removal of transient contaminants can often be achieved by thorough washing with a soap or detergent but the inclusion of a bactericidal agent reduces the time required and increases the safety of the procedure.

REFERENCES

Adair F W, Geftic S G, Gelzer J 1969 Resistance of *Pseudomonas* to quaternary ammonium compounds I. Growth in benzalkonium chloride solution. Applied Microbiology 18: 299–302

Adams R M 1972 Photoallergic contact dermatitis to chloro-2-phenylphenol. Archives of Dermatology 106: 711–714

Anderson K, Keynes R 1958 Infected cork closures and the apparent survival of organisms in antiseptic solutions. British Medical Journal 2: 274–275

Ayliffe G A J, Collins B J, Lowbury E J L 1966 Cleaning and disinfection of hospital floors. British Medical Journal 2: 442–445

Bassett D J C 1971a The effect of pH on the multiplication of a pseudomonad in chlorhexidine and cetrimide. Journal of Clinical Pathology 24: 708–711

Bassett D J C 1971b Common-source outbreaks. Proceedings of the Royal Society of Medicine 64: 980–986

Bassett D J C, Stokes K J, Thomas W R G 1970 Wound infection with *Pseudomonas multivorans*. A water-borne contaminant of disinfectant solutions. Lancet i: 1188–1191

Bean H S, Farrell R C 1967 The persistence of *Pseudomonas aeruginosa* in aqueous solutions of phenols. Journal of Pharmacy and Pharmacology Supplement 19: 183S–188S

Berkelman R L et al 1984 Intrinsic bacterial contamination of a commercial iodophor solution: investigation of the implicated manufacturing plant. Applied and Environmental Microbiology 47: 752–756

Blank I H 1969 Action of soaps and detergents on the skin. The

Practitioner 202: 147–151

Brandrick A M, Newton J M 1967 An investigation into the interaction between iodine and bacteria. Journal of Applied Bacteriology 30: 484–487

British Standards Institution 1960 Method for Laboratory Evaluation of Quaternary Ammonium Compounds. British Standard 3286: 1960

Brown P, Gibbs C J Jr, Amyx H L, Kingsbury D T, Rohwer R G, Sulima M P, Gajdusek D C 1982 Chemical disinfection of Creutzfeldt-Jakob disease virus. New England Journal of Medicine 306: 1279–1282

Burdon D W, Whitby J L 1967 Contamination of hospital disinfectants with *Pseudomonas* species. British Medical Journal 2 : 153–155

Butcher H R, Ballinger W F, Gravens D L, Dewar N E, Ledlie E F, Barthel W F 1973 Hexachlorophene concentrations in the blood of operating room personnel. Archives of Surgery 107: 70–74

Cantor A, Shelanski H A 1951 A 'capacity' test for germicidal action. Soap and Sanitary Chemicals 27: 133–135

Chen J H S, Koski T A 1983 Methods of testing virucides. In: Block S S (ed) Disinfection, sterilization, and preservation, 3rd edn. Lea & Febiger, Philadelphia, ch 49, p 981

Cheung H Y, Brown M R W 1982 Evaluation of glycine as an inactivator of glutaraldehyde. Journal of Pharmacy and Pharmacology 34: 211–214

Clark R P 1983 Formaldehyde in pathology departments. Journal of Clinical Pathology 36: 839–846

Cockcroft W H, Roberts F J, Davis F A 1965 Contamination of bactericidal agents. Canadian Medical Association Journal 93: 820–821

Collins F M, Montalbine V 1976 Mycobactericidal activity of glutaraldehyde solutions. Journal of Clinical Microbiology 4: 408–412

Crémieux A, Fleurette J 1983 Methods of testing disinfectants. In: Block S S (ed) Disinfection, sterilization, and preservation, 3rd edn. Lea & Febiger, Philadelphia, ch 46, p 918

Curley A, Hawk R E, Kimbrough R D, Nathenson G, Finberg L 1971 Dermal absorption of hexachlorophane in infants. Lancet ii: 296–297

Czerkowicz T J 1983 Methods of testing fungicides. In: Block S S (ed) Disinfection, sterilization, and preservation, 3rd edn. Lea & Febiger, Philadelphia, ch 50, p 998

Dally K A, Hanrahan L P, Woodbury M A, Kanarek M S 1981 Formaldehyde exposure in nonoccupational environments. Archives of Environmental Health 36: 277–284

Davies A, Bentley M, Field B S 1968 Comparison of the action of Vantocil, cetrimide and chlorhexidine on *Escherichia coli* and its spheroplasts and the protoplasts of Gram positive bacteria. Journal of Applied Bacteriology 31: 448–461

Death J E, Coates D 1979 Effect of pH on sporicidal and microbicidal activity of buffered mixtures of alcohol and sodium hypochlorite. Journal of Clinical Pathology 32: 148–153

Drew R T, Laskin S, Kuschner M, Nelson N 1975 Inhalation carcinogenicity of alpha halo ethers. 1. The acute inhalation toxicity of chloromethyl methyl ether and bis(chloromethyl) ether. Archives of Environmental Health 30: 61–69

Editorial 1983 Formaldehyde and cancer. Lancet ii: 26

Favero M S, Carson L A, Bond W W, Petersen N J 1971 *Pseudomonas aeruginosa:* growth in distilled water from hospitals. Science 173: 836–838

Frederick J J, Corner T R, Gerhardt P 1974 Antimicrobial actions of hexachlorophene: inhibition of respiration in

Bacillus megaterium. Antimicrobial Agents and Chemotherapy 6: 712–721

Gard S 1959 Theoretical considerations in the inactivation of viruses by chemical means. Annals of the New York Academy of Sciences 83: 638–648

Gélinas P, Goulet J 1983 Neutralization of the activity of eight disinfectants by organic matter. Journal of Applied Bacteriology 54: 243–247

Gilbert R J, Watson H M 1971 Some laboratory experiments on various meat preparation surfaces with regard to surface contamination and cleaning. Journal of Food Technology 6: 163–170

Gillespie W A, Lennon G G, Linton K B, Phippen G A 1967 Prevention of urinary infection by means of closed drainage into a sterile plastic bag. British Medical Journal 3: 90–92

Gorman S P, Scott E M 1976 Evaluation of potential inactivators of glutaraldehyde in disinfection studies with *Escherichia coli*. Microbios Letters 1: 197–204

Gorman S P, Scott E M 1977 A quantitative evaluation of the antifungal properties of glutaraldehyde. Journal of Applied Bacteriology 43: 83–89

Gorman S P, Scott E M, Russell A D 1980 A review. Antimicrobial activity, uses and mechanism of action of glutaraldehyde. Journal of Applied Bacteriology 48: 161–190

Green B L, Litsky W 1974 The use of sodium sulfite as a neutralizer for evaluating povidone-iodine preparations. Health Laboratory Science 11: 188–194

Gross A, Cofone L, Huff M B 1973 Iodine inactivating agent in surgical scrub testing. Archives of Surgery 106: 175–178

Guinness M, Levey J 1976 Contamination of aqueous dilutions of Resiguard disinfectant with *Pseudomonas*. Medical Journal of Australia 2: 392

Hegna I K 1977 An examination of the effect of three phenolic disinfectants on *Mycobacterium tuberculosis*. Journal of Applied Bacteriology 43: 183–187

Holloway C E, Dean F H 1975 ^{13}C-NMR study of aqueous glutaraldehyde equilibria. Journal of Pharmaceutical Sciences 64: 1078–1079

Kayser A, Ploeg G van der 1965 Growth inhibition of staphylococci by sodium thiosulphate. Journal of Applied Bacteriology 28: 286–293

Kelsey J C, Maurer I M 1967 The choice of disinfectants for hospital use. Monthly Bulletin of the Ministry of Health 26: 110–114

Kelsey J C, Maurer I M 1974 An improved (1974) Kelsey-Sykes test for disinfectants. Pharmaceutical Journal 213: 528–530

Kimbrough R D 1973 Review of the toxicity of hexachlorophene, including its neurotoxicity. Journal of Clinical Pharmacology 13: 439–444

Kopelman A E 1973 Cutaneous absorption of hexachlorophene in low-birth-weight infants. Journal of Pediatrics 82: 972–975

Kundsin R B, Walter C W 1957 Investigations on adsorption of benzalkonium chloride U.S.P. by skin, gloves, and sponges. Archives of Surgery 75: 1036–1042

Lee J C, Fialkow P J 1961 Benzalkonium chloride — source of hospital infection with Gram-negative bacteria. Journal of the American Medical Association 177: 708–710

Linton K B, George E 1966 Inactivation of chlorhexidine ('Hibitane') by bark corks. Lancet i: 1353–1355

Longworth A R 1971 Chlorhexidine. In: Hugo W B (ed) Inhibition and destruction of the microbial cell. Academic Press, London, ch 3B, p 95

Lowbury E J L 1951 Contamination of cetrimide and other fluids with *Pseudomonas pyocyanea*. British Journal of Industrial Medicine 8: 22–25

Lowbury E J L, Lilly H A 1973 Use of 4% chlorhexidine detergent solution (Hibiscrub) and other methods of skin disinfection. British Medical Journal 1: 510–515

Lowbury E J L, Lilly H A, Bull J P 1963 Disinfection of hands: removal of resident bacteria. British Medical Journal 1: 1251–1256

Lustig F W 1963 A fatal case of hexachlorophane ('pHisoHex') poisoning. Medical Journal of Australia 1: 737

MacKinnon I H 1974 The use of inactivators in the evaluation of disinfectants. Journal of Hygiene 73: 189–195

Malizia W F, Gangarosa E J, Goley A F 1960 Benzalkonium chloride as a source of infection. New England Journal of Medicine 263: 800–802

Martin T D M 1969 Sensitivity of the genus *Proteus* to chlorhexidine. Journal of Medical Microbiology 2: 101–108

Martin-Bouyer G, Lebreton R, Toga M, Stolley P D, Lockhart J 1982 Outbreak of accidental hexachlorophene poisoning in France. Lancet i: 91–95

Maurer I M 1969 A test for stability and long term effectiveness in disinfectants. Pharmaceutical Journal 203: 529–534

Maurer I M 1978 Hospital hygiene, 2nd edn. Edward Arnold, London

McGucken P V, Woodside W 1973 Studies on the mode of action of glutaraldehyde on *Escherichia coli*. Journal of Applied Bacteriology 36: 419–426

Morris S, Gibbs M, Hansman D, Smyth N, Cosh D 1976 Contamination of aqueous dilutions of Resiguard disinfectant with *Pseudomonas*. Medical Journal of Australia 2: 110–111

Munton T J, Russell A D 1970 Effect of glutaraldehyde on protoplasts of *Bacillus megaterium*. Journal of General Microbiology 63: 367–370

Munton T J, Russell A D 1973 Interaction of glutaraldehyde with spheroplasts of *Escherichia coli*. Journal of Applied Bacteriology 36: 211–217

Nash T, Hirch A 1954 The revival of formaldehyde-treated bacteria. Journal of Applied Chemistry 4: 458–463

O'Flynn J D, Stickler D J 1972 Disinfectants and Gram-negative bacteria. Lancet i: 489–490

Plotkin S A, Austrian R 1958 Bacteremia caused by *Pseudomonas* sp. following the use of materials stored in solutions of a cationic surface-active agent. American Journal of Medical Sciences 235: 621–627

Plueckhahn V D 1973 Hexachlorophane and skin care of newborn infants. Drugs 5: 97–107

Powell H, Swarner O, Gluck L, Lampert P 1973 Hexachlorophene myelinopathy in premature infants. Journal of Pediatrics 82: 976–981

Prince H N, Nonemaker W S, Norgard R C, Prince D L 1978 Drug resistance studies with topical antiseptics. Journal of Pharmaceutical Sciences 67: 1629–1631

Rubbo S D, Gardner J F, Webb R L 1967 Biocidal activities of glutaraldehyde and related compounds. Journal of Applied Bacteriology 30: 78–87

Rubbo S D, Stratford B C, Dixson S 1960 'Self-sterilization' of chemically treated blankets. Medical Journal of Australia 2: 331–332

Russell A D 1972 Comparative resistance of R$^+$ and other strains of *Pseudomonas aeruginosa* to non-antibiotic antibacterial agents. Lancet ii: 332

Russell A D, Furr J R 1977 The antibacterial activity of a new chloroxylenol preparation containing ethylenediamine tetraacetic acid. Journal of Applied Bacteriology 43: 253–260

Sierra G, Boucher R M G 1971 Ultrasonic synergistic effects in liquid-phase chemical sterilization. Applied Microbiology 22: 160–164

Simmons N A, Gardner D A 1969 Bacterial contamination of a phenolic disinfectant. British Medical Journal 2: 668–669

Stickler D J 1974 Chlorhexidine resistance in *Proteus mirabilis*. Journal of Clinical Pathology 27: 284–287

Stickler D J, Thomas B 1980 Antiseptic and antibiotic resistance in Gram-negative bacteria causing urinary tract infection. Journal of Clinical Pathology 33: 288–296

Thomas M E M, Piper E, Maurer I M 1972 Contamination of an operating theatre by Gram-negative bacteria. Examination of water supplies, cleaning methods and wound infections. Journal of Hygiene 70: 63–73

Walker A S, Inderlied C B, Kingsbury D T 1983 Conditions for the chemical and physical inactivation of the K. Fu. strain of the agent of Creutzfeldt-Jakob disease. American Journal of Public Health 73: 661–665

Ware G C 1958 Dilutions without tears. Journal of Applied Bacteriology 21: ix

Wear J B Jr, Shanahan R, Ratliff R K 1962 Toxicity of ingested hexachlorophene. Journal of the American Medical Association 181: 587–589

Willard M, Alexander A 1964 Comparison of sterilizing properties of formaldehyde-methanol solutions with formaldehyde-water solutions. Applied Microbiology 12: 229–233

Wiseman D 1971 The effect of cetyltrimethylammonium bromide on the cytochrome system of *Escherichia coli*. Journal of Pharmacy and Pharmacology Supplement 23: 257S–258S

Wishart M M, Riley T V 1976 Infection with *Pseudomonas maltophilia* hospital outbreak due to contaminated disinfectant. Medical Journal of Australia 2: 710–712

Wlodkowski T J, Speck W T, Rosenkranz H S 1975 Genetic effects of povidone-iodine. Journal of Pharmaceutical Sciences 64: 1235–1237

Wright E S, Mundy R A 1960 Defined medium for phenol coefficient tests with *Salmonella typhosa* and *Staphylococcus aureus*. Journal of Bacteriology 80: 279–280

Yodaikin R E 1981 The uncertain consequences of formaldehyde toxicity. Journal of the American Medical Association 246: 1677–1678

FURTHER READING

Block S S (ed) 1983 Disinfection, sterilization, and preservation, 3rd edn. Lea & Febiger, Philadelphia

Russell A D, Hugo W B, Ayliffe G A J (eds) 1982 Principles and practice of disinfection, preservation and sterilization. Blackwell, Oxford

12

Strategy in sterilization and disinfection

The account of sterilization and disinfection that has been given in the preceding chapters began with an introductory survey of the agents and apparatus and the conditions required for maximum efficiency of biocidal action. It concludes now with an equally brief summary of the ways in which sterilization and disinfection have been organized in hospitals to ensure maximum efficiency at reasonable cost. This has been achieved by transferring the responsibility for sterilization from staff located in different areas of the hospital to a special department where trained staff are employed and expensive equipment can be fully utilized. New technology has also played an important part in ensuring that the provision of sterile equipment fulfils its role within the broader context of infection control. The use of chemical disinfectants cannot be controlled in the same way but the formulation and propagation of a clearly defined hospital policy, which covers the selection of products and the correct methods of using them, enhances achievement of the intended result. It also reduces the likelihood that solutions which are used incorrectly will become a breeding ground for pathogenic bacteria.

STERILIZATION

The first system that was developed in the United Kingdom supplied sterile glass syringes to a group of hospitals in the Portsmouth area (Darmady et al, 1957). This specialized service was discontinued when presterilized syringes became available commercially but it was followed by the development of expanded facilities for the production of sterile instruments, textiles and many other types of equipment used in operating theatres, wards and diagnostic departments. A modern sterilizing department may serve only the hospital in which it is located, a group of neighbouring hospitals or a wider region within the hospital administration system.

The production of a wide variety of medical devices in large numbers is now undertaken by industry, where the efficiency of the sterilization processes can be controlled with greater precision than is· possible in hospitals. The trained hospital staff can therefore concentrate their expertise on sterilization of reusable equipment. Commercial products that are commonly termed 'disposables' are intended to be used once only and then discarded. Strategy on the part of the hospital administration is required to balance the convenience of these items against the economic factors involved in their use (Armstrong & Lockett, 1973).

Three types of hospital sterilizing departments have been established:

1. Central sterile supply departments (CSSD)
2. Theatre sterile supply units (TSSU)
3. Hospital sterilization and disinfection units (HSDU).

Central Sterile Supply Departments (CSSD)

The aim of a CSSD is 'to provide for all departments of the hospitals served ... reliably sterilized articles, including disposables, when and where required as economically as possible under conditions which can be properly controlled' (Joint Committee of the Central and Scottish Health Services Councils, 1967). The main advantages of centralized sterilization are:

1. The capacity of the sterilizers and other equipment can be fully utilized
2. Specially trained staff are employed for the management of the department and the supervision and operation of the sterilization processes
3. Preparation and packaging methods can be standardized.

Design of the department

The sterilizing department is planned around its functions of decontaminating and cleaning reusable articles, preparing and packing them for sterilization and operating the steam, dry heat and gas sterilizers. A large store for the sterilized packs is an essential part of the department, which may also be responsible for their transportation to the departments where they are used and for collecting used items for reprocessing.

Although the general layout of the department depends on the size and configuration of the available space, the work flow pattern always proceeds from the reception area, where the used articles are cleaned, through the clean area where the packs are prepared, to the sterilizers and finally to the store from which they are distributed.

The reception area is large because it must accommodate sinks for manual cleaning, an instrument washing machine or washer-sterilizer, an ultrasonic cleaner for instruments that are delicate or difficult to clean and a drying cabinet for anaesthetic tubing. Generous space is also required for cleaning and storage of the vehicles and containers that are used for transportation of supplies in the hospital (Wells, 1976a, b). The staff room should be separate from the one used by staff who work in the clean areas.

The preparation and packaging area includes work benches for sorting, examining, packing and wrapping articles received from the cleaning section. It also receives linen from the laundry; if this is folded in the sterilizing department, it should be done in a separate room to avoid dissemination of fibres. A glass topped table, lit from below, is useful for examining the integrity of surgical drapes as they are folded. Shelves or cupboards are required for the storage of bulk supplies for inclusion in composite packs.

A fully equipped department is provided with steam, dry heat and gas sterilizers of adequate capacity to cope with the volume of work. Prevacuum steam sterilizers are required for most of the work load. Ethylene oxide sterilizers should be accompanied by an adjacent aeration cabinet. This is not yet a standard requirement for low-temperature steam and formaldehyde sterilizers, although the need to eliminate formaldehyde residues is now recognized. Packs from steam and gas sterilizers should be aired before they are transferred to the store.

The store for sterilized goods may occupy one-third of the floor space in the department (Lee, 1972). It should be clean, dry and well ventilated but free from draughts that could result in contamination of packs wrapped in paper or cloth. The maintenance of sterility depends primarily on the conditions in which they are stored rather than the time that has elapsed since sterilization. Packs which must be kept in the CSSD store or in ward stores for unpredictable emergencies should be placed in clean plastic bags after steam or gas sterilization. Commercial products should also be retained in a layer of secondary packaging (a shelf storage carton) until they are required for use.

Distribution of supplies

Three systems may be used for the delivery of supplies from the sterilizing department to the ·operating theatres and wards:

1. The whole day's supply is replaced
2. The supply is topped up, replacing only the packs that have been used
3. The ward requisitions its requirements.

The second alternative is usually favoured; the first is wasteful and the third leads to hoarding which could defeat the policy of using the packs in rotation.

The manner in which used articles are returned to the sterilizing department depends on the policy of the department but the most convenient method is to enclose them in a waterproof bag or spill-proof container without rinsing them or adding disinfectant. Rinsing instruments in operating theatre annexes carries a risk of contaminating nurses' hands with potentially pathogenic microorganisms.

Theatre Sterile Supply Units (TSSU)

TSSUs were originally sited within the operating theatre complex and operated by theatre staff. However, opinion is now in favour of locating them near the CSSD, where articles can be processed by staff who are specialists in sterilization and have been instructed in the recognition and care of the instruments (Scott, 1973). The principal items sterilized in a TSSU are preset instrument trays (Bowie et al, 1963) and special instrument packs which are used to supplement them.

Hospital Sterilization and Disinfection Units (HSDU)

An HSDU is an extension of the TSSU in which bulky equipment, such as anaesthetic apparatus, mechanical ventilators, suction apparatus and infant incubators, is disinfected. Methods of disinfection may involve the use of formaldehyde vapour in a special cabinet (Babb et al, 1981) which is designed to accommodate the anaesthetic machine and separate parts of the breathing circuit or to provide for cycling of ventilators during disinfection. A suitable ethylene oxide sterilizer may also be used. An alternative method for disinfecting ventilators uses nebulized hydrogen peroxide (Ayliffe et al, 1984).

The HSDU must accommodate separate work flow patterns for sterilization and disinfection and a modular system arranged around a central communication corridor has been described (Scott, 1973).

Staff levels and training

The staff establishment for sterilizing departments in British hospitals includes the following levels:

1. Manager or superintendent
2. Supervisors or charge hands
3. Assistants.

The services of a maintenance engineer and a consultant microbiologist are also required. Special education and training of staff at all levels is essential and should be undertaken before appointment or promotion. The manager/superintendent should be expert in departmental management and familiar with the principles and practice of sterilization. Supervisors and charge hands should be skilled in the operation of all types of sterilizers and able to recognize when problems occur. They should also provide in-service training for the assistants, with the aid of an appropriate training manual (Holmes, 1974; Institute of Sterile Services Management, 1984).

DISINFECTION

The properties of several types of chemical disinfectants have been described in Chapter 10 and the factors which may determine their effectiveness in use have been discussed in Chapter 11. However, alternative methods must also be considered when formulating a policy for the rational use of disinfection in a hospital. Disinfection by hot water or steam is the principal alternative to liquid chemical disinfectants, but ultraviolet radiation and formaldehyde vapour fumigation have certain limited applications.

Disinfection by moist heat

Hot water or steam in the temperature range 65–100°C (usually 70–75°C) is lethal to all types of microorganisms except resistant bacterial spores. Other advantages over chemical disinfectants are the low cost of heat and the lack of residues on the materials treated.

Hot water is generally used because it is readily available. Clean articles, such as cystoscopes, may be immersed in a thermostatically controlled water bath (Francis, 1961), if precautions are taken to avoid trapped air within tubes and to prevent a treatment cycle in progress from being interrupted by the addition of more articles.

This method is suitable for delicate instruments which may be damaged by mechanical agitation but machines which combine washing and disinfection by heat in the same cycle have been designed for anaesthetic apparatus, bedpans and urinals, glassware, hospital linen and, in special circumstances, eating and drinking utensils. After a preliminary rinse with cold water, the articles are washed with a hot solution containing a suitable detergent and disinfection is carried out at an automatically controlled temperature for an adequate time during the rinsing stage.

Low-temperature steam at 70–75°C is a more efficient disinfectant than hot water because of the latent heat which is released when it condenses on cool objects. However, its use is more restricted because it must be produced in a chamber which can be operated below atmospheric pressure. A low-temperature steam and formaldehyde sterilizer may be used in a shortened cycle without the addition of formaldehyde. If such a machine is available, it is the ideal method for disinfection of endoscopic instruments when time is not available for sterilization.

Disinfection by ultraviolet radiation

Utraviolet radiaton, at wavelengths between 240 nm and 280 nm, is biocidal to all microorganisms if they are brought within close range of a germicidal lamp for an adequate time and are not protected by accompanying material which acts as a barrier to penetration. These requirements restrict the use of ultraviolet light as a disinfectant to room air, clear water and clean surfaces which are in the direct path of the radiation. The need for installation of germicidal lamps in areas where aseptic treatment or other procedures are carried out has declined with the installation of improved ventilation systems which are capable of reducing the bacterial content of air in occupied rooms to a low level. The use of ultraviolet water 'sterilizers' must be discouraged. If they are properly maintained and correctly operated, they produce water containing very few viable microorganisms. However, sterile water in closed containers is required for the sophisticated surgical procedures that are now used. Surface disinfection by ultraviolet radiation is useful in laboratory safety cabinets and in small rooms where aseptic manipulations, such as pouring agar plates, are carried out. In these situations, the lamps are turned on when the cabinet or room is unoccupied. Direct exposure to ultraviolet radiation is extremely irritant to the eyes but the radiation is not transmitted through glass.

Disinfection by formaldehyde vapour

Formaldehyde fumigation of rooms is a cumbersome and hazardous procedure of doubtful efficiency and its use in hospitals has been almost entirely discontinued in favour of surface cleaning methods. It is sometimes used in an attempt to kill bacterial spores in the ventilation systems of new operating theatres but this would be unnecessary if the ducts were protected from dustborne contamination while awaiting installation. If fumigation is justified in particular circumstances (e.g. decontamination of laboratories where vaccines against dangerous animal viruses are prepared, or where specific-pathogen-free animals are reared), expert advice should be sought because the method of generating the vapour from the concentrated formalin solution and the control of temperature (above 20°C) and relative humidity (60–80 per cent) are critical to the success of the operation.

Disinfection by formaldehyde vapour in uncontrolled conditions is inadequate for hospital equipment. Specially designed cabinets for decontamination of anaesthetic machines, respirators and infant incubators may be useful, but they are expensive and their efficacy has not yet been well documented in the medical or scientific literature.

Policies for disinfection in hospitals

The concept of formulating a policy for the selection and application of chemical disinfectants in hospitals was introduced by Kelsey & Maurer (1967). Their recommendations have been frequently repeated and reemphasized, (Maurer, 1978; Ayliffe et al, 1984) and are now widely practised to achieve the benefits of greater efficiency and reduced cost.

The development of a policy to suit a particular hospital is initiated by conducting a comprehensive survey of all departments and preparing a list of products that are currently purchased and the purposes for which they are used. The list provides a basis for eliminating the use of disinfectants when:

1. Sterilization is required
2. Disinfection by hot water or steam can be carried out
3. The use of an antimicrobial agent is unnecessary.

All instruments that penetrate tissues or blood vessels, or come in contact with delicate mucous membranes or wounds, must be sterilized. Some types of articles that can be disinfected by pas-

teurization have already been mentioned; the method should also be used for disinfection of manual and mechanical cleaning equipment (e.g. mops, buckets and the tanks of wet scrubbing machines) and of stock bottles when they are refilled with diluted disinfectants. Situations in which the use of a chemical disinfectant is unnecessary are exemplified by the general cleaning of the hospital environment. It has been demonstrated by Ayliffe et al (1967) and other investigators that the benefit of including an antibacterial agent in the cleaning solution is restricted to the short period of wet contact. Residual disinfectant which may remain on the floor is inactive in the dry state and does not retard the rate or decrease the level of recontamination in areas where uncontrolled movement of people and equipment occurs. Much of the equipment used in hospital wards, including infant isolettes, can also be rendered safe by efficient cleaning unless it has been used by an infected patient.

The next step towards the development of a policy is to itemize the purposes for which a chemical disinfectant is required. These may be divided into three categories:

1. Disinfection of hospital equipment
2. Disinfection of the hospital environment
3. Disinfection of skin and mucous membranes.

The selection of an appropriate type of disinfectant for each purpose, and the concentration at which it should be used, can now be made. No single type is suitable for all purposes but the aim is to reduce the number of products and different concentrations to a minimum.

Disinfection of hospital equipment

A phenolic disinfectant is appropriate for decontamination of used instruments (with the exception of those which are contaminated with blood or exudates from a suspected hepatitis B carrier or patient) and for use in discard jars in bacteriological laboratories. When the presence of hepatitis B virus is considered to be a risk, a chlorine disinfectant used at a concentration of 0.5–1 per cent (5000 — 10 000 p.p.m.) available chlorine is recommended for disinfection of blood-stained articles that withstand the high concentration. Alkaline glutaraldehyde must be substituted for metal instruments.

Disinfection with glutaraldehyde is also recommended for endoscopic instruments, such as cystoscopes and laparoscopes, in the short time available between the use of the same instrument for successive patients. These instruments should be sterilized by ethylene oxide when time is available but immersion in a solution of glutaraldehyde for 10 hours is an acceptable substitute if the recommended method cannot be used. Other types of chemical disinfectants which have restricted use in the equipment category are ethyl alcohol, 80 per cent v/v (for thermometers and ampoules), and a weak chlorine disinfectant (125 p.p.m.) for infant incubators after use by an infected patient.

Disinfection of the hospital environment

A phenolic disinfectant or a chlorine compound is suitable, depending on the types of microorganisms that are likely to be present, for disinfection of floors, walls, furniture and fittings in areas where immunodeficient or other susceptible patients are nursed and for contaminated areas in other locations. Phenolics are usually recommended but a strong chlorine preparation (5000—10 000 p.p.m.) should be used for cleaning up blood spills. Lower concentrations of available chlorine (e.g. 1000 p.p.m.) are adequate for disinfecting beds, baths or taps and 200 p.p.m. is sufficient for sanitization of cleaned benches in the hospital kitchen. Ethyl alcohol, at the usual concentration of 80 per cent v/v, may be used on clean trolley tops and the interior of laboratory safety cabinets.

Disinfection of skin and mucous membranes

Alcoholic solutions of chlorhexidine or povidone-iodine are recommended for disinfection of surgical operation and venepuncture sites. If an aqueous solution must be used in the operating theatre, povidone-iodine is recommended. Ethyl or isopropyl alcohol is appropriate for skin disinfection before routine injections because residual action is not required.

A wider selection of preparations is available for disinfection of the hands of surgical teams and ward staff. Surgical disinfection requires the reduc-

tion of the resident skin bacteria to a low number in addition to removal of transient contaminants. This can be achieved by regular use of a bactericidal skin cleanser containing 4 per cent w/v chlorhexidine or an iodophor that contains 0.75 per cent available iodine. A hexachlorophene emulsion may also be used safely for regular handwashing by adults but it lacks immediate action after occasional use. Alcoholic chlorhexidine (0.5 per cent w/v, in 95 per cent ethyl alcohol) has been reported to be even more efficient than a chlorhexidine skin cleanser when applied to clean, dry hands (Lowbury et al, 1974).

Similar methods for disinfection of the hands may be used by staff in wards, nurseries and diagnostic departments. Although transient surface contaminants on the skin can be removed with a high degree of efficiency by thorough washing with soap and water, a bactericidal cleanser containing chlorhexidine or povidone-iodine should be used because bacteria acquired by contact with patients may be pathogens. Although a washing time of at least 2 minutes is required for surgical disinfection, 15–30 seconds may achieve a satisfactory result in the ward situation. The frequency of hand washing can be reduced by the direct application of an alcoholic solution, containing 0.5 per cent w/v chlorhexidine and skin conditioners, to the hands if they have not been soiled.

Aqueous solutions must be used for disinfection of mucous membranes or cleansing of contaminated wounds and abrasions. Dilute aqueous chlorhexidine (0.02 — 0.05 per cent w/v) is used for urinary catheterization and bladder irrigation and a stronger solution (0.5 per cent) may be used in oral surgery, in conjunction with an alcoholic solution for preparation of the adjacent skin. An aqueous solution containing cetrimide and chlorhexidine is an efficient, non-toxic wound cleanser. Caution should be exercised, for reasons explained in Chapter 10, in the application of iodine preparations to mucous membranes.

Administration of a disinfection policy

The successful implementation of a disinfection policy depends on the provision of information to the staff throughout the hospital, especially persons who are responsible for putting it into practice or supervising others who do so. The responsibility for preparing dilutions should be centralized and placed under the supervision of a pharmacist. The solutions that are distributed to wards and departments should be ready for use and clearly labelled to identify the type of disinfectant. The concentration should be stated as weight/volume (w/v) whenever possible; if this cannot be done, the identity of the concentrated solution should be stated, together with the degree of dilution by volume (v/v). All of the precautions which have been discussed in Chapter 11 should be taken during the preparation and use of the solutions to avoid access of bacterial contaminants and prevent their multiplication. Fresh solutions should be prepared daily whenever possible or presterilized solutions should be used.

Selection of brands of disinfectants

The disinfection policy should include clear directions concerning the types and brands of products which have been selected for use. An alternative product may be nominated in the policy but changes must not be made unless they are authorized by the Infection Control Committee. Hospital staff at several levels and in many departments are subject to pressure from manufacturers' representatives to try a new product but the claims should be validated by an expert before a disinfectant that is performing satisfactorily, as indicated by regular In-use tests, is replaced. Even if In-use tests have revealed that a solution has supported growth of bacteria, the cause may be found in the methods of preparation or use and might not be due to a deficiency in the product.

It is sometimes difficult for hospital staff to interpret the information that is provided by the manufacturer to validate a new product and the advice of a microbiologist who understands the method of evaluation should be sought. The matter may be clarified easily if a standard requirement for the performance of hospital grade disinfectants is in existence. Any disinfectant which has passed the Kelsey-Sykes capacity test, conducted in an authorized testing laboratory, will give a satisfactory performance of bactericidal action at the concentration recommended for use. The selection of a type or brand can then be made on the basis of

other properties, such as compatibility with materials with which it may come in contact during use or the risk of harm to the user or the articles treated. Cost-effectiveness is usually the deciding factor if two products appear to be similar in other respects. It is most unwise for bacteriologists to attempt the occasional evaluation of products in hospital laboratories because special skills and regular practice are required.

REFERENCES

Armstrong K N, Lockett A G 1973 Long-range planning for disposables. Health and Social Service Journal 83: Supplement 1–14
Ayliffe G A J, Coates D, Hoffman P N 1984 Chemical disinfection in hospitals. Public Health Laboratory Service, London
Ayliffe G A J, Collins B J, Lowbury E J L, Babb J R, Lilly H A 1967 Ward floors and other surfaces as reservoirs of hospital infection. Journal of Hygiene 65: 515–535
Babb J R, Bradley C R, Ankrett D I 1981 Formaldehyde disinfection unit. Sterile World 3 (5): 16–17
Bowie J H, Campbell I D, Gillingham F J, Gordon A R 1963 Hospital sterile supplies: Edinburgh pre-set tray system. British Medical Journal 2: 1322–1327
Darmady E M, Hughes K E A, Tuke W 1957 Sterilization of syringes by infra-red radiation. Journal of Clinical Pathology 10: 291–298
Francis A E 1961 Use of a pasteurizing water bath for disinfection of cystoscopes. Journal of Urology 86: 679–682
Holmes E M 1974 Career prospects and training needs in sterile supply/TSSU departments. Journal of the Association of Sterile Supply Administrators 2(4): 17–19
Institute of Sterile Services Management 1984 A training handbook for sterile supply staff. London
Joint Committee of the Central and Scottish Health Services Councils 1967 Central sterile supply departments. National Health Service HM (67) 13
Kelsey J C, Maurer I M 1967 The choice of disinfectants for hospital use. Monthly Bulletin of the Ministry of Health 26: 110–114
Lee K S 1972 Problems involved in the distribution and store-keeping of C.S.S.D. packs. Journal of the Association of Sterile Supply Administrators 1 (1): 5–6
Lowbury E J L, Lilly H A, Ayliffe G A J 1974 Preoperative disinfection of surgeons' hands: use of alcoholic solutions and effects of gloves on skin flora. British Medical Journal 4: 369–372
Maurer I M 1978 Hospital hygiene, 2nd edn. Edward Arnold, London
Scott S R B 1973 Sterile supplies and Harness hospital development. Journal of the Association of Sterile Supply Administrators 2 (2): 12–13, 17
Wells L L 1976a Programming a cental service Part 1. Journal of the Association of Sterile Supply Administrators 4(5): 14–16
Wells L L 1976b Programming a central service Part 2. Receiving, decontamination and cleaning area. Journal of the Association of Sterile Supply Administrators 5 (2): 10–12

Index